Com...

Community Psychology

Theory, Method, and Practice

South African and Other Perspectives

EDITOR *Mohamed Seedat*

CONSULTING *Norman Duncan*
EDITORS *Sandy Lazarus*

OXFORD
UNIVERSITY PRESS

OXFORD
UNIVERSITY PRESS

Great Clarendon Street, Oxford OX2 6DP

Oxford University Press is a department of the University of Oxford.
It furthers the University's objective of excellence in research, scholarship,
and education by publishing worldwide in

Oxford New York

Athens Auckland Bangkok Bogotá Buenos Aires Calcutta
Cape Town Chennai Dar es Salaam Delhi Florence Hong Kong Istanbul
Karachi Kuala Lumpur Madrid Melbourne Mexico City Mumbai
Nairobi Paris São Paulo Shanghai Singapore Taipei Tokyo Toronto Warsaw

with associated companies in Berlin Ibadan

Oxford is a registered trade mark of Oxford University Press
in the UK and certain other countries

Published in South Africa
by Oxford University Press Southern Africa, Cape Town

Community Psychology: Theory, Method, and Practice
South African and Other Perspectives

ISBN 019 571922 0

© Oxford University Press 2001

The moral rights of the author have been asserted
Database right Oxford University Press (maker)

First published 2001

Copy-editor: Ethné Clarke
Designer: Mark Standley
Indexer: Jeanne Cope

Published by Oxford University Press Southern Africa
PO Box 12119, N1 City, 7463, Cape Town, South Africa

Set in 10.5 pt on 14 pt Adobe Caslon by PeterMac
Reproduction by PeterMac
Cover reproduction by The Image Bureau
Printed and bound by Creda Communications

The authors and publishers gratefully acknowledge permission to reproduce
material in this book. Every effort has been made to trace copyright holders,
but where this has proved impossible, the publishers would be grateful for
information which would enable them to amend any omissions in future
editions.

Abridged table of contents

contents

SECTION III

Practice in community psychology   213

list of contributors

Rashid Ahmed, Psychology Department, University of the Western Cape, PO Box x17, Bellville, 7535

Arvin Bhana, Psychology Department, University of Durban-Westville, Private Bag x54001, Durban, 4000

Brian John Bishop, School of Psychology, Curtin University, GPO Box U1987, Perth, 6845, Australia

Robert Alexander Butchart, Institute for Social and Health Sciences, University of South Africa, PO Box 1087, Lenasia, 1820

Jackie Cock, Sociology Department, University of the Witwatersrand, Private Bag 3, WITS, 2050

Cheryl de la Rey, Department of Psychology, University of Cape Town, Private Bag, Rondebosch, 7701

Neil Murray Drew, School of Psychology, Edith Cowan University, 100 Joondalup Drive, Joondalup, 6027, Australia

Norman Duncan, Psychology Department, University of Venda, Private Bag x5050, Thohoyandou, Northern Province

Dave Edwards, Department of Psychology, University of Zululand, Private Bag x1001, Kwa-Dlangezwa, 3886

Adrian Thomas Fisher, School of Psychology, Victoria University, GPO Box 14428, MCMC, Melbourne, 8001, Australia

Kerry Gibson, Child Guidance Clinic, University of Cape Town, Private Bag, Rondebosch, 7701

Brandon Hamber, Centre for the Study of Violence and Reconciliation, PO Box 30778, Braamfontein, 2017

JW Pretorius-Heuchert, Department of Psychology, Allegheny College, 520 North Main Street, Meadville, PA, 16335, USA

Anil Kanjee, Education and Training Assessment Studies Unit, Human Sciences Research Council, Private Bag x41, Pretoria, 0001

Kevin Kelly, Psychology Department, Rhodes University PO Box 94, Grahamstown, 6140

Johan Kruger, Psychology Department, University of South Africa, PO Box 392, Pretoria, 0001

Sandy Lazarus, Educational Psychology Department, University of Western Cape, Private Bag x17, Bellville, 7535

Stanley Lifschitz, Psychology Department, University of South Africa, PO Box 392, Pretoria, 0001

Mahomed Rafiq Lockhat, Psychology Department, University of the Western Cape, Private Bag x17, Bellville, 7535

Thulani Masilela, Centre for the Study of Violence and Reconciliation, PO Box 30778, Braamfontein, 2017

Dinesh Mohan, Centre for Biomedical Engineering, Indian Institute for Technology Delhi, Hauz Khas, New Delhi, 110016, India

Victor Nell, Institute for Social and Health Sciences, University of South Africa, PO Box 1087, Lenasia, 1820

Corinne Oosthuizen, Psychology Department, Rand Afrikaans University, PO Box 524, Auckland Park, 2006

Anthony Linguim Pillay, Department of Psychology, Midlands Hospital Complex, PO Box 370, Pietermaritzburg, 3200

Charles Potter, Psychology Department, University of the Witwatersrand, Private Bag 3, WITS, 2050

Mohamed Seedat, Institute for Social and Health Sciences, University of South Africa, PO Box 1087, Lenasia, 1820

Christopher Conrad Sonn, School of Psychology, Edith Cowan University, 100 Joondalup Drive, Joondalup, 6027, Australia

Elizabeth Sparks, School of Counselling, Boston College, Chestnut Hill, MA, 02167, USA

Leslie Swartz, Child Guidance Clinic, University of Cape Town, Private Bag, Rondebosch, 7701

Martin Terre Blanche, Psychology Department, University of South Africa, PO Box 392, Pretoria, 0001

Mary van der Riet, Psychology Department, Rhodes University, PO Box 94, Grahamstown, 6140

Ashley van Niekerk, Institute for Social and Health Sciences, University of South Africa, PO Box 406, Cape Town, 7764

Preface

Although the idea of this book was mooted repeatedly in discussions with colleagues over the past ten years, the project was only initiated four years ago in January 1997, which coincided with the Islamic month of Ramadaan. Whereas January is conventionally associated with recommitment to unfinished and new projects, Ramadaan is a period of intense self-reflection and heightened awareness about the disenfranchised and their struggles for human rights and independence in a pluralistic world. Thus this book and its initiation are an extension of my own personal and shared reflections about the struggles for intellectual independence and creativity that ultimately must serve the interests of the marginalized in our society. So as I proceeded to co-ordinate and lead the editing of the book I wanted to ensure that it represented more than just an academic exercise. I wanted the book and its development to embody the principles of community fellowship, mutual exchange, self-reflective dialogue, and a collective struggle to forge innovative modes and systems of knowledge production.

Even though I did not explicitly articulate these principles I thank all the contributors for intuitively engaging them, especially those who took an active interest in the book's development and served as peer reviewers with a blend of sensitivity and intellectual excellence. I thank all the contributors for making the development of the book an enjoyable and enriching experience. Aside from the opportunity to harness my own editorial skills, I learnt more about the demons that continue to threaten to find a home in many hearts and the outer despotic tendencies that occasionally surface to undermine the organic fellowship of community psychologists and social scientists.

I extend a special thanks to Norman Duncan and Sandy Lazarus for approaching their tasks as consulting editors with grace, astuteness, and unparalleled passion. They remained a fountain of inspiration throughout. A hearty thanks to Gail Barton, who liaised closely with Victor Peteke and Lenah Mautjana to prepare the book manuscript with care and meticulous attention to detail. Gail's love for quality nurtured this book to completion. I thank Eloise Wessels for maintaining an interest in the book and for her assuring support. A special thank you to Leanne Martini who guided this book through the final review and publication phase. A hearty note of appreciation to Robert Plummer and Ethné Clarke for bringing editorial excellence to the book.

A warm note of gratitude to all my very dear friends, wife Alicia, sons Aziz and Zaheer, and family who as always provided the supportive, containing, and embracing milieu from which I continue to pursue my passions and wrestle with the hidden demons and visible despots.

Finally, I wish to dedicate this book to my late paternal aunt Khadija, who joined the world of angels on 22 August 1999, and whose life of perseverance, patience, and devotion to family and God kindles and re-kindles my own quest for nourishment in and outside of community psychology. I hope that this book, which encompasses years of work and the commitment of so many scholars, will ultimately inspire the virtues of perseverance, patience, and honest enquiry as we continue in our search for emancipatory theories, methods, and praxis.

Mohamed Seedat
December 2000
Ramadaan, 1421
Johannesburg

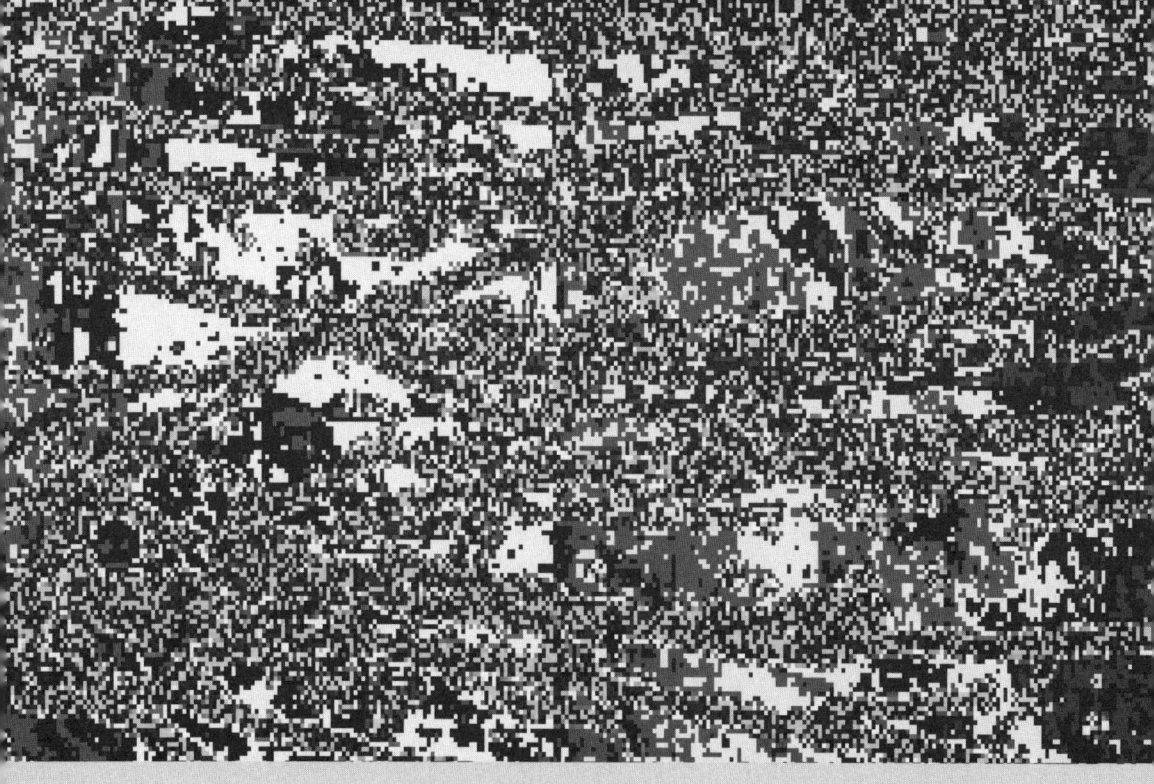

Introduction

Community
Psychology

1 Community psychology: theory, method, and practice

Mohamed Seedat
Norman Duncan
Sandy Lazarus

Study objectives

By the end of this chapter you should:
- be familiar with the scope and contents of this book;
- begin to understand the distinguishing features of community psychology theory, method, and practice in South Africa; and
- be able to formulate initial questions about the achievements and challenges inherent in community psychology in South Africa.

1 Introduction

Community psychology tends to be defined by its philosophy, ideological assumptions, and approach, and is concerned with:
- extending mental health services to all citizens, in particular the historically unserved, underserved, and oppressed;
- transforming the way in which the genesis and development of psycho-social problems are conceptualized and understood;
- providing a contextual analysis that takes cognizance of social issues and addresses environmental stressors;
- radicalizing the praxis of psychological service delivery to include prevention initiatives; and
- redefining the role of psychologists towards a broader public health portfolio that embraces the functions of advocacy, lobbying, community mobilization, community networking, and policy formulation (Lazarus and Seedat, 1996).

The juxtaposing of 'community' and 'psychology' is another defining feature that places the accent on the psyche of the collective, and conveys ideas about an academic activist agenda seeking to reform, redirect, or revolutionize the theory, method, and

3

practice of psychology in the interest of disadvantaged groups. Understandably then, the appeal of community psychology arises from its origins and radical underlying philosophy. This radical agenda is perhaps pronounced in the southern hemisphere where community psychology tended to emerge and burgeon during periods of profound sociopolitical conflict and resistance to oppression. Even though in North America community psychology was formalized during the period of civil rights struggles there, 'the climate was conducive to taking stands on social issues and there was new funding for innovative programs directed at disenfranchised groups' (Mulvey, 1988, p. 81).

Community psychology in the northern hemisphere has tended to assume an accommodationist position seeking greater influence within the mainstream fraternity without necessarily challenging the restrictions and outcomes imposed by exploitative economic arrangements and dominant systems of knowledge production. The European Network of Community Psychology (ENCP), for example, does not explicitly address the issue of theoretical and methodological ethnocentrism in their statement of objectives. Instead, the ENCP seeks to promote community psychology within the wider discipline of psychology, perhaps inadvertently excluding an analysis of the possible restrictions imposed by the general discipline on the theory, method, and praxis of community psychology (Arn et al., 1998).

In contrast, in the southern hemisphere (for example, in South Africa and Latin America), community psychology came to be associated with broad democratic movements seeking to dismantle oppressive state structures and ideological state apparatuses, which were also embodied in the disciplinary practices of the social and medical sciences during the previous colonial and apartheid eras. In South Africa, community psychology as it formally emerged in the 1980s embraced a radical challenge to the discriminatory foundation, theory, method, and practice of psychology. Community psychology was accordingly identified as the 'promise' that would 'liberate' South African psychology from the discriminatory approaches and hegemonic and epistemological domination evident in Euro-American psychology (Seedat, 1993).

Now, more than a decade later, as we engage in co-ordinating and editing this volume, we are in a privileged position to reflect on the achievements and challenges inherent in the theory, method, and practice of community psychology in the south of Africa and other parts of the southern hemisphere, such as Australia.

Has community psychology delivered on its promise? Has it transcended the epistemological domination of Northern psychology? Has it developed distinctive methods to promote its epistemological foundations and commitment to social praxis? Has it earned any discernable distinctions, and what kind of influence does it enjoy at the level of theory, method, and practice? This volume, while taking into account the work of the many distinguished scholars in the field of psychology, seeks to answer some of these and other such questions with honesty and clarity. Below, by way of introducing the scope and nature of this volume, we shall attempt to present some of our own critical reflections on a few of these questions and other challenges inherent in community psychology theory, method, and practice, with the explicit intention of encouraging you, the reader, to formulate your own critical questions as you engage with the contents of this volume. We hope that these reflections, as well as the contents of this volume, will also serve as a foundation for your attempts to arrive at your own answers to the above-mentioned questions.

A close reading of particularly the first section of this volume reveals that, despite its indisputable accomplishments, community psychology in South Africa still has to achieve both distributive equality and distributive sufficiency. According to Gordon and Shipman (1988), distributive equality addresses issues of political representation and social justice. Distributive sufficiency requires us to go beyond issues of sharing and to examine questions of need: *Are our theoretical and methodological frameworks and associated intervening processes sufficient to promote the well-being of the marginalized sectors of society?* That there is a minority of black African contributors to this volume points to issues of distributive equality. In South Africa, the underrepresentation of black Africans, in particular to the process of knowledge production in psychology, and the social sciences in general, requires us to question these issues (Seedat, 1993). The need to bring about distributive equality calls on us to wrestle with questions about how to address the silences and distortions still so evident in the institutions of knowledge production: *Is the act of academic writing still the purview of professionals located in universities? How do we collaborate with community spokespersons at the level of authorship? Does the inclusion of community*

voices at authorship level represent an act of tokenism? As we proceed to ponder these questions it is clear that we are challenged to reconsider our ideas about community participation, engagement, and control. It is also clear that community psychology has not even begun to approach distributive sufficiency in any serious way. For instance, *does community psychology theorize about how psychological liberation may be achieved through the process of empowerment and collective struggle? Has it sufficiently integrated radical perspectives into its theoretical formulations? And how does it conceptualize community?*

The social action model, among the most radical perspectives in community psychology, suggests, for example, empowerment of the underclasses within the existing socio-political order of society. The emphasis on what occurs in oppressed communities, rather than on the interactions between them and the wider social context, implicitly accords community empowerment more immediate value than the transformation of the broader processes and structures that perpetuate social inequities. By not challenging the existing economic order, the notion of community empowerment, in this sense, allows a few individuals and small groups to gain better access to the exploitative free-market system (Seedat, Cloete, and Shochet, 1988). Also, because community empowerment often becomes an end in itself, in South Africa, for example, the racial-cum-cultural divisions brought about by the apartheid ideology may easily be recreated and reinforced. Both the mental health and social action models choose the community to be their unit of intervention. For the mental health model a geographical catchment area is often synonymous with community. For the social action model, on the other hand, community is a geographically as well as politically defined locality. A geographical catchment area, defined as community, is a vehicle for collective struggle and change. Communities are therefore to be cherished, sustained, and supported. The implicit appeal to be sensitive to communities is similar to the calls of cross-cultural psychology for cultures to be respected and protected (Butchart and Seedat, 1990; Seedat and Nell, 1990).

Psychologists calling for cultural and community sensitivity implicitly accept predetermined ideologically laden values that indicate what professionals, cultures, and communities should strive for. Because communities and cultures are judged to be good, they should be protected and sustained. This means that community psychology recreates instrumental reasoning, which uncritically accepts the 'existing object world as given' (Horkheimer, 1974; Shotter, 1975). Instrumentally reasoned interventions are directed at the achievement of predetermined goals, without first examining the reasons for striving towards the goals and interrogating whose long-term interests and values will be advanced through their attainment (Butchart and Seedat, 1990).

The uncritical usage of the concepts 'community' and 'culture' by many mainstream psychologists often masks their functions as euphemisms for terms such as 'race' and 'ethnicity' in South Africa. In the recent past, in order to avoid their provocative connotations, the apartheid state abandoned the terms 'race' and 'ethnic groups', and substituted them for 'community' and 'cultural groups'. The term 'community' retained its positive connotation and was employed to maintain the legacy of segregation and to produce new divisions where necessary. For instance, groups historically referred to as 'tribes' were categorized as 'communities' and people classified as 'Indian' and 'Coloured' in terms of the anachronistic Population Registration Act were referred to as people of the 'Indian' and 'Coloured' communities (Bozzoli, 1987; Butchart and Seedat, 1990; Thornton and Ramphele, 1988). Once these terms were applied at a national level, they were used to allocate resources along 'ethno-community' lines, with each 'ethno-community' responsible for the management of its 'own' resources. Within the framework of apartheid discourse, the term 'community' ultimately became a means of reinforcing and legitimizing inequalities and disadvantaging blacks further. Thornton and Ramphele (1988) suggest that when they are required to provide for their own needs, communities with the least resources will have the most difficulty in contributing to direly needed facilities. Conversely, communities that have been historically favoured will have no problem in providing a small percentage of their income for commonly used facilities.

The uncritical usage of the term 'community' by social action psychologists recreates a context for the sedimented ideological biases of apartheid to be reproduced inadvertently in the very ideas and interventions that are planned to undermine them. Although community psychology, and in particular the social action model, communicates a philosophical commitment to proactive theorizing and practice, it too suffers from paradoxes that accompany endeavours to develop a liberatory psychology. Even though community psychology remains part of the movement within psychology that encourages an examination of the assumptions of the discipline and the adoption of new ideas, it has failed to incorporate adequately the agendas of several social movements representing, among others, the working class, children, feminists, and anti-racists.

More than a decade ago, Mulvey (1988), in tracing the commonalities between feminist thinking and community psychology, offered some explanations for the failure of community psychology to integrate radical perspectives, and its consequent complicity in the perpetuation of old reactionary practices under new labels. Aside from the lack of awareness within community psychology about the natural fit between itself and feminism, Mulvey (1988) cites four other main reasons for the peripheralization of critical perspectives in community psychology. Firstly, community psychology theory, which includes macro-level variables, systems analyses, and ecological thinking, tends to be presented in vague and global terms without interventions or practical applications, or both, at the level of praxis being clearly defined. Secondly, community psychology theory sometimes fails to take cognizance of how people are limited by institutional structures. (This criticism is echoed in Hamber, Masilela, and Terre Blanche's chapter in this volume.) For example, 'empowerment' and 'systems ana-

lysis' are examined very vaguely without any theoretical explication of how, and in whose interest, non-personal dimensions operate. Thirdly, even though community psychology endorses particular admirable principles in the formative stages of the discipline, these are rarely applied to specific real-world conditions that are structured by phenomena such as the global proliferation of weapons of war, poverty, racism, and sexism. Fourthly, because 'community psychology is a profession and as such seeks to maintain itself and protect its turf' (Mulvey, 1988, p. 81), it may be constrained in its quest to develop alternative theories that are inclusive of marginalized world-views and perspectives and the struggle for psycho-social liberation.

All of the above observations point to the massive challenge that confronts those involved in the development of community psychology, particularly where there is a quest to retain and further develop its commitment to social transformation, especially in terms of addressing the needs of the historically unserved, underserved, and oppressed. Within this context, the development of the theory, method, and practice of community psychology in South Africa, as in North America and elsewhere, is an unfinished project.

2 Outline of the contents of this volume

To enhance the coherence of the various contributions to the present volume, as well as for ease of reading, the volume has been organized into four thematic sections. A brief outline of the contents of these sections follows.

2.1 Section I: Theoretical and paradigmatic considerations

The first section, which includes six chapters, discusses historical developments and paradigmatic perspectives in the field of community psychology. In Chapter 2 Pretorius-Heuchert and Ahmed present the reader with a succinct, contextual framework within which to study the subsequent chapters. The lucid definition of community psychology and its associated roles in this chapter points to the multiplicity of perspectives and challenges characterizing this discipline. This plurality of perspectives and challenges is evident in the subsequent chapters contained in this volume.

The challenges inherent in establishing relevance for South African psychology are taken up by Swartz and Gibson in Chapter 3. They examine the contextual pressures that enable and limit the development of community psychology theory and practice in South Africa and implicitly approach the search for disciplinary distinctiveness in a conciliatory manner. Swartz and Gibson argue that, despite the apparent schism between the established theories and practices of psychology, and aspects of the new local variants of community psychology, community psychology practice may well still benefit from conventional psychological ideas. Consequently, they caution against a total break from conventional psychology. Echoing the views of Bernal (1985) and Mulvey (1988), they contend that the development of community psychology in South

Africa requires risks and innovation. Thus, for Swartz and Gibson 'the challenge we face is the challenge of creating new things'.

In Chapter 4 Hamber, Masilela, and Terre Blanche offer a Marxist orientation to community psychology analysis, theory, and practice. Consequently, they problematize the theory and practice of psychology evident within a capitalist framework and so accentuate the connection of community psychology to the material base of society. They challenge the reader to consider the hegemonic influences of the free-market economy on the discipline and wider practices of psychology, and highlight the associated ambiguities. They argue that despite the noble intentions of community psychology, it is sometimes still trapped in its tendency to individualize, idealize, and relativize psycho-social problems. Even though psychologists, by virtue of their class location, may be part of the problem, Hamber et al. posit that it is the very same class position that paradoxically privileges psychologists to access critical tools and understandings about their roles and limitations in the promotion of society's mental health.

Chapter 5 by Ahmed and Pretorius-Heuchert examines the notions of social change that operate as a central premise of community psychology, informing the theory, method, and practice in the discipline. Favouring a critical socio-historical perspective, Ahmed and Pretorius-Heuchert problematize common ideas about social change held in community psychology. The two authors assert that, despite the commitment of community psychology to social change, the associated conceptualizations are insufficient in that they are primarily 'evolutionary rather than revolutionary'. Thus, they reinforce the analysis provided by Hamber et al. in Chapter 4 and call for a closer integration of a Marxist framework in community psychology. It is recommended that this chapter be read in conjunction with Chapter 4.

In Chapter 6 Pillay and Lockhat extend the paradigmatic boundaries and invite us to examine specific models for rendering services to children. In presenting various delivery approaches, they also review the scope and nature of child mental health disorders in South Africa and provide an exposition of the economic issues affecting delivery. In view of the multiplicity of extant approaches and considerations about appropriateness, Pillay and Lockhat propose a hybrid delivery approach that is an amalgamation of the community mental health and primary health care models. If maximum benefit is to be derived from the insights contained in Chapter 6, the chapter should ideally be read in tandem with Chapter 2 by Pretorius-Heuchert and Ahmed.

In Chapter 7 Lifschitz and Oosthuizen extend our theoretical lenses by linking the theory and practice of community psychology to a specific cultural context. They break with traditional academic writing by assuming a personal approach to telling their story about the formation and re-formation of a healing community. In this narrative, they place the accent on how the process of struggle shapes and reshapes communities as well as the context necessary for healing. In their view, no a priori theory or paradigm can possibly predict or substitute for the experiences of those involved in community interventions. The readers are challenged to

resist the tendency towards imposing theoretical frameworks that may be reductionist and inadequate for understanding a community's experiences.

2.2 Section II: Methodological considerations

Section II, which discusses methodological concerns in the field of community psychology, consists of three chapters. In Chapter 8 Bhana and Kanjee encourage an examination of the relationship between methodology and epistemology; that is, the philosophy of how we know what we know. The values underlying each epistemological position frame the choice of specific methods. Consequently, these authors posit, it becomes necessary to scrutinize whether existing methods fulfil the requirements of distributive sufficiency in the field. Bhana and Kanjee seem to suggest that methodological eclecticism can assure sufficiency provided the selected methods are appropriate for specific purposes and contexts. However, they remain mindful of the difficulties inherent in conducting community psychology research and the challenges that accompany attempts at forging methodological sufficiency and representivity.

In Chapter 9 Kelly and Van der Riet are clear in their choice of methodology and so examine the foundations, processes, and methods of the participatory research (PR) approach. They take a critical view of the characteristics evident in PR, the idea of research as praxis, and the relationship between PR and community control and decision making. They also analyse the processes involved in initiating PR, fostering

9

community engagement in the research endeavour, and enabling critical reflections in contextual research. Even though planning for real and participatory rural appraisal are useful methods for encouraging community collaboration, these authors remind us that the real challenge lies in forging hybrid methodologies that incorporate local knowledge. The creation of such hybrids obviously challenges our understanding and ideas of science.

These challenges are further accentuated by Potter and Kruger in Chapter 10, which is the last chapter in this section and discusses issues pertinent to programme evaluation. Potter and Kruger extensively and critically review the field of programme evaluation, highlighting its current status and associated methodologies and applications. When read alongside the other chapters in this section, we discern that the challenges perhaps converge around questions of ideology, the relationship between politics and knowledge creation, and contested world-views. How and why we produce and disseminate knowledge depend on our world-views, which logically then requires us to examine the philosophy, purpose, and history of science as we know it and all its variants today.

2.3 Section III: Practice in community psychology

In Section III, which examines community psychology practice within the South African context, we note that despite the theoretical, methodological, and contextual restrictions that scholars alert us to, community psychologists in South Africa – like many of their peers elsewhere – have forged innovative roles and associated applications that endeavour to transcend the limitations of the individual orientation. Community psychologists have intervened to address several key priority psycho-social areas, discerning a role for themselves in the promotion of safety; in the development of a culture of accountability where criminal justice systems have failed; in reconstructing gendered identities; in upholding gender equality; in empowering marginalized caregivers; and in policy formulation.

In Chapter 11 Butchart and Kruger reveal the synergistic potential of forging links between community psychology and public health when promoting safety at an aggregate level. They show how the public health methodology of epidemiology and associated concepts of incidence, prevalence, morbidity, and mortality can usefully complement the systems and process focus of community psychology to foster injury prevention within low-income and marginalized communities. Mohan, in Chapter 12, extends this perspective by alerting us to the nuances and complexities inherent in adopting a public health focus in safety promotion in low-income countries. This author argues that education campaigns cannot by themselves reduce injury. The complex socio-economic, technological, and cultural profiles of low-income countries warrant more than a simple adaptation of technologies and methodologies developed in high-income contexts. Among the many innovative safety promotion measures that require consideration, Mohan recommends the establishment of consumer protection courts and rapid data-gathering and assessment techniques.

In Chapter 13 Nell picks up the key arguments from the two preceding chapters to examine the applicability of the public health approach in situations where the criminal justice system, including policing, has become dysfunctional and inept. The uncritical adoption of a public health approach without adequate efforts to foster a culture of accountability and effective policing may well undermine the safety-promotion agenda in low-income countries. Nell appeals to the activist agenda of community psychology in his analysis of how the discipline's methodologies and technologies may be applied to engender accountable and effective policing. Community psychology, Nell argues, can make its best contribution by addressing the root causes of suffering and transforming those contexts that produce adversity in the first place.

How should gun violence be approached? Is it a public health or criminal justice issue? In Chapter 14 Cock addresses these and other vexing questions on the subject of gun violence. Gun violence has reached crisis proportions in contemporary South Africa, and the way out of this situation, according to Cock, lies in the development of a localized anti-militaristic ethos and transformative feminism that transcends the boundaries of individualized therapy and state-driven policy formulation. Cock keenly addresses the linkages between gender identities, power, and violence. Like Nell (Chapter 13), she challenges community psychology to extend its activist agenda, and goes further to encourage us to redefine our analytical prisms to include 'Utopian thinking' and 'multiple streams' in our theoretical and applied formulations.

Whereas Cock sensitizes us to the gendered nature of identities, De la Rey, in Chapter 15, examines the relationship between gender, social inequality, mental health, and mental health service provision. In addressing a marginalized area of activity within community psychology in general, De la Rey expounds on the benefits of a consciousness-raising approach to groupwork when intervening to promote gender equality. While De la Rey extols the value of groupwork and implicitly demonstrates the commonalities between community psychology and feminism, she emphasizes the importance of using groupwork alongside a multiplicity of other strategies. The usefulness of consciousness-raising groupwork as intervention strategy is augmented if it is used alongside other macro-level and multi-sectoral initiatives addressing gender equality.

In Chapter 16 Duncan and Van Niekerk examine the logic, context, processes, and outcomes associated with a multi-leveled psycho-educational programme designed to harness the well-being of pre-school children. Framed within a community psychology perspective, the programme operationalizes the concept of empowerment through training programmes for care-givers of pre-school children. Following Swartz and Gibson (Chapter 3), these authors also examine some of the tensions evident in their programme. Even though participants fared well in paper and pencil examinations and showed an increased awareness of pre-school children's psycho-social, emotional, and intellectual needs, an initial evaluation revealed that there is little indication of the 'multiplier' effect in the form of the envisaged social action by the trainees. The tendency among trainees to define themselves as psychotherapists in training and the associated power differential between the trainers and trainees are among the many challenging issues that Duncan and Van Niekerk attempt to evaluate in their assessment of the value of their work with care-givers of pre-school children.

In Chapter 17, the concluding chapter of this section, Lazarus employs personalized case material to help us understand the role, challenges, and skills inherent in working at a social policy level. Whereas most of the chapters in this section tend to favour bottom-up actions, Lazarus demonstrates the merits of engaging the macro-social policy level. Lazarus demystifies the processes and dynamics associated with social policy formulation work that otherwise remains inaccessible and inexplicable to community and academic activists. Despite the value of working at social policy level, Lazarus alerts us to the dangers of regarding policy work as a panacea for community activism, and emphasizes the need for community psychologists to continue operating as critical analysts, providing critical commentary on policy developments insofar as they may or may not advance a culture of human rights.

2.4 Section IV: Perspectives from elsewhere

In Section IV, which presents views on trends and practice in community psychology in non-South African settings, we are transported to Australia and the United States, where community psychology originated under somewhat different circumstances to those in South Africa.

In Chapter 18, Bishop, Sonn, Fisher, and Drew reflect on the fluid state of the discipline in Australia and demonstrate the extent to which the philosophy of North American community psychology has become universalized. Yet its techniques and methods are sometimes amenable to adaptation to suit local applications. While scholars may debate the wisdom of adapting North American techniques for local situations, the case examples provided by Bishop et al. offer instructive lessons on how the theory, method, and practice of community psychology may be synergized to promote local development in an ethical and responsible manner. Some of the more important questions raised in this chapter include: Does the adaptation of North American community psychology deny us in South Africa, and the South in general, the opportunity to develop and forge our own indigenous forms of psychology? If so, can our localized psychology be free of the ideological, philosophical, and epistemological influences of the American discipline? Furthermore, are we suggesting that there are multiple culturally constructed conceptual worlds that are stratified by unequal power relationships, and therefore have very little hope of intersecting in any real way?

In Chapter 19, the final chapter of this volume, Sparks, like Mulvey (1988), points us to the many barriers to the activist orientation and the commitment of community psychology to championing the plight of the marginalized. Despite its early reformist orientation, the growth of the community mental health movement in the United States has been stymied by fiscal constraints arising from legislative changes informed by political conservatism, an underplanned and undercoordinated de-institutionalization process, and the uncritical introduction of managed care. Ironically, despite the core tenets of community psychology that place the focus squarely on the mental health of the collective and the deleterious impact of uncaring environments, interventions in practice often place the accent on the individual and his or her family. Marginal attention is accorded to socio-economic issues relating to housing, unemployment, poverty, and transportation. The ecological and social action perspectives tend to enjoy marginal application within the discipline as a whole. Pretorius-Heuchert and Ahmed, and Ahmed and Pretorius-Heuchert in Chapters 2 and 5, respectively, also articulate this view. Sparks warns against too much reliance on governmental or other large single sources of funding. The development of economic independence is cardinal in efforts to uphold epistemological and philosophical independence, which places the emphasis on the disenfranchised and marginalized peoples of the North and South.

By way of a conclusion we wish to stress that this book represents a celebration of the diverse yet interlinked works of some primarily South African based psychologists struggling to attain epistemological autonomy, uphold theoretical pluralism, and forge innovative and inclusive methodologies. This book also reflects the struggles of these psychologists to transcend rhetorical platitudes and to define applications that permit global thinking within the purview of local action. After a careful study of this book you will no doubt appreciate that community psychology remains an incom-

plete project. So we invite you, the reader, to celebrate the achievements and insights of all the contributors to this book as you prepare to take up the call to develop your own innovative solutions to the many unanswered questions this book raises.

References

ARN, D., STIEGER, C., LOBNIG, H., GUSCHEL-BAUER, H., and FRYER, D. (1988). European network of community psychology. *Journal of Community and Applied Social Psychology*, 8(6), 429–431.

ASARIA, M. I. (1984). Science: Western prerogative or Muslim priority. *Afkar Inquiry. Magazine of Events and Ideas*, 1(2), 4.

BERNAL, G. (1985). A history of psychology in Cuba. *Journal of Community Psychology*, 13(1), 222–235.

BOZZOLI, B. (1987). *Class, community and ideology: The evolution of South African society.* Johannesburg: Ravan Press.

BULHAN, H. A. (1989). *Family therapy in the urban trenches: Dialectics of oppression and therapy.* Unpublished manuscript.

BUTCHART, A. and SEEDAT, M. (1990). Within and without: Images of community and implications for South African psychology. *Social Science and Medicine*, 31(10), 1093–1102.

DOKECKI, P. R. (1992). On knowing the community of caring persons: A methodological basis for the reflective-generative practice of community psychology. *Journal of Community Psychology*, 20(1), 26–35.

GORDON, E. W. (1988). *Human diversity and pedagogy.* New Haven: Yale University.

GORDON, E. W. and SHIPMAN, S. (1988). *Human diversity and pedagogy.* In E. W. Gordon and Associates (Eds.), *Human diversity and pedagogy.* New Haven: Yale University.

HORKHEIMER, M. (1974). *Eclipse of reason.* New York: Seabury Press.

LAZARUS, S. and SEEDAT, M. (1996). *Community psychology in South Africa.* Paper presented at the fifth biannual conference of the Society for Community Research and Action, Chicago.

MCGUIRE, W. (1981). *A contextualist view of psychology*. Unpublished document, Yale University.

MUDIMBE, V. J. (1988). *The invention of Africa: Gnosis, philosophy and the order of knowledge*. USA: Indiana University Press.

MULVEY, A. (1988). Community psychology and feminism: Tensions and commonalties. *Journal of Community Psychology*, **16**(1), 70–83.

NGUGI WA THIONG'O. (1986). *Decolonising the mind: The politics of language in African literature*. Zimbabwe: Zimbabwe Publishing House.

SARDAR, Z. (1984). The need for Islamic science. *Afkar Inquiry. Magazine of Events and Ideas*, **1**(2), 47–48.

SEEDAT, M. (1993). *Topics, trends and silences in South African psychology 1948–1988: Ethnocentrism, crisis and liberatory echoes*. Unpublished doctoral thesis, University of the Western Cape.

SEEDAT, M., CLOETE, N., and SHOCHET, I. (1988). Community psychology: Panic or panacea. *Psychology in Society*, **11**, 39–54.

SEEDAT, M. and NELL, V. (1990). Third world or one world: Mysticism, pragmatism and pain in family therapy in South Africa. *South African Journal of Psychology*, **20**(3), 141–149.

SHOTTER, J. (1975). *Images of man in psychological research*. London: Methuen.

STANFIELD, J.H. (1985). The ethnocentric bias of social science knowledge production. *Review of Research in Education*, **12**(2), 320–331.

THORNTON, R. and RAMPHELE, M. (1988). The quest for community. In E. Boonzaier and J. Sharp (Eds.), *South African keywords: The uses and abuses of political concepts*. Cape Town: David Philip.

WYN DAVIES, M. (1986). Islamising the behavioural sciences. *Afkar Inquiry. Magazine of Events and Ideas*, **3**(7), 54–58.

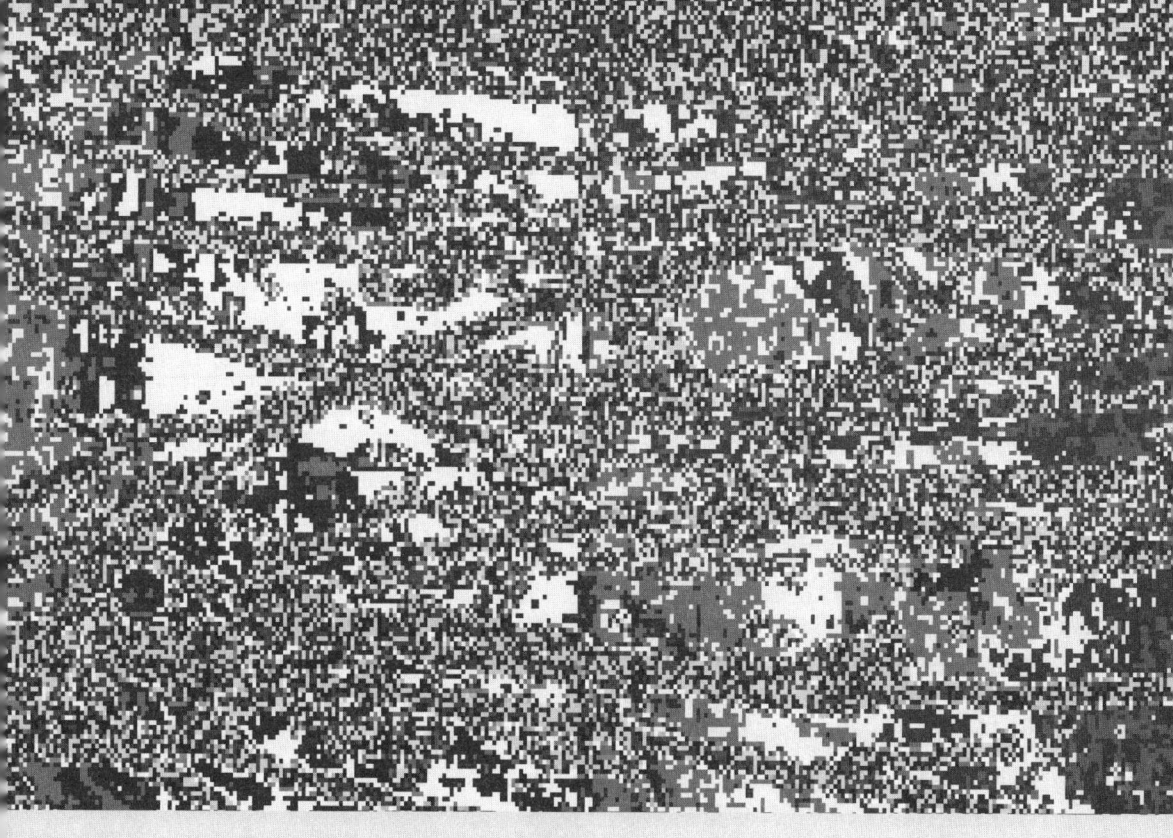

SECTION I

Theoretical and
paradigmatic
considerations

2

Community psychology: past, present, and future

JW Pretorius-Heuchert
Rashid Ahmed

'Power concedes nothing without a demand'
Frederick Douglass 1855/1969 (Bulhan, 1985, p. 278).

Study objectives

When you have completed the material in this chapter, you should be able to:
- give an accurate description of what the discipline of community psychology entails;
- discuss how Frederick Douglass's maxim 'nothing is conceded without a demand' applies to community psychology;
- discuss the current role of community psychology;
- describe how the different perspectives in community psychology can influence what psychologists working within these perspectives do;
- describe and differentiate between mental health demands, socio-political demands, and academic and professional demands in the development of community psychology;
- differentiate between 'prevalence' and 'incidence' in epidemiological research;
- describe who works in communities, from the community psychology perspective;
- discuss the historical reasons for the development of community psychology;
- discuss the role that community psychology can play in South Africa's future; and
- discuss what the main objections to mainstream psychology are.

1 Introduction

When Frederick Douglass wrote that 'nothing is conceded without a demand' he was talking about his own, and the African-American, struggle for liberation. However, his statement is also an appropriate summary of the history and development of community psychology. In most countries in the world community psychology was developed in response to oppressive systems and

17

often in contrast to existing helping services. As a discipline, community psychology was developed in response to three broad demands: (1) a demand for appropriate services for people who could benefit from psychological intervention; (2) a socio-political demand for the effective use of psychology in the fight against oppression (or to help the victims of oppression); and finally, (3) a demand from within psychology for a more relevant psychology at the levels of application, theory, and research. Invariably these demands led to a focus on social change as a final goal and outcome. The role these demands played in the development of community psychology will be considered throughout this chapter and book, in which we will look at what the role and place of community psychology are, and the historical development of the field in South Africa and other countries. We will also consider social change as a model for community psychology in post-apartheid South Africa.

In this age of psychology we are becoming increasingly aware of the frailty of the human psyche, particularly within the context of oppressive systems, and the associated resilience of people and communities who survive, and often thrive, despite the odds against them. Psychologists, other professionals, community leaders, and the general public are confronted with the great need for psychological services in South Africa and in other countries. Community psychology is often seen as a means of providing these services, while working for social change and attempting to understand the needs of people and communities.

During the apartheid era the prevailing socio-political and economic context in South Africa was one of strict racial segregation, violent oppression of the majority, and economic exploitation and deprivation of labour. This led to a racially stratified society, with whites living under so-called First World conditions with colonial privileges, and blacks living under so-called Third World conditions of poverty, oppression, and exploitation. South Africa is a low- to middle-income country, but the racially skewed distribution of wealth ensures that most whites live as if in a highly industrialized country, leaving most blacks in conditions similar to that of a non-industrialized country. These socio-political and economic factors were obviously detrimental to the physical and mental well-being of all South Africans. The long-term negative psychological effects of oppression, especially on the oppressed, but also on the oppressor, have been explicated in the writings of Frantz Fanon (1967a, 1967b, 1967c; 1968), Hussein Bulhan (1985), and others. Material conditions of the majority of South Africans were appalling and many people were living under conditions of extreme deprivation. Seedat (1984) demonstrates how the policies of apartheid were designed to systematically 'cripple the nation'. Several psychologists responded to the need to address social factors impinging on the mental well-being of communities. Community psychology, particularly the social action approach, provided the means to act.

The racial stratification referred to above was also evident in the provision of mental health services and in the responses of communities to apartheid. Most whites either accepted and supported apartheid, or at least complacently benefited from the privileges it afforded them. Most blacks resisted in whatever overt or covert way they could. Balancing the extent and nature of resistance against the need for survival are crucial factors that are always evident in the decisions people make about responding to oppression. Community psychology provided a legitimate vehicle, which was acceptable to mainstream psychology, for some psychologists to take socio-political action. For others, however, this legitimacy was incidental and community psychology provided a revolutionary weapon in the struggle for democracy and human liberation.

2 What is community psychology?

Community psychology can be described as a heterogeneous branch of psychology and no single definition can accurately capture the complexities inherent in its theory and praxis. There is also no consensus among the different paradigms in the discipline about a single definition for the field. The different approaches to community psychology, for example mental health, social action, ecological, and organizational, and the different perspectives within these approaches presented in this text, will demonstrate the heterogeneous nature of community psychology.

Generally speaking, a central premise of community psychology is 'the importance of developing theory, research, and intervention that locates individuals, social settings, and communities in sociocultural context' (Trickett, 1996, p. 209). This means

that community psychology regards whole communities, and not only individuals, as possible clients. There is an awareness of the importance of the interaction between individuals and their environments, in terms of causing and alleviating problems. The approach is based on group organization; community strengths, dynamics, resources, and competencies; the empowerment of individuals, groups, and communities (Kroeker, 1995; Perkins and Zimmerman, 1995); the prevention and alleviation of psychological symptoms; and the elimination of individual and socio-political conditions that produce psychological symptoms. This is usually achieved through social action by individuals, communities, or community psychology professionals aimed at changing material conditions and socio-political policies and systems. In addition to the above, community psychology also evaluates psychological intervention, and the impact of interventions on communities and individuals. Recently the promotion of 'wellness' or 'well-being' has also begun to be accepted as one of the goals of the mental health paradigm of community psychology (Cowen, 1997). Although there is no single definition of community psychology, it is fair to say that all the approaches in community psychology have the common goal of improving the human condition and promoting psychological well-being. This goal is achieved by applying knowledge and methods of study, research, intervention, and evaluation from the broader disciplines of psychology and the social sciences in community or organizational contexts.

Although community psychology is currently a sub-division of the field of psychology, its intimate and comprehensive involvement in the broader community necessitates a much larger theoretical and practical base than only psychology. Community psychology is therefore located largely in psychology, but also in mental health, public health, psychiatry, politics, anthropology, history, archeology, environmental studies, sociology, and other fields.

3 What is currently accepted as the role of community psychologists?

The different approaches in community psychology usually circumscribe the role of the community psychologist working from a particular perspective. Thus, a community psychologist working from the mental health perspective will most likely work in a community mental health centre, offering psychological services such as psychotherapy to clients, or designing and implementing mental illness prevention programmes. A community psychologist working from a social action perspective may assist neighbourhood organizations in communities to mobilize against drug traffickers, or against biased police action, or in favour of a safe playground. A community psychologist from the ecological perspective, however, may be involved in doing research on the impact of economic changes in a community or how a 'sense of community' is established (Plas and Lewis, 1996). A community psychologist from an organizational perspective may be involved in multicultural sensitivity training in an organization or an

intrapersonal empowerment project in the workplace (Spreitzer, 1995). Very few psychologists, however, adhere to only one perspective. Most community psychologists use parts of different theories in their everyday practice.

There are many people involved in communities, and the field that community psychologists work in is claimed by many, but not owned by any. Clinical psychologists, counselling psychologists, community psychologists, psychiatrists, mental health workers, activists, counsellors, consultants, community organizers, psychiatric nurses, and social workers are all active in the field, and there is often very little distinction between what they all claim to do. For a discussion of the different roles and origins of some of the above professions, the reader may consult Sarason (1976). This list of community workers is by no means exhaustive, and there are also other organized groups such as sociologists and anthropologists, cops and gangs, teachers and preachers, and a myriad of others involved in some communities. These groups are differentiated by the different perspectives, motives, and value systems underlying their involvement in a community. What most of them have in common is a willingness to take action to improve the quality of life of the community. However, professionals sometimes tend to disagree about disciplinary boundaries and the associated areas of specialization. Community psychology is no exception. For example, alleviation of psychological distress is one of the specialization areas of community psychology, but Nell (1994) points out that the medical professions, mainly physicians and nurses, in

South Africa have colonized psychological distress. He argues strongly in favour of a demedicalization of psychological distress. Community psychology represents an attempt to work across, and within, many disciplines, combining the knowledge and practices of many fields. Practitioners of community psychology therefore also come from many disciplines.

4 Historical overview of the origins of community psychology

It is often said that psychology has a short history, but a long past. The better part of this statement refers to the roots of psychology, namely philosophy, religion, and other disciplines. Its relatively short history refers to the fact that psychology was only formally established about a hundred years ago. The field of psychology was formally established in Europe in the 1800s when the individual was exalted. Since then, the theory and practice of mainstream psychology has concentrated on the functioning of the individual. As a result, most of the work done by psychologists has been to help individuals to adapt to life – be it to their personal psychological existence, their biological drives, or their social and political circumstances. In addition, most psychologists still operate from the medical model where the professional provides remediation for individual deficits by promoting intrapsychic change, instead of empowering the individual to affect systemic change, where necessary. Mainstream psychology is largely

a conservative discipline that, actively or passively, omits to work for change and tends to thereby support the status quo.

Community psychology, on the other hand, has an even shorter history of about thirty years, and an even longer past. Ever since the first humans organized themselves into groups, and a sense of belonging to a group, working together towards a common goal, and caring for one another was established, community psychology has been at work. This sense of community stood people in good stead until the Industrial Revolution and its concomitant individualization, alienation, and exploitation of workers. Capitalist systems are in essence individual-oriented systems, and generally oppose collective ideas, movements, and groups. This aspect of capitalism has entered every area of human endeavour, including the relatively new academic disciplines such as psychology (see Hamber, Masilela, and Terre Blanche's Chapter 4 in this volume). The discipline of community psychology is in some way a formalization or professionalization of the age-old wisdom of people living together. Some would say community psychology represents an appropriation or colonization.

Community psychology came about at a time when there was a greater awareness of the benefits of collective action. This awareness came about primarily in response to oppression and the restriction of civil liberties, an understanding of the detrimental effects of an over-reliance on individuality, and an acceptance of the potential benefits of mass intervention and prevention of distress. In addition, there was also an increasing awareness of the limits of traditional methods of psychological treatment, mostly psychotherapy to individuals who had the means, and chose to have therapy, or else custodial care of severely mentally disturbed individuals. Another major source of dissatisfaction with the traditional approach was that it was largely based on the medical model that saw psychological problems as 'illnesses' based in the individual, with very little understanding of the complex environmental forces contributing to the establishment of psychological problems. It should be remembered that the United States of America, in particular, was at the time of the formal establishment of community psychology, during the 1960s, under pressure to respond to demands from human rights activists to attend to social inequalities such as poverty, discrimination, civil rights, racism, and sexism. A more cynical interpretation of the events that led to the establishment of community psychology is that governments saw the economic benefits that may be gained by discharging large numbers of patients from psychiatric hospitals and shifting the burden of care from the state to the community (Pretorius, 1988).

De-institutionalization and community psychology

An important historical mental health related event was the process of de-institutionalization. This legal mandate in the USA forced professionals and communities to provide community-based services to the thousands of long-term patients discharged from psychiatric hospitals. The pressure to release patients came at an opportune time when the liberal social and professional climate of the 1960s was supportive of a mass release of patients into the community. Unfortunately, in many cases, the community was not ready, willing, able, resourced, or prepared for this event, and this led to the 'not in my backyard' type of opposition to mental health facilities being established in neighbourhoods (Takahashi and Dear, 1997). As a result most ex-patients soon made their way back to hospitals and jails, or ended up destitute and on the streets (Pretorius, 1988). (Also see Sparks' Chapter 19 in this volume.)

In South Africa the ideas and principles of community psychology and de-institutionalization have also, and are still being, applied. For example, Hillbrow Lodge, a halfway house of Sterkfontein Psychiatric Hospital, was established in 1975 in an effort to reintegrate long-term psychiatric patients into the community. Current educational efforts to mainstream children with special needs involve the application of two important principles of the mental health perspective of community psychology. These are the principle of de-institutionalization, which keeps children out of special schools and in the regular classrooms, and the principle of the 'least restrictive environment', which allows people to function at their highest level.

The realization that hospitals were

often ineffective, inefficient, expensive, overcrowded, and poorly staffed with poorly trained personnel that provided little more than custodial, and many would say abusive or inhumane, care, also led to de-institutionalization. Long-term hospitalization is also often harmful to eventual community reintegration. Furthermore, patients in psychiatric hospitals were traditionally treated and socialized as irresponsible, helpless, and powerless. Very few skills needed to survive independently were acquired in traditional psychiatric hospitals. A decrease in patient numbers was also caused by the discovery of psychotropic medication. This meant that people could 'safely' be discharged because medication was keeping them tranquil and under control. Straight-jackets and padded isolation cells were therefore no longer needed.

Many of the ideas behind de-institutionalization were good, but the motives and methods were often questionable. The poorly planned mass discharge of patients left many individuals, families, and communities vulnerable, and the lack of funding for community facilities suggested an economic motive, rather than the best interest of the patients or the communities. The care of people with psychological or psychiatric problems remains one of the main challenges for community psychologists.

It is generally accepted that the official birth of community psychology occurred at a conference in Swampscott, Massachusetts, USA, from 4 to 8 May 1965. One of the aims of the conference was to reflect on 'the place of psychology in the community mental health movement' (Heller and Monahan, 1977, p. 3). The participants at the Swampscott conference concluded that psychology had a definite role to play in this area. Heller and Monahan (1977) state that social problems have many causes, and propose that psychological solutions, as well as social or political ones, should be considered. It was nonetheless clear that psychology saw a new role for itself, namely expanding its scope to include work in, with, and for the community.

The community mental health movement reflects both the theoretical understandings mentioned above, as well as a process set in motion by new legislation and financial realities in the USA in the late 1950s and early 1960s.

Historical context and reasons underlying the need for the development of community psychology

1 Large numbers of people with psychological problems.
2 Too few people who could help.
3 Not enough financial and physical resources to ensure the provision of help.
4 Too few people with problems sought help from traditional mental health systems.
5 Traditional mental health services provided inefficient, ineffective, and inappropriate services.

6 Traditional mental health services functioned on a waiting basis, rather than a seeking and preventing basis.

7 Societal factors, e.g., apartheid, oppression, and poverty caused psychological problems and stressors.

8 A need for intervention in the larger system was indicated.

9 Prevention, rather than remediation, became a priority.

10 The struggle against apartheid and oppression demanded that psychologists apply their knowledge and skills towards liberation.

The development of community psychology thus served many disparate purposes:

1 It addressed mental health needs in a more effective and appropriate way than traditional, mainstream psychology and psychotherapy.

2 It provided the opportunity to develop a more relevant psychology.

3 It was used as an excuse by some to co-opt and neutralise activist psychologists, while deflecting criticisms of mainstream psychology and at the same time passing the responsibility and costs of mental health services to communities.

4 It provided a 'safe haven' and effective vehicle for those fighting for social change and the improvement of the human condition.

5 Socio-polical demands

5.1 Socio-political factors in the USA

Socio-political changes in the USA, particularly those brought about by the civil rights movement, combined with economic factors, were perhaps the primary catalysts that influenced events in favour of the development of community psychology in the 1960s. The successful insistence on equal political, social, and legal rights for ethnic, social, and political minority communities in the United States, together with widespread consciousness raising and an acceptance of egalitarian values, led people to look at other oppressed groups such as the hospitalized and incarcerated mentally ill. The mechanisms of oppression and liberation also apply to the treatment of those diagnosed as mentally ill. Ignorance, fear, and bias against the mentally ill led to their ostracization, isolation, and oppression. Through community psychology, attempts have been made to bring them back into the mainstream where, as a collective, we are forced to face the challenges of mental illness. The struggle for civil rights for these groups led to many changes in the oppressive laws in the United States, as well as the establishment of several progressive laws under the Democratic Party government of the United States. An example was the legislation to fund the building of mental health centres to provide mental health services in communities instead of removing people who needed help to distant and isolated hospitals. The *Zeitgeist*, or spirit, prevailing at that particular time and place was a dualistic application of Frederick Douglass's maxim that 'nothing is conceded without a demand' – perhaps best embodied by Malcolm X and the Black Consciousness movement, together with the application of Mahatma Gandhi's principles of non-violent resistance through mass civil disobedience and social action, best embodied by Dr Martin Luther King's Utopian 'I have a dream' vision for an integrated, free, and fair society.

Oppressors have always used psychological means to terrorize citizens into submission. In the early 1960s the discipline of community psychology was for the first time formally used as a weapon in the fight against socio-political oppression. Community psychology was established in part to counter the abuses of poverty, racial discrimination, and insufficient mental health services in the USA, and to mobilize for liberation, especially in countries in South America (Montero, 1996) and in South Africa.

5.2 Socio-political factors in South Africa

All the factors mentioned above were also relevant in South Africa. However, South Africa was characterized by greater need, fewer resources, fewer progressive psychologists to work for change, and a much more repressive system. The system of apartheid severely compromised the mental health of all South Africans, including the professional lives of psychologists in terms of their practice and training (Berger and Lazarus, 1987).

South Africa has been the scene of many struggles for liberation for hundreds of years. More recently, however, the National Party ruled South Africa (from 1948 to 1994) and a system of racial segregation, referred to as 'apartheid', was legalized, implemented, and enforced. Blacks were denied the right to vote and there existed a tremendous disparity in political, social, and economic circumstances between the black majority and the white minority.

There was national and international opposition to the system of apartheid, which took many forms. In the late 1950s and early 1960s, after the Sharpeville massacre and the infamous Treason Trial, the Pan African Congress, the African National Congress, and others embarked on an armed struggle to obtain liberty for all South Africans. This struggle was met with intensified repression by the apartheid state, which in turn led to intensified resistance by the oppressed. This active resistance led to the Soweto uprisings of 1976, initially by schoolchildren, followed by workers and students. These uprisings were met with increased violence, massacres, detentions, police torture, bannings, and other forms of repression. This violent reaction to the demand for liberty and civil rights had as a result a more focused and successful armed struggle and an increase in international pressure on the South African government. South African society in the 1970s and 1980s was also marked by a period of intensified resistance from different sectors in civil society. This had as a result the formation of the United Democratic Front (UDF) and the National Forum (NF) in 1983. These organizations consisted of a broad coalition of anti-apartheid forces in

South Africa, and included a range of organizations, from civic to religious bodies, all united in their opposition to apartheid.

In the struggle against apartheid, every person, every group, and even every academic discipline were called upon to contribute and to apply their knowledge and skills towards the liberation of South Africa. A small number of South African psychologists heeded this call and tried to apply the principles of psychology in the fight against oppression, as well as in caring for the victims of this violent system. Psychology was also used to bring about social change in South American countries (Montero, 1996) and in the United States.

5.3 The emergence of community psychology as a mechanism to bring about social change in South Africa

It was during this period of struggle that a small number of psychologists more actively and visibly challenged mainstream psychology and its complicity with apartheid. There was an attempt at developing a critical psychological discourse, as reflected in the title of the 'alternative' journal *Psychology in Society*. There was also organizational engagement through non-governmental organizations in the health and welfare sector. Various organizations, such as Psychologists Against Apartheid and the Organization for Alternative Social Services in South Africa (OASSSA), two organizations of mental health activists, professionals, and students, were established locally and abroad to coordinate concerted resistance against apartheid from within the mental health field.

Mainstream psychology in South Africa, however, remained fixed in the traditional mode of psychology. The debate over the relevance, or irrelevance, of psychology in South Africa is still going on. (See the chapter by Swartz and Gibson, Chapter 3 in this volume, and also Anonymous (1986); Berger and Lazarus (1987); Bodibe (1994); Dawes (1986); Mauer, Marais, and Prinsloo (1991); Michelson (1994); and Perkel (1988).) This debate often centres on South African psychologists' individual-centred practice preferences (Bassa and Schlebusch, 1984), and their lack of community involvement and activism in working for social change.

Community psychology was used in this context as an attempt to make psychological theory and practice 'relevant' for the South African context. Seedat (1990) reviewed articles that appeared in *Psychology in Society* between 1983 and 1988, and according to his thematic categorization 14,9 per cent dealt with the theme of 'Community Psychology', the second highest percentage frequency after the theme 'Materialist and Ideology Critiques' (21,3 per cent). Community psychology was seen by some professionals as an alternative to mainstream approaches. Seedat, Cloete, and Shochet, (1988) considered this issue more fully and argued that community psychology is a contested area and, depending on professionals' vested interests and class locations, could be linked either to an agenda of social change or a mechanism to absorb the challenges posed to mainstream psychology. In their view the latter may serve to keep the discipline intact and maintain the status quo.

Community psychology, then, was one attempt to develop a more 'relevant' psychology in South Africa during the 1980s and early 1990s. Two important achievements need to be highlighted here. Firstly, some professionals took an overt political position by opposing apartheid. Secondly, there was an attempt at developing theory and practice relevant to the oppressed and exploited majority in South Africa. While these were important achievements, certain problems remained. Most professionals were white and middle class and there was a silence around issues related to racism, political violence, and collective action (Seedat, 1990). It is argued that a 'relevant' psychology needed to address these issues as well.

6 Mental health demands

It is difficult to determine the extent of the need for psychological help in South Africa. This is due to the lack of current, relevant data from South Africa because there is no comprehensive mental health information management system. To get an idea of what the need for psychological intervention may be, we can extrapolate from epidemiological research that determines the rate and distribution of different disorders in a community (see Butchart and Kruger in this volume, Chapter 11). Kessler et al. (1994) report that 48 per cent of the population of the United States has at least one diagnosable mental disorder during their lives. If the rates are similar in South Africa, and Reeler (1993) states that there is reason to believe that they are, this would mean that about eighteen million South Africans may be in need of psychological intervention at some point

in their lives. Another indicator could be the known prevalence rate (how many people have a particular disorder) for specific, serious, and debilitating disorders, such as schizophrenia, which is generally accepted to be about 1 per cent of any population. This means that there are about 380 000 schizophrenics who may be in need of services in South Africa. These statistics give one an idea of the extent of psychological services that may be needed in South Africa, if one accepts the traditional definitions of mental health and mental illness, and if one can accurately extrapolate from data generated in other countries. (See Pillay and Lockhat's Chapter 6 in this volume for a detailed discussion on the community mental health service needs for children.)

Only a fraction of the people needing psychological services seek and get treatment at any given time. There are many reasons for this, such as a lack of services, particularly in the rural areas, very few black psychologists, language and cultural barriers, and societal norms that lead to psychological services being perceived as irrelevant or inappropriate. Due to a traditional, or medically based, perspective, as well as limited staff, most workers in the helping sector in South Africa function in a waiting mode, where people with existing problems seek out their services, if available and affordable. A seeking mode of service delivery, on the other hand, takes services to the people that may need them, but more importantly also identifies potential problems and initiates preventative actions. In the context of our special circumstances, which includes recovery from a particularly vicious and oppressive political dispensation, extreme poverty on a massive scale, crime, violence, and a historical time period characterized by uncertainty and change, there are probably millions of people in need of psychological help in South Africa.

Kentridge (in Michelson, 1994), for example, states that more people died in an area in KwaZulu-Natal in an eighteen-month period than in twenty years of violent conflict in Northern Ireland. Michelson (1994) reports a post-traumatic stress disorder (PTSD) incidence rate of 87 per cent in a sample of people displaced by political violence in the same area. If one considers the thousands of displaced people alone, an 87 per cent incidence rate may indicate great distress in many other communities as well. PTSD is a long-term disorder and often has a very negative impact on the people who care for the victim. Witnessing violence also has a significant negative effect on people (Farrel and Bruce, 1997). The snowball effect of the lack of treatment for these victims exponentially increases the need for services.

The effectiveness of individual, one-on-one psychotherapy was questioned at the time. In addition, it was also clear that few people had access to, or could afford, individual therapy, and the community perspective raised the hopes of more affordable and accessible mental health care, particularly for the poor and poorly educated groups who were often excluded from receiving psychotherapy. Fundamental questions about the validity of diagnosis and the understanding of mental illness from a medical model or disease perspective were also asked. In particular, the individually based explanatory system used to account for psychological distress was questioned

and an awareness of societal and environmental contributing factors was developing. The long-term psychological effects of discrimination, poverty, and oppression were especially targeted for study and intervention.

Emotional health, and emotional problems, are still a concern of many psychologists, including community psychologists. De-institutionalization and the 'least restrictive environment' are also still guiding principles in the field. However, if traditional psychology and psychotherapy, if deemed effective or appropriate, are to be used to alleviate the problems mentioned above, it would mean that many thousands of psychologists would have to have been trained by now. But, as in the USA, South African psychologists are realizing that 'no mass disorder afflicting humankind is ever eliminated or brought under control by attempting to treat affected individuals, or by attempting to train individual practitioners in large numbers' (Albee, 1983, p.4). What is the alternative? Many psychologists have sought the answer to this question in the field of community psychology, and specifically in the social action model of community psychology. The fact that community psychology aims at mass interventions, trains and uses large numbers of people for interventions, and purports to prevent psychological problems before they arise makes it an attractive alternative to traditional individual psychotherapy where one person is seen at a time.

7 Academic and professional demands

Mental health needs and the civil rights *Zeitgeist* converged with the establishment's economic interests in the development of community psychology as a compromise between revolutionary psychologists and the status quo. There are several other examples where community psychology has, rightly or wrongly, been accused of blunting the initial radicalism of progressive psychology. Since it was accepted as a branch of psychology, community psychology has been under pressure to become more mainstream and to tone down its political radicalism and activism. This pressure often relates to the criticism of being unscientific, which is regarded as a mortal sin in mainstream psychology. So, since its inception community psychology has been under threat of co-option, rejection for being too radical, or criticism for not being radical enough. Finding a common voice and protecting itself from being used for nefarious purposes have proven impossible, and perhaps undesirable. Hence the different approaches, perspectives, and underlying philosophies in the current discipline. The debate on the relevance of community psychology and the need for radical solutions to social problems continues unabated, as is evident from several chapters in this text (see Hamber, Masilela, and Terre Blanche, Chapter 4; and Swartz and Gibson, Chapter 3, in this volume).

The academic discipline of psychology consists of many areas of interest for the hundreds of thousands of psychologists world-wide. In the United States the American Psychological Association (APA) has, in addition to a division for community psychology, forty-seven other separate divisions (Morris, 1996). The Psychological Society of South Africa (PsySSA) has nine divisions, but none for community psychology, yet. Although community psychology uses many of the principles of the broader discipline, it also has some fundamental differences with what is considered mainstream psychology.

7.1 A brief critique of mainstream or traditional psychology

There have been a wide range of criticisms against mainstream psychological theory and practice, both nationally (see, for example, Nicholas and Cooper, 1990) and internationally (see, for example, Ibáñez and Íñiquez, 1997; Serrano-Garcia, Lopez, and Rivera-Medina, 1987; Serrano-Garcia, 1994). These criticisms raise fundamental challenges to mainstream theory and practice, and alternative paradigms linked to an agenda of social change, such as community psychology (Rappaport, 1977; Serrano-Garcia et al., 1987), have been preferred as alternatives.

It is not possible to fully explore all of the issues raised but hopefully this brief discussion captures the main thrust of the arguments without oversimplifying them. At the outset it is important to stress that many of the issues discussed are related, but the headings are used to organize the information more meaningfully.

The main criticisms of mainstream psychology are related to the following:

1   The appropriateness of a natural science methodology based on positivism as a framework for psychology.

2   At the ideological and political level the role that psychological theory and practice play in producing and maintaining oppressive and exploitative social relations. This refers to the role of psychology in maintaining power and unequal relationships.

3   The unwillingness or inability to consider social, historical, and political dimensions in psychological discourse and practice.

Each of these is discussed in turn below.

7.1.1 Psychology as a science

There have been fundamental challenges to psychology's epistemological, philosophical, and ideological framework (Moll, 1983; Serrano-Garcia et al., 1987; Spears, 1997). The dominant tradition in psychology has been the positivist approach. Positivism holds that there is an objective reality that can be discovered by the neutral scientist (Moll, 1983). In this conception the scientist/practitioner is a neutral, value-free individual whose role it is to objectively gather data in the pursuit of truth or knowledge. Knowledge is gained by following established scientific procedures based on a natural science methodology.

The positivist approach has been vigorously challenged as an inadequate framework for human subjectivity. Criticisms are aimed at its underlying assumptions about science and humans, its ahistorical and acontextual approach, and the role of the scientist/practitioner in knowledge production. Instead of natural science methodology, Serrano-Garcia et al. (1987) argue for the use of alternative methodologies and different theoretical frameworks, because a positivist framework neglects the social and historical dimensions of human subjectivity. There have also been numerous calls for social contextual understandings of the human experience (Serrano-Garcia et al., 1987; Spears, 1997). Values and social needs should therefore inform the field, direct priorities, and form the context for understanding and valuing human subjectivity.

The positivist assumption of a neutral, value-free scientist/practitioner has in recent years been the subject of consistent critique. According to Rappaport (1977) neutrality is itself a political position. Being neutral and not challenging an oppressive system means that the oppression is allowed to continue unchecked. Therefore being neutral means support for the status quo by allowing it to continue. Claiming neutrality not only supports prevailing capitalist values, but also discourages socio-political activism and action. Professionals therefore need to be aware of their own subjectivity in terms of values and beliefs, and to be critical of the meta-theoretical and epistemological assumptions underlying their work. As Spears (1997) suggests, scientists also need to be critical of their interventionist role in knowledge production.

The positivist assumption that science is a quest for truth has been similarly challenged. Post-modernist thought challenges the idea of a single, objective truth and emphasises multiple understandings of reality. Multiple truths should, however, not lead to extreme relativism, where oppressive ideologies are reproduced by allowing other views while undermining them at the same time as subjective relativism. The aim of post-modernism should be seen as supporting and encouraging hidden voices and liberating our understanding from the positivist constrictions of a single truth. It can be argued that positivism in fact distorts truth and serves to mask unequal social relations. Within community psychology, Reiff (1977) and Serrano-Garcia et al. (1987) argue for the use of knowledge for social change rather than some esoteric scientific pursuit of truth.

7.1.2 Psychology, ideology, and power

How is psychology implicated in producing and maintaining oppressive and exploitative social relations? Professionals within the discipline find themselves in a relatively powerful position in society and may take active steps to retain this power. They may do this by openly aligning themselves with those in power (Nicholas and Cooper, 1990) or by being involved in scientific activities that perpetuate existing social relations – for example, the professionals who were engaged in research that supported the apartheid state in South Africa. Professionals' interventions and the knowledge they produce may also unwittingly maintain relations of domination by, for example, helping and encouraging people to adapt to oppressive situations, instead of equipping and encouraging them to change the situation. Thompson (1990) refers to ideology as a set of beliefs that can either be used to maintain or used to challenge relations of power.

Psychological knowledge and practice as well as its silences, that is, what is not addressed, may be viewed as ideological, in the sense that they serve to maintain power and domination. Marxists would argue that all knowledge that does not reveal economic and class domination serves to maintain relations of domination inherent in capitalism. A Marxist critique would include traditional psychology as a discipline and body of knowledge that does not reveal economic and class domination. (See Chapter 4 by Hamber, Masilela, and Terre Blanche in this text for more on a Marxist community psychology.)

7.1.3 Psychology and social change

There has always been a tension in psychology, and in philosophy before the establishment of psychology, with regards to the extent that people are influenced by their biology, as opposed to their environment. This relates to the old nature/nurture debate. The position one takes in this debate will determine how one sees change. If you adhere to the nature/biology perspective, you would probably see change as localized in the individual, but if you support the nurture/environment perspective, you would probably think that society needs to change if you want to affect the individual. As has been indicated before, psychology has been an individual-centred discipline. After the Swampscott Conference, however, psychology tried to emphasize communities and social change. While this emphasis was new for psychologists and psychology, the value of communities had been known in different forms throughout the ages. Spaulding and Balch (1983), for example, document the history of primary prevention in communities since the early 1900s.

In South Africa, formal community-based interventions also occurred long before the official birth of community psychology. The study of South Africa's 'poor white' population, conducted for the Carnegie Report in the 1920s, is an example of an early community-oriented research and intervention project. The importance of this report lies not only in its comprehensiveness, but also serves as an example of how information is used politically. This five-year study and five-volume report was dedicated to study and help an already privileged section of the South African population, while no such work was commissioned to study the disenfranchised majority. We should remember that psychology, and community psychology in particular, is never politically neutral and that there are usually conservative or progressive agendas, as well as conservative agendas masquerading as progressive agendas at play in any community psychology endeavour. (Chapter 19 by Sparks in this volume illuminates the intricate relationship between politics, legislation, funding, ideology, and practice in community psychology.)

The social change perspective argues that an individual-centred psychology is not only inappropriate and ineffective, but could be counter-productive in that it impedes social advancement and can be used to mollify and thus oppress people.

8 Post-apartheid South Africa, social change, and challenges for community psychology

The first democratic post-apartheid election of 1994 resulted in an overwhelming victory for the African National Congress, and the people of South Africa. One of the major tasks facing the present government is addressing the inequities of the past and building a democratic society. The changing global economy (Hoogvelt, 1997), the collapse of communism in Eastern Europe, and changing material conditions nationally have also provided new obstacles in the task of social transformation in South Africa.

There is enormous debate as to what constitutes social transformation. Two key elements of this debate are, firstly, the mechanisms in South Africa that guarantee both individual and group rights and freedom, that is, democratization and political freedom. The second, related element refers to addressing historical disadvantage in order to establish a more just and democratic society.

With the new South African Constitution and reforms in the legal system, both democratization and political freedom are largely achieved and ensured. Addressing historical disadvantages should ensure that sectors and groups who were previously discriminated against and marginalized achieve equality in the new social order. In order to achieve this, the principles of access, redress, and equity need to be attended to. Access refers to establishing mechanisms by which groups can have recourse to previously denied resources; redress refers to the attempt to correct historical imbalances in power and resources; and equity refers to achieving parity, fairness, and equality in the distribution of power and resources.

An equitable distribution of power and resources, and increasing democratization and political freedom are two indices of social transformation. However, there are different views with regard to these indices. While the more obvious disparities are the economic and political ones, there are still ideological and social differences evident in the 'Rainbow Nation', particularly in terms of power and people's world-views, that need to be synergized. Social change therefore involves both a political and ideological struggle (Simon, 1982). Furthermore, while the universal franchise and a new constitution are crucial for social change, they do not guarantee change (Badat, 1994). What is also needed is active citizen participation at the many different levels that will enable citizens to contribute to the process of change.

What can psychology contribute to this process of restitution, nation-building, reconciliation, and reconstruction, while continuing to attend to the needs of the victims of the previous system, redressing past neglects, and attending to new concerns and crises? Clearly, community psychology provides theories and practices that can be used for the mass interventions needed in the transformation of oppressive systems. By working towards social change, community psychology can assist in the political and ideological challenges ahead, and it can facilitate greater citizen participation. It can

provide a more relevant psychology, and appropriate and effective social services, and facilitate the process of social change in the move to a post-apartheid South Africa where there is an improvement in the well-being of all South Africans.

South Africa is a unique social laboratory where universal issues of different cultures, languages, and contexts can be resolved. So, an added challenge for community psychology in South Africa could be to see South Africa as a microcosm of the world and use the opportunities South Africa presents to work towards solving global problems in psychology and other fields.

Perhaps the most important contribution to social change that community psychology can make in South Africa is to help develop a sense of community in a country steeped in decades of conflict and animosity. According to Plas and Lewis (quoting Sarason, 1976, p. 109) this sense of community will include developing the 'perception of similarity to others, an acknowledged interdependence by giving to, or doing for others what one expects from them, the feeling that one is part of a larger dependable and stable structure'. In other words, community psychology should contribute towards building a secure and stable society from the fragments left by apartheid.

Exercises

1 Form a panel of experts with four other people in your class. Your task is to make a recommendation to your class with regards to the community-based treatment options that should be

considered for a patient who has been in a psychiatric hospital for many years. The patient is not a risk to society, or to him-/herself, but he/she needs supervision and care.

2 Political activism is a controversial issue in community psychology. Form two teams in your class to debate the arguments in favour of psychologists including political action in their work, and the arguments against such activism.

3 The president of South Africa has asked you to propose a plan that can be used to address any psychological or mental health issue of national concern. If your plan is accepted, government support and funding will be provided. Identify the issue you will propose, and write out a four-page motivation indicating why this problem should be addressed, and how you propose to address it.

4 What is an important issue in your community that can benefit from some type of intervention? What contributions can psychologists make to help alleviate this issue? Discuss your ideas with two other people and reach consensus about what the most important issues and the most immediate needs are.

5 What, in your opinion, can make psychology more relevant to the needs and experiences of the majority of South Africans? What content would you include in a training programme for psychologists? After careful

consideration and discussion with your class, prepare a model curriculum for the training of psychologists.

6 What social change is most necessary in the post-apartheid South Africa? What can you, as a psychologist, do to work towards that change? What do you need to prepare yourself for functioning as a social change agent? Write out a five-year plan that will ensure that you get the qualifications or experiences necessary for that role.

References

ALBEE, G. W. (1983). Foreword. In R. D. Felner, L. A. Jason, J. N. Moritsugu, and S. S. Farber (Eds.), *Preventive psychology: Theory, research and practice.* New York: Pergamon.

ANONYMOUS. (1986). Some thoughts on a more relevant or indigenous counselling psychology in South Africa: Discovering the socio-political context of the oppressed. *Psychology in Society,* 5, 81–89.

BADAT, S. (1994). Creating new political space. *DSA in Depth: Reconstructing Education,* 15–16.

BASSA, F. M. and SCHLEBUSH, L. (1984). Practice preferences of clinical psychologists in South Africa. *South African Journal of Psychology,* 14, 118–123.

BERGER, S. and LAZARUS, S. (1987). The views of community organisers on the relevance of psychological practice in South Africa. *Psychology in Society,* 7, 2–6.

BODIBE, R. C. (1994). *The need for a third voice in South African psychology.* Paper presented at the Psychology and Societal Transformation Conference, University of the Western Cape, January 1994.

BULHAN, H. A. (1985). *Frantz Fanon and the psychology of oppression.* New York: Plenum.

COWEN, E. L. (1980). The community context. In

M.P. Feldman and J. Orford (Eds.), *The social psychology of psychological problems* (pp. 311–335). New York: Plenum.

COWEN, E. L. (1997). On the semantics and operations of primary prevention and wellness enhancement (or will the real primary prevention please stand up?). *American Journal of Community Psychology, 25*(3), 245–256.

DAWES, A. R. L. (1986). The notion of relevant psychology with particular reference to Africanist pragmatic initiatives. *Psychology in Society, 5*, 28–48.

DOUGLASS, F. (1855/1969). *My bondage and my freedom.* New York: Dover.

FANON, F. (1967a). *Black skin, white masks.* New York: Grove.

FANON, F. (1967b). *A dying colonialism.* New York: Grove.

FANON, F. (1967c). *Towards the African revolution.* New York: Grove.

FANON, F. (1968). *Wretched of the earth.* New York: Grove.

FARREL, A. D. and BRUCE, S. E. (1997). Impact of exposure to community violence on violent behaviour and emotional distress among urban adolescents. *Journal of Clinical Child Psychology, 26*(1), 2–15.

HELLER, K. and MONAHAN, J. (1977). *Psychology and community change.* Homewood, IL: Dorsey.

HOOGVELT, A. (1997). *Globalisation and the post colonial world: The new political economy of development.* London: Macmillan Press.

IBÁÑEZ, T. and ÍÑIQUEZ, L. (Eds.). (1997). *Critical Social Psychology.* London: Sage.

KESSLER, R. C., MCGONAGLE, K. A., ZHAO, S., NELSON, C.B., HUGHES, M., ESHLEMAN, S., WITCHEN, H. U., and KENDLER, K. S. (1994). Lifetime and 12-month prevalence of DSM III-R psychiatric disorders in the United States. *Archives of General Psychiatry, 51*, 8–19.

KROEKER, C. J. (1995) Individual, organisational, and societal empowerment: A study of the processes in a Nicaraguan agricultural co-operative. *American Journal of Community Psychology, 23*(5), 749–765.

MAUER, K. F., MARAIS H. C., and PRINSLOO R. J.

(1991). Psychology: The high road or the low road? *South African Journal of Psychology, 21*(2), 90–96.

MICHELSON, C. L. (1994). Township violence, levels of distress, and post-traumatic stress disorder, among displacees from Natal. *Psychology in Society, 18*, 47–55.

MOLL, I. (1983). Answering the question: What is psychology? *Psychology in Society, 1*, 59–77.

MONTERO, M. (1996). Parallel lives: Community psychology in Latin America and the United States. *American Journal of Community Psychology, 24*(5), 589–216.

MORRIS, C. G., (1996). *Psychology: An introduction.* (9th ed.). Upper Saddle River, NJ: Prentice Hall.

NELL, V. (1994). Critical psychology and the problem of mental health. *Psychology in Society, 19*, 31–44.

NICHOLAS, L. J. and COOPER, S. (Eds.). (1990). *Psychology and apartheid.* Cape Town: Vision.

PERKEL, K. A. (1988). Towards a model for a South African clinical psychology. *Psychology in Society, 10*, 53–75.

PERKINS, D. D. and ZIMMERMAN, M. A. (1995). Empowerment theory, research and application. *American Journal of Community Psychology, 23*(5), 569–579.

PLAS, J. M. and LEWIS, S. E. (1996). Environmental factors and sense of community in a planned town. *American Journal of Community Psychology. 24*(1), 109–144.

PRETORIUS-HEUCHERT, J. W. (1988). *Free to be hungry and homeless.* Unpublished paper, Boston University.

RAPPAPORT, J. (1977). *Community psychology, values, research and action.* New York: Holt, Rhinehart and Winston.

REELER, A. P. (1993). Psychological disorders in primary care: Cross-cultural comparisons. *Psychology in Society, 17*, 19–34.

REIFF, R. (1977). Ya gotta believe. In I. Iscoe, B.L. Bloom, and C.D. Spielberger, (Eds.), *Community psychology in transition: Proceedings of the National Conference on Training in Community Psychology* (pp. 107–125). Washington, DC: Hemisphere.

SARASON, S. B. (1976). *The psychological sense of community: Prospects for a community psychology*. San Francisco: Jossey-Bass.

SEEDAT, M. (1984). *Crippling a nation*. London: International Defence and Aid Fund.

SEEDAT, M. (1990). Programmes, trends and silences in South African psychology 1983–1988. In L. J. Nicholas and S. Cooper (Eds.), *Psychology and apartheid* (pp. 22–49). Cape Town: Vision.

SEEDAT, M. A., CLOETE, N., and SHOCHET, I. (1988). Community psychology: Panic or panacea. *Psychology in Society*, 11, 39–54.

SERRANO-GARCIA, I., LOPEZ, M. M., and RIVERA-MEDINA, E. (1987). Toward a social-community psychology. *Journal of Community Psychology*, 15, 431–446.

SERRANO-GARCIA, I. (1994). The ethics of the powerful and the power of ethics. *American Journal of Community Psychology*, 22(1), 1–20.

SIMON, R. (1982). *Gramsci's political thought: An introduction*. London: Lawrence and Wishart.

SPAULDING, J. and BALCH, P. (1983). A brief history of primary prevention in the twentieth century: 1908 to 1980. *American Journal of Community Psychology*, 11(1), 59–80.

SPEARS, R. (1997). Introduction. In T. Ibáñez and L. Íñiquez (Eds.), *Critical social psychology* (pp. 2–10). London: Sage.

SPREITZER, G. M. (1995). An empirical test of a comprehensive model of intrapersonal empowerment in the workplace. *American Journal of Community Psychology*, 23(5), 601–630.

TAKAHASHI, L. M. and DEAR, M. J. (1997). The changing dynamics of community opposition to human service facilities. *Journal of the American Planning Association*, 63(1), 79–94.

THOMPSON, J. B. (1990). *Psychology, society and subjectivity: An introduction to German critical psychology*. London: Routledge.

TRICKETT, E. J. (1996). A future for community psychology: The contexts of diversity and the diversity of contexts. *American Journal of Community Psychology*, 24(2), 209–235.

3

The 'old' versus the 'new' in South African community psychology: the quest for appropriate change[1]

Leslie Swartz

Kerry Gibson

Study objectives

The objectives of this chapter are:
- to develop an understanding of some contextual challenges and pressures that influenced the development of community psychology in South Africa;
- to explore how both old and new theories and methods in psychology may be helpful to community psychologists in the South African context; and
- to explore some of the complexities involved in the well-known community psychology dictum of 'giving psychology away'.

1 Introduction

In developing an appropriate form of psychological practice in South Africa, there has been an acknowledged tension between the established theories and practices of the discipline and the thrust towards entirely new ways of thinking and working. This chapter is an attempt to re-examine some aspects of the new local forms of community psychology from a critical perspective that draws from some of the older theoretical ideas and established practices in psychology. In this sense it is also an attempt to bridge the apparent schism between the old psychology and the new, and argues instead that conventional psychological ideas may yet have something to offer to South African community psychology practice. Through a recognition of the complexity underlying the apparently straightforward tenets of community psychology in the local context, some ideas about what might constitute appropriate practice are considered.

2 The crisis of relevance in the 'old' psychology

There is often a sense that local forms of community psychology can, and should, represent a total break with conventional or First World psychological theories and practices. This perception has partly arisen out of the particular way in which some branches of progressive psychology have developed historically in South Africa (Swartz, Gibson, and Swartz, 1990). The major transformations that have taken place in local psychology were in many ways given impetus by the political turmoil of the 1980s. There was a clear recognition in these times that the traditional consulting room practices of clinical psychology were not reaching the large numbers of people who were affected psychologically by the war in the streets. Further, it was argued that ideas developed in rarefied Western countries would be unable to understand or account for people's needs in the apparently unique political context of apartheid (Vogelman, 1986). It was clear that psychologists needed to link more closely with community organizations, to think more clearly about prevention, and to broaden the range of their interventions (Swartz, Dowdall, and Swartz, 1986). There is no question that at the time there was much wrong with the practice and theory of clinical psychology. The academic discipline was dominated by a banal obsession with what was easily countable, easily testable, and hence, often, the most trivial. The clinical practices had undergone little change from their origin in settings quite unlike our own and there had been little attempt to even begin to evaluate the extent to which these might be appropriate for the local context. Against this background there was a real need for critical thinking about the role of psychology and particularly a need to separate, not only from the mindlessness of the past, but also from the active employment of psychological ideas in the furtherance of conservative ideologies (Swartz et al., 1990).

Ironically, as psychologists sought radically to re-think their role, the political struggles of the 1980s, which constituted the background to their thinking, were dominated by the rhetoric of war rather than talk of psychological pain, suffering, and reflection. A contributor to a local progressive psychology journal argued against psychology, labelling it a middle-class enterprise, and saying that 'the oppressed must act' (Anonymous, 1986). These sentiments, while strongly expressed here, were not out of keeping with the general crisis of relevance within the social sciences. The myths of neutrality within academia and the helping professions were being strongly challenged. With this, attention was being drawn to the way in which psychological theories and practices, both wittingly and unwittingly, had contributed to silences and omissions in the understanding of political issues such as oppression (Ingleby, 1981).

In addition to this, the ideology of non-racialism, so central to some dominant branches of progressive academic thinking, was often profoundly anti-psychological in its application. Social scientists, for example, were strongly engaged in the important work of demonstrating that 'race' and 'culture' were social constructions and not immutable realities 'out there'; they were not determined either by biology or essence (Sharp, 1988). The reality of living through these labels, not simply as they affected material circumstances but also as they affected identity and every aspect of psychological development, was obscured (Swartz, 1996). Talk of the experience of differences between groups of people on the basis of social categories like race, culture, and social class became politically dangerous talk. Part of what had been lost by these particular interpretations of progressive thought was the contribution black consciousness had made, and continues to make, to our understanding of psychological processes of enculturation and oppression. Within this approach, resistance to racial oppression is recognized as fundamental to the liberation of the individual from internalized oppression (Bulhan, 1985; Fanon, 1970). While a too simplistic merging of the relationship between the social and the individual can be criticized (Seedat, Cloete, and Shochet, 1988), this approach does point to the importance of race as a defining feature of identity and psychological experience.

This view was reflected in some attempts to transform psychology by mainly black psychologists (Nicholas and Cooper, 1990). This potentially powerful challenge to conventional psychology was, however, marginalized by the dominance of white psychologists in both mainstream and other progressive health and mental health organizations (Manganyi, 1991). Ironically, the split between the progressive black psychologist groups and the so-called non-racial progressive groupings, which were largely white, seemed to mirror the racial divisions

of apartheid both groups were seeking to challenge. The inadequacies of conventional psychology on the one hand and a divided progressive movement on the other created particular difficulties in the attempt to invent a more appropriate kind of psychology for the South African context.

The typical undergraduate essay question in university courses at the time was: 'Is psychology relevant in South Africa?' The short answer, if you wanted a first, was 'no'. This nihilism about psychology and about its application in the broader South African context was reinforced by several other factors. The first was the mechanistic and a-contextual tradition in many psychological theories, which did not sit well with the recognition of the fundamental importance of the political context as a defining feature of people's lives in South Africa. The effects of the political context were most clearly visible in the high levels of political violence in the 1980s, which became a point of mobilization for progressive psychology (Swartz et al., 1990). Of particular relevance to this concern with the psychological effects of violence were the theories of stress and trauma internationally, and in the United States in particular. Young (1995) has demonstrated how the category of post-traumatic stress disorder, far from being an apolitical 'discovery' of the 1980s, in fact medicalizes and renders politically safe many of the tensions in the United States in the post-Vietnam period. Post-traumatic stress theory, with its emphasis on discrete events and its neglect of issues of power, did not seem to work here in the context of ongoing oppression and deprivation. So local psychologists experienced a sense of being cut off in their work from what was happening in the mainstream of theories that might account for the relationship between traumatic social conditions and psychological distress.

The second factor that caused doubt about whether there were existing capacities within psychology that could be used to develop a relevant community practice was the reality that most South African psychologists were white and trained to work with middle-class patients, from similar backgrounds to their own. Psychotherapeutic work in psychiatric hospitals, practically the only places where there were any contact with black patients, was all but nonexistent, as Manganyi (1991) has shown. Black colleagues from within the profession, furthermore, made a strong case as to why white psychologists could never properly connect with oppressed black communities. The experience of many white psychologists of being out of their depth in contexts and with people profoundly unfamiliar seemed to reinforce the sense that there was little that conventional skills and knowledge could offer in dealing with the needs of most South Africans. These anxieties about the apparent inadequacies of conventional psychology were further heightened by criticisms from both within and beyond the boundaries of the profession. There were concerns that by offering psychological help to disadvantaged communities, psychologists would be increasing the demand for their help, which existing services could not begin to cope with (Floyd, 1986).

From very different quarters there was another concern, namely, that the imposition of psychology in these contexts was simply a way of extending the medical gaze, a mechanism of the production of desire and hence of social control (Foucault, 1973a, 1973b). In this view, which is influenced also by the anti-psychiatry movement of the 1960s and 1970s, attempts to broaden the influence of psychology become at base attempts to place boundaries and controls around people, and to interfere with and police their lives in an elaborate form of surveillance masquerading as service. There is much that is useful theoretically in this view, especially insofar as it forces us to concede that psychology is a value-laden and potentially oppressive enterprise centrally concerned not with unconditional positive regard, as the Rogerians would have it, but with the production and reproduction of a particular moral order. In spite of the usefulness of this position in terms of critique, its post-modernist relativism added further to the paralysis and doubt that seemed to be a part of the attempts to develop new and appropriate forms of psychological theory and practice.

All of these factors conspired to create a climate in which psychologists, who were seeking to establish a new, relevant, and politically acceptable psychology, felt less and less able to even evaluate objectively the capacities and skills that they already possessed. There was often a sense that with so many problems inherent in conventional models of psychological thought and practice, all aspects of this work needed to be abandoned and something entirely new established in its place.

3 The 'new' psychology

The 'new' psychology differed from the 'old' in almost all important respects. It rejected professionalism in favour of community participation; elitist academic knowledge in favour of lay understanding; and the consulting room in favour of community-based interventions. The 'new' psychology was, and is, about trying out new roles, breaking rules, and finding out things that could never have been discovered in the confines of the consulting room. This new psychological role was similar to what Rappaport (1996) has called a 'boundary spanning' and involved taking on a range of different functions and roles such as advocate, consciousness raiser, consultant, and activist. It was about being engaged in the world in such a way that the usual trappings of professional psychology, and especially the rarefied version of professional psychology as value-neutral and separate from the world, were abandoned.

There is, however, a strong tradition within psychology of attempting to reinforce appropriate boundaries between and around people. This tradition comes from at least two theoretical sources – systems theory and psychodynamic theory. The argument for reinforcing boundaries rests essentially on the idea that it is within safe limits that growth will occur optimally. Children need to know what the rules are of the society into which they are being enculturated, for example, and adults can develop creatively only when they feel safe about the world. Stress researchers have shown, furthermore, that dramatic life changes, posi-tive or negative, are commonly associated with difficulties in adjustment, and that negative events that are difficult to predict and control are far more problematic to deal with than events that are predictable and controllable (Dohrenwend and Dohren-wend, 1974).

The second part of this chapter aims partly to show how cognizance of both these approaches in psychology – those of the 'new' psychology of boundary-crossing and the 'old' psychology of boundary-making – might be helpful in contributing towards the development of an appropriate local form of community psychology. In particular, it looks at the way in which some of the central tenets of the 'new' psychology might benefit from some of the theoretical and practical tools taken from both the established body of knowledge in psychology and the more marginalized progressive traditions within progressive psychology itself. In suggesting a fusion between these various traditions we critically examine community psychology's ideas on the dissemination of psychological skills, community participation, holistic primary health care, and cultural integration.

3.1 Who gets to be a psychologist?

One of the cornerstones of the 'new' psychology, with its emphasis on community participation and the democratization of knowledge, is the community health worker. The term community health worker (CHW) has many meanings, but in the current context it is used to refer to people who are not formally trained in the health field but who, with a relatively brief training, are put to work, generally in their own communities, in order to improve community health. In line with the Alma Ata Declaration of the World Health Organization (WHO) (1978), CHWs are seen to form part of comprehensive primary health care; a system emphasizing physical, mental, and social well-being, and with an accent on curative, promotive, and preventive care. In South Africa, the late 1980s saw a huge increase in the number of community health workers in line both with the WHO goal of health for all by the year 2000, and in keeping with moves in progressive circles to democratize health care.

A complex ideology surrounds the community health worker vision. Some have argued that CHWs are second-rate health care providers for poor people, but those in favour of the CHW vision support it largely on the basis that the strengths of CHWs lie precisely in the fact that they are not alienated from their communities by professional trappings (see Berman, Gwatkin, and Burger, 1987, and Walt, 1990, for a summary of these debates). Being part of communities, CHWs are in touch with the norms and needs of their communities, and are in a unique position to design culturally appropriate interventions. (See Duncan and Van Niekerk's Chapter 16 in this volume.)

A major problem with CHW programmes internationally, though, is the high turnover of staff, and the concern in the late 1980s with how psychologists could support the CHW movement in this country and help prevent this high turnover. Binedell (1991) interviewed CHWs in Cape Town, and discovered some key factors leading to burnout

amongst them. Firstly, there was considerable role overload. In the context of scarce resources, CHWs were acting as preventive, promotive, and curative health workers, and also as consultants on any number of social and practical matters, such as intervening in disputes and helping to complete application forms for hire purchase. Within the ideology of holistic health care, all of these functions can legitimately be seen as part of health promotion, but the load on the person fulfilling all these functions is very great. Secondly, CHWs operating in a context of abject poverty are often called upon to assist with the material needs of their community. The CHWs generally are not well paid themselves, but the material needs around them and their desire to respond to them can be overwhelming. A further factor concerns the CHW being a member of the community, known to everybody. This leads to a situation where the boundary between work and private life dissolves. CHWs are called upon at all hours of the day and night and are never really off duty. Their private lives are often inseparable from their working lives.

This suggests a need to re-examine the assumptions of the 'new' psychology about the ease with which community-based workers can be expected to take on the health and mental health needs of their communities. Although the idea of a CHW having an organic relationship with the community and 'naturally' being able to understand the community is attractive, this romantic view flies in the face of everything we know about the efficacy of psychological healing. Psychological treatment depends precisely on the fact that there are boundaries between practitioner and client, and on the power differential between practitioner and client. Although there is an impressive literature on how this power differential can be abused (Ingleby, 1981), there is little debate about the need for boundaries between practitioner and client, for both the client's needs and those of the practitioner. In attempting to 'give psychology away' (Miller, in Orford, 1992), we were perhaps divorcing the idea of teachable psychological skills from our understanding that these skills operate best within a specific context. This realization does not imply a call to retreat to the consulting room. However, it can inform our approach to assisting CHWs to be comfortable with not being able to be all things to all people, to be able to say no to requests at times, and to take time off for themselves. CHWs have often found it very hard to form boundaries because they see their role as being available to the community as far as possible. It has been a difficult and at times painful process to assist them to develop more of an ethos of self-care; something we have always regarded as very important for psychologists.

The organicist idea that CHWs automatically are in touch with and understand all the health and social needs of their communities is also problematic. Research by Binedell (1993) showed that CHWs in Cape Town were well aware of the difficulty of disruptive mental health problems that involved violence or bizarre behaviour, but reported that depression, for example, did not exist. Some of the workers were operative in an area where epidemiological research the previous year had shown a prevalence of depression among elderly women of 44 per cent. The reported absence of depression in such areas by CHWs cannot be attributed to different cultural practices in the labelling of disorders, as Binedell had used a careful vignette method to ensure that the behaviour described to the CHWs was congruent with actual behaviour observed by clinicians in Cape Town. What was clear from this research was that under conditions of enormous workload in deprived circumstances, CHWs could simply not afford to uncover or give priority to psychological states that did not bother anyone else. Paradoxically, many of these states are easily dealt with, without the use of complex professional skills or medication.

3.2 Whose knowledge counts?

The previous case study suggests the need for more attention to be paid to the process of disseminating knowledge to people who do not have training in psychology or a related field of mental health. In the context of the thrust towards the democratization of knowledge it is often felt incorrect to acknowledge the value of professional knowledge, which was perhaps too quickly dismissed as common sense or the mystification of lived experience. Ironically, the early attempts to disown professional knowledge, which were aimed at establishing a sense of equality with communities, were often experienced by those communities as an attempt to withhold knowledge from them (Swartz and Swartz, 1986).

Romantic notions of 'the community' are of course profoundly disrespectful towards members of that community, principally because they gloss over and ignore conflict and power differentials in that community. The marginalization of black consciousness ideas in some dominant progressive discourses, for instance, also meant that important issues concerning the necessary conditions for the empowerment of black people did not receive sufficient attention. In essence this romanticization of community glosses over an important factor: that access to knowledge is not, for obvious political and economic reasons, equally spread across society. This can lead to some dilemmas for psychology in particular. Locally, we have had to struggle over and over again with conflicts between our own ideas on child and spouse abuse, and those of dominant members of communities.

The issue of divisions in communities becomes even more stark when one considers the negotiations involved in determining health and psychological needs. For example, it is well known that mental illness and mental handicap can place very great burdens on communities because these conditions are often stigmatized and feared. Thus we have found in a number of contexts a reluctance on the part of community representatives to engage with these issues. Our responsibility in the field of community clinical psychology is often precisely to those people who will not in the usual course of events be identified as needy or deserving by members of their own communities.

3.3 Who participates in community participation?

The question of community participation also has important psychological sequelae

and antecedents, and is not naturally a feature of a supposedly homogeneous community (Petersen et al., 1997). Benjamin (1994) set up a highly successful group for known psychiatric patients and their families as part of the Mamre Community Health Project in the Western Cape. Her evaluation research showed very impressive results for those who attended, with low rates of relapse of mental illness. Importantly this research showed that however useful the intervention was, those psychiatric patients who were most debilitated by their symptoms were unable to make use of the group. For them, even to attend the group was just too difficult.

It is far too easy in the current context of attention to community participation in health care to forget about the constituency who cannot participate, by virtue of their condition, as other people can. As we quite appropriately attempt to stretch resources by working more and more in group and workshop settings, and in the contexts of prevention and promotion, it is important not to forget those who will always be on the margins of society. Understanding this involves a return to less popular ideas about the real impact of psychological as well as social conditions on people's capacities to engage actively in their own lives.

3.4 Integration or marginalization of psychological issues?

Much of the focus of community psychology has been on the integration of psychology into primary health care. Both in terms of the adequate use of scarce resources, as well as the emphasis on accessibility, primary health care has appeared to be the most viable setting for the development of an appropriate community-based psychology (Freeman, 1992). This notion involves a commitment to cross old boundaries, which distinguished the physical from the psychological, and to treat the whole person.

Miller and Swartz (1990, 1991) have shown how the use of clinical psychology in health care can, paradoxically, marginalize rather than integrate psychological issues. They refer to a neurology ward in which a psychologist was employed where the world of the emotions began to be seen to be the professional domain of the psychologist, and other staff were relatively disempowered from providing psychological support. Another example is that of a boy referred to a psychologist for assessment for medication or psychotherapy on the grounds that he was depressed. The boy was Xhosa-speaking and when the psychologist began her interview with him through an interpreter it emerged that the boy was very lonely in the ward as nobody could communicate with him. The solution was simple: to arrange for Xhosa-speaking nursing staff to spend what time they could with him. As a result, his 'depression', which was in fact a psychological label masking inequities in access to appropriate health care on the basis of language, disappeared. There are enormous dangers in the use of psychology in the health care context to reify, individualize, and depoliticize other issues.

Marginalization of another type has been highlighted by Van der Walt (1996). Her research, which was intended as an evaluation of an intervention programme offered to nurses in primary care clinics dealing with tuberculosis (TB), found that in one of the clinics the idea that patients could benefit from counselling was taken on enthusiastically. What this meant in practice, though, was that patients who were already attending the clinic every weekday for daily observed treatment of their TB were asked to come back on another occasion to attend a support group and receive counselling. In this arrangement, counselling and support came to be viewed as specialized activities separate from the business of most of the medical personnel. The interweaving of psychological factors with every aspect of medical care and health promotion is hidden when we view psychology simply as another speciality with its own sphere of operation. It can be argued that when psychologists with relatively little self-reflection train a host of other practitioners in counselling skills, all that may result is a slightly larger pool of semi-skilled counsellors. One real job for psychology in primary health care is to help nurses be better nurses, and other practitioners to be better practitioners. Part of this work lies in providing support for practitioners so that they have the emotional space to continue with their work in a humane way. Packages of easily transferable 'skills' may therefore not be the answer.

4 Bringing the 'old' and the 'new' together: the role of the community psychologist

The research reviewed above suggests that the tenets of the 'new' psychology are

45

fraught with complexity and contradiction that are not always evident in the rhetoric around the need for an appropriate local form of psychology. It is clear that the attempt to disseminate psychology into community contexts is a task that requires an understanding not just of political imperatives but also of psychological processes. If the community psychologist's role is not simply to give away simplified packages of psychological skills that empower communities to deal with their own mental health problems, what then is their role?

Increasingly, in response to these kinds of questions, psychologists working in communities have begun to return to existing psychological theories to account for the ways in which the attempts to democratize, to change, and to integrate psychology into communities have not always been successful. Van der Walt (1996), for example, has begun to explore the utility of psychodynamic notions of transference, countertransference, and projective identification in understanding nurse-patient behaviour, while Gibson (1996) uses a similar approach to understanding the process of training teachers in psychological skills. This suggests that the psychologist's role in providing assistance at the primary care level may lie in giving due regard to the complex feelings evoked not only by work in health care but by the fleeting yet intense intimacy of practitioner-client relationships.

This view appears to be confirmed by previous research in which it was found that primary care practitioners may tend to overestimate the presence of a psychological component among patients consulting them for medical care (Rumble et al., 1996).

The researchers found a significant difference between what the practitioners had estimated on interview and their actual records of psychological cases. The estimates of psychological cases were higher than the recorded cases.

There are many ways to interpret the data, but the important point here is that the emotional experience of the practice of primary care, especially under deprived conditions, seems to take on a significance over and above what could be measured as a simple count of psychological cases seen. An implication of this for the appropriate integration of psychological work into primary health care is the need to cross boundaries and train health care workers themselves. This is a difficult idea to sell to a medical system that, though committed in principle to comprehensive primary health care, is nevertheless constructed theoretically on the biomedical belief that a speciality involves expertise in a discrete area of patient care. It is easy to talk about holistic health care, but the extent of adjustment that is needed to implement holistic care becomes apparent only when those aspects that have traditionally been marginal force us to reconsider how we think about people.

The psychologist's role in this kind of work might best be described as that of a consultant. Consultation here refers to the range of activities that psychologists undertake in making their skills and knowledge available to front-line workers in their direct work with clients and communities. This can include anything from case discussion to training and support work. Ideally, however, a consultative relationship implies a co-operative partnership between psychologists and other workers, which results in a jointly constructed approach to the needs of clients. There is considerable literature on the subject of consultation in mental health, but as Holdsworth (1994) in her research has shown, the dominant American approach to this area fails to account for the psychological factors involved in this process. There are a range of reasons for this, but some relate to a confusion between respect for the consultee, which is clearly necessary, and the blanket assumption that consultees are coping and are unaffected by the emotional aspects of their work, which clearly cannot be true, if consultees are really people like the rest of us. Holdsworth was able to show that in the South African context of deprivation and oppression in particular, psychological consultation that excludes the psychological needs of the consultee simply cannot work.

This research idea was developed further by Maw (1996), who has interpreted psychodynamic theory in the context of South African political realities to develop an approach to assessment of the suitability of both the consultant and the consultee for the consultation relationship. Psychological consultation at its best, she has shown, involves a process that allows for adequate consideration of how painful South African divides of race, class, gender, and language affect who we are and how we work. Psychological support involves allowing the space for all those issues to be held within the boundaries of a consultation relationship and allows them to be explored painfully, but safely. The parallels between this process and the process of individual therapy cannot be ignored, and there may

be many aspects of this kind of work from which the 'new' psychology can draw.

In understanding the complexity of these relationships it is important also to return to the previously taboo area of culture and identity. It is noteworthy that in debates about appropriate psychology and community work in South Africa, scant attention has been paid to the language issue. This is particularly ironic given the centrality of language in all mental health intervention. The adoption of eleven official languages in South Africa signals hope for the country and brings with it enormous challenges. In the health and social service sector the dream exists that language will no longer be a boundary in the way of appropriate care. However, the vast majority of psychologists in South Africa speak no indigenous languages apart from Afrikaans. The construction of language issues as either unimportant or marginal to the real practice of mental health care is somewhat bizarre. Every day people in South Africa are excluded from specific forms of psychological intervention simply on the basis of the languages they do, or do not, speak.

Drennan (1996a, 1996b), a psychologist at a local psychiatric hospital currently doing research in this area, has found that asking questions about language in an institution is tantamount to raising issues about the very identity of that institution. The language question appears to be inextricably linked with investments from all sides in specific areas of professional power and resistance. It is by no means clear, as one would have thought, that for both multilingual practitioners and for those who cannot communicate with patients, the prospect of all staff being able to converse directly with all clients and patients would be welcomed. In exploring the language issue in mental health care we have a valuable opportunity to examine the ways in which a situation that all parties agree is unsatisfactory has come to be a site of often unspoken rivalries and struggles for power. Clinicians and clientele alike struggle with a situation in which clients are misunderstood and marginalized by systems that have been constructed historically to exclude certain languages. Until multilingualism constitutes an important part of the agenda for progressive community psychology, there is little means of forging meaningful and complex partnership relationships between professional psychologists and communities.

5 Important issues and future directions in local community psychology

At this time in history, community psychologists in South Africa are no longer faced only with the demands of struggle politics, and with defining themselves as being outside the boundaries of the mainstream. The challenge we face is the challenge of introducing new ways of thinking. Struggle politics was all about how successfully we could stop things. The boycott was raised to a fine art. The transition from being good at stopping things to being able to construct a new order and to take responsibility for whatever we construct is not easy. The role of creative authority is often far more difficult than that of marginal, though often

powerful, antagonist against the status quo. For generations South Africa has been devoid of almost any legitimate authority, which reinforces the tendency to conflate any authority with oppressive authority. It is difficult to take on responsibility; it is difficult to take on the risk of constructing new approaches and to withstand the inevitable criticism that innovation demands.

In a psychological sense, the task we face in South Africa is that of growing up, and often in the absence of appropriate models of the adult role. Many service organizations are currently torn apart by strife concerning the very identity of who we are in a world in which we have suddenly become the parents and can no longer be the rebellious children. The politically necessary subversion of the power relationships along age lines in the struggle period has left us with questions about how to be adults. Our concern for democracy has led us to be reluctant to acknowledge differences where they do exist – differences in both outlook and competence.

Community clinical psychology has a role to play in helping communities and organizations take on the responsibilities, the challenges, and the pleasures of authority, and to assist psychologists in acknowledging the painful differences that divide us. It is, however, equally important for us as psychologists to accept our own power: to claim our existing knowledge base and to reinforce it where that is necessary.

Exercises

1 Read through the contents pages of any local South African psychology journal published between the years 1985 and 1990. List the kinds of topics covered by papers in this journal.

1.1 What seem to be the primary concerns of psychologists in this period of transition?

1.2 What areas appear to have received little or no attention?

1.3 What do you think should have been the central issues to have been addressed during this period of time?

2 Use one or more of the following questions to generate group discussions:

2.1 Do disadvantaged communities need psychologists?

2.2 Is it fair to ask disadvantaged communities to help themselves?

2.3 Who should psychology be 'given away' to?

2.4 Can black psychologists work effectively with white communities (and vice versa)?

2.5 What would some of the advantages and disadvantages be of working as a community health worker with people you know? Picture yourselves working with your friends and neighbours to help you answer this question.

2.6 What sort of person do you think would make a good community health worker?

Note

1 Portions of this chapter are adapted from 'Crossing or creating boundaries: challenges in clinical psychology in the community', an inaugural lecture by Leslie Swartz, University of Cape Town, 16 October 1996.

References

ANONYMOUS. (1986). Some thoughts on a more relevant or indigenous counselling psychology in South Africa: Discovering the socio-political context of the oppressed. *Psychology in Society*, 5, 81–89.

BENJAMIN, E. (1994). *Coping with mental illness: A case study in initiating a support group in Mamre.* Unpublished MA thesis, University of Cape Town.

BERMAN, P. A., GWATKIN, D. R., and BURGER, S. E. (1987). Community-based health workers: Head start or false start towards health for all? *Social Science and Medicine*, 25, 443–459.

BINEDELL, J. (1991). *Community health workers talk about their work.* Presented at the Association for Sociology of Southern Africa Conference, University of Cape Town, July 1991.

BINEDELL, J. (1993). *Methods and madness: Researching community health workers' perceptions of mental illness in Khayelitsha and Nyanga.* Unpublished MA thesis, University of Cape Town.

BULHAN, H. A. (1985). *Franz Fanon and the psychology of oppression.* New York: Plenum Press.

DOHRENWEND, B. and DOHRENWEND, B. (Eds.). (1974). *Stressful life events: Their nature and effects.* New York: John Wiley and Sons.

DRENNAN, G. (1996a). Counting the cost of language services in psychiatry. *South African Medical Journal*, 86, 343–345.

DRENNAN, G. (1996b). *Institutional obstacles to equitable access to psychiatric services in the Western Cape.* Paper presented at the conference: Communication for the Health Professional in a Multi-lingual Society, University of Natal, Durban, 11 July 1996.

FANON, F. (1970). *Black skin, white masks.* London: Paladin.

FLOYD, L. (1986). *Psychological problems presenting to primary health care clinics in Soweto.* Paper presented at the Apartheid and Mental Health:

OASSSA National Conference, Johannesburg, 17–18 May 1986.

FOUCAULT, M. (1973a). *Madness and civilization*. New York: Vintage.

FOUCAULT, M. (1973b). *The birth of the clinic: An archaeology of medical perception*. New York: Vintage.

FREEMAN, M. (1992). *Providing mental health care for all in South Africa: Structure and strategy*. Paper No. 24. Johannesburg: Centre for Health Policy, University of the Witwatersrand.

GIBSON, K. (1996). Working with children in violence: The therapeutic classroom. *Psychoanalytic Psychotherapy in South Africa*, 4(2), 19–31.

HOLDSWORTH, M. (1994). *Consultation and training challenges at the Mamre community health project*. Unpublished MA thesis, University of Cape Town.

INGLEBY, D. (Ed.). (1981). *Critical psychiatry*. Harmondsworth: Penguin Books.

MANGANYI, N. C. (1973). *Being black in the world*. Johannesburg: Sprocas/Ravan.

MANGANYI, N. C. (1991). *Treachery and innocence: Psychology and racial difference in South Africa*. Johannesburg: Ravan.

MAW, A. (1996). *The consultation relationship as a complex partnership*. Unpublished MA thesis, University of Cape Town.

MILLER, T. and SWARTZ, L. (1990). Clinical psychology in general hospital settings: Issues in interprofessional relationships. *Professional Psychology: Research and Practice*, 21, 48–53.

MILLER, T. and SWARTZ, L. (1991) Integration or marginalization: Clinical psychology as a strategy for dealing with psychosocial issues in a South African neurosurgery ward. *Sociology of Health and Illness*, 13, 293–309.

NICHOLAS, L. and COOPER, S. (Eds.). (1990). *Psychology and apartheid: Essays on the struggle for psychology and the mind in South Africa*. Johannesburg: Vision/Madiba.

ORFORD, J. (1992). *Community psychology: Theory and practice*. Chichester: John Wiley and Sons.

PETERSEN, I., BHAGWANJEE, A., PAREKH, A., GIBSON, K., GILES, C., and SWARTZ, L. (1997). Community mental health care: Ensuring community participation. In D. Foster, M. Freeman., and Y. Pillay (Eds.), *Mental health policy in South Africa* (pp. 55–68). Cape Town: MASA.

RAPPAPORT, J. (1996). *Keynote address presented to the conference:* Child and family well-being: Strategies for community partnerships and mental health training, University of Cape Town, January 1996.

RUMBLE, S., SWARTZ, L., PARRY, C., and ZWARENSTEIN, M. (1996). Prevalence of psychiatric morbidity in the adult population of a rural South African village. *Psychological Medicine*, 26, 997–1007.

SEEDAT, M., CLOETE, N., and SHOCHET, I. (1988). Community psychology: Panic or panacea. *Psychology in Society*, 11, 39–54.

SHARP, J. (1988). Introduction: Constructing social reality. In E. Boonzaier and J. Sharp (Eds.), *South African keywords: The uses and abuses of political concepts* (pp. 1–16). Cape Town: David Philip.

SWARTZ, L. (1996). Culture and mental health in the rainbow nation: Transcultural psychiatry in a changing South Africa. *Transcultural Psychiatric Research Review*, 33, 119–136.

SWARTZ, L., GIBSON, K., and SWARTZ, S. (1990). State violence in South Africa and the development of a progressive psychology. In N. C. Manganyi and A. du Toit (Eds.), *Political violence and the struggle in South Africa* (pp. 234–264). London: Macmillan.

SWARTZ, S., DOWDALL, T., and SWARTZ, L. (1986). Clinical psychology and the 1985 crisis in Cape Town. *Psychology in Society*, 5, 131–138.

SWARTZ, S. and SWARTZ, L. (1986). *Negotiation of the role of mental health professionals: Workshops for pre-school teachers, Cape Town 1985–1986*. Paper presented at the Apartheid and Mental Health: OASSSA National Conference, Johannesburg, 17–18 May 1986.

VAN DER WALT, H. (1996). *Health systems reform: Towards an understanding of different responses to in-service training*. Unpublished paper, Medical Research Council.

VOGELMAN, L. (1986). *Apartheid and mental health*. Paper presented at the Apartheid and Mental Health: OASSSA National Conference, Johannesburg, 17–18 May 1986.

WALT, G. (Ed.). (1990). *Community health workers in national programmes: Just another pair of hands*. Philadelphia: Open University Press.

WORLD HEALTH ORGANIZATION (WHO). (1978). *Primary health care: Report of the international conference on primary health care, Alma Ata, USSR, 6–12 September, jointly sponsored by the WHO and UNICEF*. Geneva: World Health Organization.

YOUNG, A. (1995). *The harmony of illusions: Inventing post-traumatic stress disorder*. New Jersey: Princeton University Press.

4

Towards a Marxist community psychology: radical tools for community psychological analysis and practice

Brandon Hamber
Thulani Clifford Masilela
Martin Terre Blanche

Study objectives

After reading this chapter and doing the exercises you should:

- have a clear understanding of basic Marxist theory and be able to apply this understanding to South African community psychology;

- be able to describe how Marxism applies to South African community psychology in relation to:

  - the status of community psychology as a critical branch of psychology;

  - the relation to the material base of society of community psychology;

  - the nature of the psychological damage done by capitalism; and

  - the problem of effective community action within a determinist framework.

1 Introduction

Community psychology is generally considered one of the more socially responsive and applied branches of psychology and thus to be more firmly embedded in the real, concrete world of daily life than most of the rest of the discipline. However, the nature of the 'real world' in which community psychology is supposed to operate is itself the subject of considerable controversy and debate. In this chapter we consider one way of understanding this world – Marxism – and draw out the implications this understanding has for the practice of community psychology. We present four basic principles of Marxism and in each case show how community psychologists already subscribe to similar ideas, as well as how Marxism could further extend their thinking and professional practice. The style of our presentation, as you will see, is deliberately polemical, as we want you to engage with Marxism as not just another theory, but as a radical challenge to psychologists to engage with communities in a fundamentally transformative way.

At this point you may well ask why we as community psychologists should bother with Marxism at all, as it has been so thoroughly discredited by the totalitarian excesses and eventual collapse of the former Soviet Union. We would concur with Hayes (1996) that the collapse of the Communist regimes in Eastern Europe, and the radical reform of Communist states elsewhere, have paradoxically re-opened spaces for applying Marxism as a critique of the capitalist world order. There is, in a manner of speaking, only a Marxism of capitalism and no Marxism of Marxism (Therborn, 1980), so that Marxist critique could never effectively be brought to bear on the forms of totalitarian government that flourished in Eastern Europe. The degree to which these states were indeed Marxist is debatable, and it may even be doubted if a form of government based on pure Marxist principles would ever be practically feasible. What Marxism does seem to provide, however, is a set of tools useful for critiquing the capitalist system, which now governs most of the world economy. Alongside the great wealth it has brought for some, especially in North America and Europe, the rise of the capitalist world order has also been accompanied (Gray, 1999) by further impoverishment of underdeveloped economies, increased financial instability of developing economies, and an ever-widening gap between the poor and the wealthy in developed economies. While community psychologists could not be expected to address or even to have a full understanding of such global processes, these processes do form the background against which our smaller-scale interventions occur. In addition, the same Marxist principles that can help us understand what is happening on a national and international level, also apply to the structure and functioning of local communities.

There are many highly technical debates within Marxism and between Marxist and other theorists, but it is possible to identify four key principles that form the cornerstone of most Marxist work. We discuss these below, in each case showing how it reflects and extends similar ideas in community psychology. We also suggest, for each principle, a number of aphorisms designed to encourage Marxist-oriented action within community psychology. These aphorisms are listed again at the end of the chapter as the 'seven radical steps' (see p. 63). We encourage you to place an enlarged copy of these steps in a prominent position at your university or workplace, and to attempt giving effect to them.

2 Reality is not what it used to be (a philosophy of suspicion)

If then the social agents experience capitalist society as something other than it really is, this is fundamentally because capitalist society presents itself as something other than it really is. . . . It is not the subject that deceives himself [sic], but reality which deceives him [sic].
(Geras, 1989, p. 79)

Marxism is in the first place a 'philosophy of suspicion'. That is, it is convinced that under the apparently benign and democratic exterior of modern life there lurk sinister forces that systematically distort our understanding of reality. However, in saying that the true essence of society is radically different from its outward appearance, Marx does not argue that this appearance is simply a delusion without foundation, but acknowledges that it is quite real, although misleading and incomplete. Marx does not merely reject appearances, but wants to understand 'the inner pattern from which these appearances derive and evolve' (Sowell, 1985, p. 7).

Much of psychology is thus from the outset already out of step with Marxism in that psychology is for the most part simply not concerned with revealing any grand truths behind the false facade of everyday life. Rather than truth, empirical psychology aims for a more modest accumulation of theories and findings, which even if taken together do not constitute the slightest challenge to the established order, but at best a kind of footnote to it. Applied psychology, on the other hand, is – with a few exceptions – concerned with assisting individuals in functioning more effectively within a given socio-political context, without ever questioning the nature of the context itself. This has been the case in South Africa, where one might have expected psychology to resist the apartheid state, as much as elsewhere.

South African clinical psychologists typically tried to provide 'non-political' services, while many psychological researchers tried to conduct their enquiries in a politically neutral, scientific manner. For example, throughout the apartheid period researchers at the National Institute for Personnel Research (NIPR), many of whom were opposed to apartheid policies, tried to keep their work out of politics by appealing to the concept of scientific objectivity. However, as has been shown by Terre Blanche and Seedat (1994), because their commitment to neutrality prevented them from analysing their own political interests, they in many cases conducted research that bolstered rather than opposed the status quo. For example, much of the research conducted at the National Institute for Personnel Research (NIPR) had to do with improving productivity, while very little had to do with improving workers' ability to negotiate better wages.

Although there are individual psychologists who opposed apartheid, and it is in fact becoming increasingly difficult to find any who admit to ever having supported it (Asmal, Asmal, and Roberts, 1996), organized opposition was very limited. Three organizations that did include psychologists opposed to apartheid were the *Organization for Alternative Social Services in South Africa* (OASSSA), which consisted largely of progressive white psychologists, the *Psychology and Apartheid Group*, which was a grouping of progressive black psychologists, and the *South African Health and Social Services Organization* (SAHSSO), an interdisciplinary health workers' organization. These organizations, despite serious disagreements among them, were united in condemning apartheid and in locating mental health within a political context.

Importantly, many psychologists belonging to these organizations were also involved in community psychology initiatives and participated in vigorous debates about whether and how community psychology could constitute an advance over mainstream clinical and scientific psychology (Seedat, Cloete, and Shochet, 1988). While these progressive community psychologists occasionally made use of Marxist ideas in developing their critique of apartheid, it is principally by starting to forge a psychology suspicious of social appearances that community psychology in South Africa is historically in league with Marxist thinking. Progressive community psychologists in the apartheid era did not always see the need explicitly to link their critique of racial oppression to class domination, which, as we will see, is a cornerstone of Marxist thinking. In the past race and class appeared to be virtual synonyms, and an understanding of racial oppression could thus in many respects substitute for an understanding of class oppression. Increasingly, however, this is no longer the case; in South Africa, reality is not what it used to be. This preceding analysis leads us to the formulation of Aphorism I: Professional and scientific 'neutrality' is a form of political partiality; to avoid politics is a form of political action.

3   Money talks (economic relations underlie everything else)

Society does not consist of individuals, but expresses the sum of interactions, the relations within which these individuals stand. (Marx, 1953, p. 265)

In conventional thought a country's economy is the sum of the entrepreneurial skills and efforts of individual actors, but according to Marxist thinking the individual (or as Marx labelled it, the 'bourgeois individual') is not the creator, but a product of the capitalist economy. Marxist theory is thus similar to psychoanalysis in that it does not take individual psychology as a given, but seeks to understand the hidden mechanisms that produce individuality, so that where Freud speaks of inner drives and intimate relations within families as the origins of psychology, Marx points to social and economic realities.

Of course there are many ideas about what makes individuals and the economy tick. People talk about these things endlessly. According to Marx, the things people say, the ideas people have about themselves and society, about right and wrong, religion, philosophy, morality, art, science, and all the institutions that have been set up around these concepts can all be traced back to material conditions. Therefore ideas such as free choice and the institution of the free market should not be judged in terms of empirical evidence of efficiency, internal coherence, or some abstract notion of morality, but should be understood in terms of the class interests they serve. Anything can be made to appear logical or good, and philosophical questions can never be settled through debate – that is just something people do to avoid facing the real conflicts of interest that underlie the points of contention.

In Marx's view there are essentially two kinds of interest in the modern world; that of the capitalists who own the 'means of production', namely, the property, machines, and finance needed to produce goods, and that of the working class, who have to sell their labour for a living. Of course there were also many other groups at the time when Marx wrote in the second half of the nineteenth century. These groups include, for example, rural peasants, the 'criminal classes', referring to those eking out a living even below the level of the working class, and the 'petty bourgeois', referring to the small-time capitalists such as traders and shopkeepers. Marx recognized that the central dynamic of the economic struggle involved the conflict of interest between capitalists, who wanted to extract as much value from workers as possible, and workers, who wanted to sell their labour as expensively as possible. Whether this dynamic is still at the centre of the global economy is debatable, but the principle established by Marx – that economic relations, which he termed the base, determine the world of feelings, ideas, and institutions, which he called the superstructure – remains a powerful counter to disciplines such as psychology, which would like to think that causality runs the other way around.

There were a few South African psychologists, principally those connected to the Psychology and Apartheid Group, OASSSA, and SAHSSO, who argued during the apartheid years that psychological and individual ill health are directly linked to where an individual is placed within society, that is, that base determines superstructure. These psychologists, who as we have seen were often involved with community psychology initiatives, criticized South African

psychology for failing to locate the individual within the social context where psychological and mental health problems occur (e.g., Anonymous, 1986; Bassa and Schlebusch, 1984; Berger and Lazarus, 1987; Dawes, 1985; Freeman, 1992; Seedat, Cloete, and Shochet, 1988; Straker, 1988; Thomas, 1987; Vogelman, 1986). They also pointed out how psychological services were almost exclusively available to whites living in urban middle-class areas (Berger and Lazarus, 1987; Freeman, 1992; Korber, 1990; Pillay and Petersen, 1996), and emphasized the need for more black psychologists and for community psychological interventions in areas previously ignored.

The tradition of locating psychological phenomena within political and economic realities, started by South African community psychologists in the 1980s, is in danger of being abandoned in post-apartheid South Africa because direct political oppression is no longer such a dominant feature of our society. Consider, for example, the work of the Truth and Reconciliation Commission (TRC), which operated between December 1995 and mid-1999 in South Africa. In the course of the TRC's operations it was argued by some mental health practitioners (Hamber, 1996a; 1996b) that there was a significant need for a mental health emphasis in relation to the TRC. It was argued that the TRC could operate as a psychologically rehabilitative mechanism because, like basic psychological theory, it aimed to go back, relive, and address past traumas so that individuals and the country could move to a healthier future. It was also acknowledged that the TRC was not a sufficient process in itself to promote individual and collective psychological rehabilitation, and that a range of psychological structures and strategies were needed to run parallel to the TRC. For example, on the individual level, even with the efforts of the TRC and victims giving testimony, the impact of the trauma of past political violence can be expected to live on for many years, and this requires the ongoing need for trauma counselling services long after the demise of the TRC process.

However, as important as these services may be to individuals, throughout the process of the TRC there was a lack of attention to the structural position of those testifying. The individuals who testified before the TRC cannot be seen as isolated 'victims of political violence' separate from the structural circumstances in which they live. In the majority of cases that appeared before the TRC the people were victimized not only because of their political affiliation and activities, but because of their structural circumstances, including their gender, their poverty, their race, and their general social marginalization. In this context, psychology has claimed a 'new' relevance in trying to pick up the pieces of shattered psyches through trauma counselling and other interventions, while ignoring the ways in which marginalized groups are structurally exposed to being re-victimized due to their unchanged social position.

It is important to realize, however, that although linking mental health problems to poverty and oppression is a first step, it does not in itself constitute a Marxist analysis of psychology and society in South Africa. Marxism entails economic determinism, but not a mechanical determinism that sees poverty as causing mental ill health, implying that people would not have psychological problems if only they were rich. Rather, it links superstructural phenomena, such as individual psyches, to a specific understanding of the economy, namely as a relationship of economic exploitation, and to a specific kind of remedial action, namely fundamental change in the structures of society.

One way of extending community psychology's understanding of the way in which the material base affects the development of society would be by making use of the idea of the 'dialectic'. Marx's theory is sometimes referred to as historical materialism or dialectical materialism, because he took Hegel's notion of the dialectic, which holds that progress occurs as a result of struggle between contradictions, and gave it a materialist twist. Hegel was an idealist in that he saw history as a process of conflict between opposing ideas, which would continually give rise to further, more sophisticated oppositions each time one idea won out over another. While Marx used Hegel's concept of the dialectical process, he saw the opposing forces as rooted in material realities (Gottlieb, 1992). Unlike Marxism, psychology often relies on an idealist interpretation of the social world, and when it does acknowledge material realities, psychology tends to slip into the stagnant materialism of biology rather than the dialectal materialism of class struggle.

Dialectics is premised on the assumption that any economic or other system, such as capitalism, contains within itself certain tensions or contradictions (for example, between the working class and the middle class) and that progress occurs when these contradictions become so acute that the system can no longer contain them and has to undergo a qualitative transformation into a new kind of system with its own set of contradictions. In this view much activity under capitalism that appears not to be directly related to economic exploitation of people, such as charity work, human rights campaigns, or community psychology initiatives, can be seen as attempts to smooth over the contradictions inherent in capitalism. Thus, rather than fighting exploitation, such efforts to uplift people and improve their lot can be seen as propping up the system. This is not to argue that human welfare activism is always wrong, but that we should be constantly aware that short-term gains are sometimes achieved at the cost of the long-term perpetuation of a system of exploitation. For example, a community psychology initiative might lead to better housing for farm workers (short-term gain) who would feel more content with their lot and therefore less likely to consider the possibility that they should share in the ownership of the land (the perpetuation of a system of exploitation).

Another way of extending community psychology's understanding of the material base of mental ill health is to understand community psychology as a form of 'township psychology'. Precisely because community psychology has started to move away from psychology's idealist tendencies, it has had to exist on the margins of the established discipline in the same way as poor black townships were built at the margins of affluent white suburbs during the apartheid years. While clinical and industrial psychology can be said to inhabit the Sandtons and

Constantias of South African psychology, community psychology inhabits the Sowetos and Cape Flats of the discipline.

The marginal position of community psychology can be positively embraced in the same way as marginalized groups such as gays and physically challenged people have seized their marginality as a source of organizational power. However, the idea of a township psychology can also be disempowering, implying a passive acceptance that the mainstream of psychology should not be concerned with socio-political issues. Furthermore, targeting 'township people' as the recipients of our well-meaning interventions runs the risk of patronization and re-colonization, and can function as a mechanism for satisfying middle-class curiosity about other people defined as exotic creatures. The statement that community psychology is 'township psychology' both reflects a state of affairs that needs to be remedied and is an expression of pride. Thus the principle of 'money talks' gives rise to three further aphorisms: Base precedes superstructure (Aphorism II); Community psychology is township psychology (Aphorism III); and Charity begins at home (Aphorism IV).

4 Damaged goods (alienation and the human subject)

In what way does the proletarian differ from the slave? . . . The slave is sold once and for all. The proletarian must sell himself by the hour or by the day. (Engels, 1847, p. 3)

For psychology, the political is always only personal, and a politics that sees the personal as rooted in social relations, as Marxism does, is usually seen as a personal problem. (Spears and Parker, 1996, p. 1)

Marx was primarily interested in the economic base, but many theorists have subsequently expanded on his ideas regarding the superstructure. Perhaps the best known of these is Louis Althusser (1971), who described how ideology is a key component of continuing class domination. He wrote:

> requires not only a reproduction of its skills, but also, at the same time, a reproduction of its submission to the rules of the established order, i.e. a reproduction of a submission to the ruling ideology for the workers, and a reproduction of the ability to manipulate the ruling ideology correctly for the agents of exploitation and repression, so that they, too, will provide for the domination of the ruling class 'in words'. (Althusser, 1971, p. 127-128)

The false ideologies of capitalism are perpetuated by means of 'ideological state apparatuses' – churches, schools, the press, and the family – while 'repressive state apparatuses' – the police, the army, the prisons system – stand ready to step in should ideological control fail. In this scheme, the discipline of psychology can be seen as nothing but an ideological state apparatus, feeding people the kinds of ideologies that emphasize the importance of individual needs and feelings, the possibility

of fulfilment in the apolitical sphere of personal relations, and the necessity for continual self-improvement that are needed to keep a free-market economy going. It is thus clear that for later Marxist theorists such as Althusser, it is no longer simply a case of base determining superstructure, but a mutual determinism in which ideological apparatuses maintain the conditions for certain forms of economic exploitation, and these forms of exploitation give rise to particular ideologies. Thus the economy is not the *only* determining factor – both economy and ideology produce what is then studied by psychology as 'real life', but which is in fact a distortion of our true human potential.

Under apartheid the victims of the system not only suffered arbitrary arrests, beatings, assassinations, and torture, but at the same time were subjected to the structural and systematic violence of poverty, malnutrition, forced removals, inferior education, urban overcrowding, and social strife in townships (Dowdall, cited in Desjarlais et al., 1995). The psychological consequences of the deprivation caused by poverty, which is the condition the majority of South Africans still find themselves in, are endless. These include the mental and physical developmental impact of poor nutrition on children and the anxiety, depression, and stress-related conditions caused by poor living conditions and occupational circumstances.

The conditions of the English working class in Marx's time were similar to those experienced by poor people in South Africa under apartheid and today. However, Marx argued that even if the majority of people had jobs and money, there is a profound sense in which they would remain damaged for as long as the capitalist system persists. The term he used for this was alienation. Alienation denotes both the process or mechanism through which the exploiters in society expropriate 'surplus value' produced by the exploited, and the manner in which this tends to turn the exploited into objects of production, alienated from their labour. According to Marxist theory only part of every worker's daily output is needed to 'maintain' him- or herself as a productive worker – one that is adequately fed, housed, and has his or her basic psychological needs seen to. The remaining output is surplus value, which is simply taken from the worker by capitalists. Thus, the capitalist mode of production degrades and depersonalizes individuals who become 'mere appendages of flesh on a machine of iron'. Modern society still relies on a large workforce and the majority of the world's poor still engage in the kind of menial work common in Marx's time, but even the more fortunate among us who are employed in white-collar occupations are often still mere cogs in a larger bureaucratic machine. Even where people might feel that they are not being economically exploited, such as in modern organizations that claim to have satisfactory working conditions, the creative act of productive labour is transformed into a possession. The worker's labour becomes a form of merchandise that can be bought and sold.

Rather than direct action to remedy our state of alienation, the capitalist economy tends to side-track individuals into what Marx called 'commodity fetishism', which

means to ascribe special, almost magical powers to consumer goods. The system encourages us to believe that we would be happy if only we could buy the latest electronic gadget, a car, a house, maybe even our own business. What the quest for such things usually leads to, however, is an even deeper entrapment in the system of alienated labour. Community psychologists sometimes imagine that poor communities would be immune from these forces and that the needs expressed by such communities would therefore somehow be more authentic. A glance at the proliferation of consumer items such as television sets in informal settlements – where electricity is provided – shows that commodity fetishism is not the exclusive preserve of the rich.

Alienation and commodity fetishism are only two of the ways in which our psyches, our understanding of our real conditions of life, and the nature of our relations with others have become distorted. Althusser (1971) argued that there is already a distortion at the very heart of who we are – our personal identities. He claimed that capitalist ideologies produce certain ready-made roles, such as housewife, charity worker, or community psychologist, into which individuals are slotted. We can think of ideologies as deliberately calling out, or as Althusser put it, 'interpellating' individuals to fill these roles. Individuals being hailed in this way experience it as if they already had the identity in question and simply recognized themselves in what was being called out, while in fact it is their socio-economic position that made them able to hear the call in the first place.

If we accept that what we thought were

59

most intimately our own, namely our personal identities, are in fact the products of economic relations and ideologies, then authentically we should experience ourselves as slaves or virtual machines and not as free agents. Paradoxically, Marx intended such a realization to be liberating, since it is precisely the ideology of the free subject, free to sell his or her labour to the highest bidder, that keeps us chained to capitalism. The capitalist form of production requires that we assert our individual freedom in order that we may be enslaved to the system. A liberal or humanist response to the problem of exploitation (and this was in fact Marx's first response) is to campaign for the restoration of individuals' rights and freedoms, but the more people are 'free to choose' under capitalism, the more efficiently the system functions. Capitalism is adept at taking all forms of dissent and incorporating them as just another commodity to be bought and sold on the free market (you bought this book on community psychology, didn't you?). The later Marx therefore insisted that true liberation could not come from empowering people by ensuring that they are accorded their due rights, as many community psychologists would want to do, but rather from a fundamental change in society, namely a working-class revolution. Thus Aphorism V: We are damaged goods spat out by the capitalist machine.

5 Making it happen (individual vs. collective agency)

The philosophers have only interpreted the world, in various ways; the point is to change it. (Marx, 1845, p. 2)

For if the last shall be first, this will only come to pass after a murderous and decisive struggle between two protagonists. That affirmed intention to place the last at the head of things, and to make them climb at a pace (too quickly, some say) the well-known steps which characterise an organised society, can only triumph if we use all means to turn the scales, including, of course, that of violence. (Fanon, 1968, p. 37)

As should be clear by now, Marxism is about nothing less than changing the world. Although community psychologists are not usually quite so ambitious, they share with Marxism an impatience with the way society is currently organized and a desire to make it different. Many of the other chapters in this book detail the small- and large-scale changes that have resulted from community psychology initiatives. (See Chapters 11 to 17.) However, change is never easy and it is often tempting to insulate oneself from the obligation to make things different. There are two ways in which community psychologists can do this. The one is to become armchair intellectuals, concerned only with describing psychological and social processes. The other is to jettison the theoretical tools afforded us by our academic training and to engage in mindless social action for its own sake. The Marxist concept of 'praxis', which entails action informed by critical social analysis, social analysis that springs from an engagement with the real world, is meant as an antidote to these two illnesses of capitalism.

A large section of professional psychology is organized around the rhetoric of scientific objectivity, which postulates an objective observer standing outside the phenomena being studied. A glance at most journals of psychology will illustrate how barren and unrelated to the real world this brand of psychology has become. Action research and similar approaches that seek to reinsert the observer into what is being observed and to bring about change rather than merely to codify, point the way to how a critical community psychology should be practised. It is important, however, not to fetishize social action, which can easily become just another form of charity. In Marx's day there were many charitable organizations trying to bring relief to the poor, but as Marx argued, in effect they were practising a form of class oppression in that they both helped disguise the consequences of oppression and continually re-emphasized the lesser worth of those they were being charitable towards.

In addition to noting the importance Marxism attaches to engaging in well-theorized social action, you may also have noticed an apparent contradiction. On the one hand Marxism is a call to action, while on the other it is unashamedly determinist. It claims that people are determined in every respect by history, politics, and economy. To complicate matters further,

Marx also maintained that history does not make people but that people make history. Marx's argument was as follows: 'Men [*sic*] make their own history, but they do not make it as they please; they do not make it under self-selected circumstances, but under circumstances existing already, given and transmitted from the past' (Marx, 1869, p. 1).

The crucial issue here is that while Marx denied individual agency, which he dismissed as a bourgeois fantasy, in some interpretations of Marx collective agency – as in the working class rising up against their masters – remains a possibility. An optimistic reading of Marxist and post-Marxist thought would suggest that people can change history by working together in groups. What brings such groups together as effective organs of change is not theoretical or professional allegiance (as would be the case, for example, for a professional association of psychologists), but shared oppression. Thus, to be true to the Marxist spirit, community psychologists, together with other professionals who want to be part of the process of change, have to join with organizations constituted by the oppressed. However, this does not mean that 'the oppressed' always know what the best solutions to social problems are – like those from the professional class, they are also the product of false ideologies – but by working together against oppression it is possible to overcome the limitations imposed by individuals' class positions. Thus, community psychologists, and students of community psychology, may become what Gramsci (1971) termed 'organic intellectuals' or, as Marx hoped, become part of that small section of the ruling class that cuts itself adrift and joins the revolutionary class. (If these issues interest you, you may want to read some of Gramsci's writings, as he was concerned not only with the relationship between the working class and intellectuals, but also more generally with how Marxist theory can be adapted to account for the way capitalism has developed since Marx.)

To 'join with the working class' we first need to accept that we are all born into a certain class in our society. For example, we may be born into the moneyed classes of northern Johannesburg, live in a smart house, and get sent to expensive schools and universities and study to become community psychologists, or we may be born as one of the rural poor in the Eastern Cape and grow up to become a migrant labourer. Although the class structure of society is far more complicated and diverse than was the case in Marx's time, the basic fact of hereditary privilege remains. Furthermore, even if we manage to move outside the realms of our class, for example, a working-class person going to university and getting a good job, there will be a tendency to turn one's back on the place where one has come from. Psychology is a professional degree and cannot but instill in those who study the subject some middle-class attitudes and cause their material interests to become aligned with those of the middle classes. In South Africa, particularly during the apartheid days, most psychologists were white, urban-based, and middle class. In essence, the profession replicated and gave access to those who were already in socially powerful positions. Today, the danger of creating professionals who are situated outside communities remains a threat, particularly as a new black élite becomes a reality.

Even if we, as middle-class community psychologists, find it possible to form alliances with working-class people, social change will still be difficult to achieve, as those who rule society will not hand over power voluntarily. Frantz Fanon (1968), who was influenced by Marx's ideas of revolution, went so far as to say, when talking about overcoming colonization, that violence was the only way to effect real change. Although times have changed since Fanon developed his ideas, the problems of colonization remain. Dependency on Western markets and foreign aid in African countries is a reality, and a process of so-called neo-colonization has developed in some, particularly African, countries. The basic argument is that after colonization was overcome and countries became liberated, the means of production have increasingly fallen into the hands of the local bourgeoisie and because of this, local people have become an 'upper class polarised against a lower class increasingly taking the form of an urban proletariat' (Wallenstein and De Braganca, 1982, p. 71). The continuation of this system of exploitation depends on what Fanon termed the intellectual laziness of the national middle class (Rhodes, 1970). To compel the privileged classes to change can therefore entail not only physical force, but also intellectual guerilla warfare aimed at dislodging the middle classes from their intellectual complacency.

Psychology has traditionally seen itself as a humanist enterprise that does not force interpretations and solutions on people, and community psychology has tended to follow the parent discipline in this, frequently acting as if communities operated or should operate on the basis of consensus. The Marxist injunction to compel the ruling classes to give up their privilege therefore runs counter to our professional socialization, while the idea of actually using violence to forcefully bring about change falls completely outside anything foreseen by humanist psychology. However, the various forms of oppression embedded in our system continue unabated, and community psychologists should ask themselves whether a romantic passivism is likely to put an end to this. Following the principle of 'making it happen' we therefore suggest two further aphorisms: Social theory without social action is barren; social action without social theory is a form of class oppression (Aphorism VI); and The ruling classes will not relinquish their privilege voluntarily; I have to decide where my allegiance lies (Aphorism VII).

The seven radical steps

1 Professional and scientific 'neutrality' is a form of political partiality; to avoid politics is a form of political action.
2 Base precedes superstructure.
3 Community psychology is township psychology.
4 Charity begins at home.
5 We are damaged goods spat out by the capitalist machine.
6 Social theory without social action is barren; social action without social theory is a form of class oppression.
7 The ruling classes will not relinquish their privilege voluntarily; I have to decide where my allegiance lies.

6 Conclusion

The teaching of Marx is all powerful because it is true. (Lenin, 1918)

It is tempting to dismiss Marxism as 'old news' or something that failed and has been superseded by the apparent successes of the new global free-market capitalism seen in the late 1980s and early 1990s. The economic crises of the late 1990s in South East Asia and elsewhere have, however, prompted many to reconsider Marxism's contribution to understanding the capitalist economy.

In this chapter we have argued that psychology is a product of this economy. Not only is the discipline a product of the economy but that which it should study, namely individual subjectivity, is also economically determined. Mainstream psychology denies both its own origins, claiming to arise as if by magic from morally neutral empirical procedures on the one hand and a concern for human welfare on the other, as well as the origins of its subject of study, treating the psyche as if it had an independent reality on a par with natural facts. Community psychology is by no means immune to these fallacies, and South African community psychologists, despite some noble efforts to engage with 'relevant' social issues, have historically fallen prey to exactly the kinds of individualizing, idealist, and relativizing tendencies that Marxism is concerned to dispel. Thus, without a Marxist analysis, individuals who are traumatized by their structural conditions are often seen as existing in an idealized psychological realm and their struggles are divorced from broader economic realities. Given the social position of psychologists as middle-class professionals, it is of course hardly surprising that this sort of distortion should occur. We cannot escape our class position. However, at the very least, it should be possible to use the intellectual tools available to us by virtue of our class position to develop a critical awareness of our own social and economic role, and of the ways in which this limits our ability to influence society's mental health.

Marx is often seen as the champion of the oppressed. However, the lasting legacy of Marx is not that he revealed the existence of oppression, but rather that he theorized the many different, often hidden, levels at which oppression is perpetuated. This includes the social, economic, political, and psychological. It is also not necessarily the case that Marxist theory is always right, as Lenin claimed, but Marx did develop a style of interrogating social reality that continues to threaten the status quo.

The purpose of this chapter was therefore not to provide answers to the problems of community psychology, or to convince you of the absolute truth of Marxist theory, but to (re-)introduce you to a particular style of critical thinking and action, which can transform the way you think of yourself as a community psychologist.

Exercises

To get the most out of this chapter we suggest that you debate the following issues:

1 Do the economic relations and material conditions of a society really determine a society's state of mental health or can mental health problems stand outside of economic relations?

2 Is community psychology about channelling resources to where the greatest needs are or about satisfying psychologists' curiosity and assuaging our guilty consciences?

3 It is wrong to give money to 'beggars'. Debate.

4 Community psychologists claim to empower people, but true empowerment would result in social revolution. Therefore, what community psychologists call empowerment is nothing more than charity. Discuss.

5 To change society, and hence some of the root causes of mental ill health, community psychologists need to voice their opposition from outside of the mainstream system. Or can change happen by working within mainstream psychology, big corporations, and government departments?

6 Community psychologists can be neutral; politics and psychology should be separated, because if psychology becomes too political no services will be provided and research results will be biased. Discuss.

7 Psychology very frequently refers to depression but rarely to oppression. Why? Who are the oppressed?

8 Psychologists have no place in bringing about social change; their role is to treat individuals. Do you disagree or agree with this statement?

9 Think of a powerful person or group of people in your community. Is there any way they can be persuaded to give up their privileges willingly?

10 F. W. de Klerk and the National Party voluntarily gave up their power during the negotiated settlement in South Africa and were not forced to do so. Discuss the relevance of the debate about this statement to community psychology practice and theory.

11 Violence begets violence and can never be condoned, especially not by a community psychologist. Discuss.

12 The numerous violent coups and liberation struggles that occurred in African states after the demise of colonialism prove that violence achieves nothing, especially not for the mental health of a country's people. Discuss.

13 The authors of this chapter are all middle-class men (some more white than others). Do you think their class, race, and gender affected the writing of this chapter? How?

References

ALTHUSSER, L. (1971). *Lenin and philosophy and other essays*. London: NLB.

ANONYMOUS (1986). Some thoughts on a more relevant or indigenous counselling psychology in South Africa: Discovering the socio-political context of the oppressed. *Psychology in Society*, (5), 81–89.

ASMAL, K., ASMAL, L., and ROBERTS, R. S. (1996). *Reconciliation through truth: A reckoning of apartheid's criminal governance*. Cape Town: David Philip.

BASSA, M. and SCHLEBUSCH, L. (1984). Practice preferences of clinical psychologists in South Africa. *South African Journal of Psychology*, 14(4), 118–123.

BERGER, S. and LAZARUS, S. (1987). The views of community organisers on the relevance of psychological practice in South Africa. *Psychology in Society*, (7), 6–23.

DAWES, A. (1985). Politics of mental health: The position of clinical psychology in South Africa. *South African Journal of Psychology*, 15(2), 55–61.

DESJARLAIS, R., EISENBERG, L., GOOD, B., and KLEINMAN, A. (1995). *World mental health: Problems and priorities in low-income countries*. New York: Oxford University Press.

ENGELS, F. (1847). *On Marx's capital*. Moscow: Foreign Language Publishing House.

FANON, F. (1968). *The wretched of the earth*. New York: Grove.

FREEMAN, M. (1992). *Providing mental health care for all in South Africa: Structure and strategy*. Paper No. 24. Johannesburg: The Centre for Health Policy, Department of Community Health, University of the Witwatersrand.

GERAS, C. (1989). Fetishism in Marx's capital. *New Left Review*, (65), p. 79.

GOTTLIEB, R. S. (1992). *Marxism: Origins, betrayal and rebirth*. New York: Routledge.

GRAMSCI, A. (1971). The intellectuals. In R. Dale (Ed.), *Schooling and capitalism* (pp. 218–223). London: Penguin.

GRAY, J. (1999). *False dawn: The delusions of global capitalism*. Great Britain: Granta Books.

HAMBER, B. E. (1996a). *The need for a survivor-centered approach to the Truth and Reconciliation Commission: Community mediation update, Issue 9*. Johannesburg: Community Dispute Resolution Trust.

HAMBER, B. E. (1996b). Sleeping dogs do not lie. *Recovery (Research & Co-operation on Violence and Rehabilitation of Young People)*, 1(3).

HAYES, G. (1996). The psychology of everyday life. In I. Parker and R. Spears (Eds.), *Psychology and society: Radical theory and practice* (pp. 153–162). London: Pluto.

KORBER, I. (1990). Indigenous healers in a future mental health system: A case for co-operation.

Psychology in Society, (14), 47–62.

LENIN, V. I. (1918). *The chief task of our times.* London: Workers' Socialist Federation.

MARX, K. (1845). *Theses on Feurbach.* Berlin.

MARX, K. (1869). *The eighteenth Brumaire of Louis Napoleon.* Hamburg.

MARX, K. (1953). *Grundrisse der Kritik der politischen Ökonomie.* Berlin.

PILLAY, Y. G. and PETERSEN, I. (1996). Current practice patterns of clinical and counselling psychologists and their attitudes to transforming mental health policies in South Africa. *South African Journal of Psychology,* 26(2), 76–80.

RHODES, R. (Ed.) (1970). *Imperialism and underdevelopment.* New York: Grove.

SEEDAT, M., CLOETE, N., and SHOCHET, I. (1988). Community psychology: Panic or panacea. *Psychology in Society,* (11), 39–54.

SPEARS, R. and PARKER, I. (1996). Marxist theses and psychological themes. In I. Parker and R. Spears (Eds.), *Psychology and society: Radical theory and practice* (pp. 1–17). London: Pluto.

SOWELL, T. (1985): *Marxism: Philosophy and economics.* London: Allen & Unwin.

STRAKER, G. (1988). Apartheid and child abuse. *Psychology in Society,* (5), 113–118.

TERRE BLANCHE, M. J. and SEEDAT, M. (1994). *Martian landscapes: The social construction of race and gender at the National Institute for Personnel Research, 1946–1984.* Paper presented at the Psychology and Societal Transformation Conference, University of the Western Cape, Cape Town.

THERBORN, G. (1980). *Science, class and society: On the formation of sociology and historical materialism.* London: Verso.

THOMAS, T. (1987). *Homelands psychosocial pathology: Impressions of a community doctor.* Paper presented to the second national conference of OASSSA on the theme 'Mental Health in Transition', University of the Western Cape, September 1987.

VOGELMAN, L. (1986). *The political economy of mental health in South Africa.* Opening address to OASSSA conference on 'Apartheid and Mental Health', Johannesburg, 17–18 May 1986.

WALLENSTEIN, I. and DE BRANGANCA, A. (1982). *The African liberation reader, Volume I.* USA: Lawrence Hill.

5

Notions of social change in community psychology: issues and challenges[1]

Rashid Ahmed
JW Pretorius-Heuchert

Study objectives

After studying this chapter you should be able to:

- define social change;
- distinguish between socio-historical and other perspectives on social change;
- discuss the assumptions about social change inherent in the different perspectives in community psychology;
- discuss the challenges facing community psychology with regard to issues of social change; and
- assess the usefulness of a socio-historical perspective on social change for community psychology.

1 Introduction

There are important differences between mainstream approaches in psychology and community psychology, which have led

Rappaport (1977; 1981) to declare that community psychology represents a paradigm shift and should be considered a social movement. From this perspective the issue of social change is a central premise for community psychology and informs its theory and practice. The historical review in Chapter 2 (Pretorius-Heuchert and Ahmed) in this volume has highlighted how community psychology promised to change:

- existing notions of science and the associated theories and paradigms;
- research methodologies and approaches;
- modes of intervention; and
- the existing psychological notions of change.

The main purpose of this chapter is to discuss critically how community psychology deals with the issue of social change. We will explore the implicit and explicit assumptions about social change inherent in community psychology and compare these with mainstream psychology's views of social change. It is argued that a Marxist or socio-historical perspective will contribute to a greater understanding of issues related to social change in community psychology. Our socio-historical perspective will also serve to raise some important challenges and address key silences in community psychology. We will therefore also discuss these challenges briefly to suggest a way forward for community psychology.

2 Social change

Lauer (1982) notes that the concept of social change is often discussed without being clearly defined, and covers everything from an attitude change to the historical evolution of societies. As the debates around its definition are beyond the scope of the present chapter the reader is referred to Nisbet (1972) and Schneiderman (1988) for a detailed discussion of the issue. For purposes of the present chapter, however, we will attempt to generate a broad working definition.

Lauer (1982) defines social change as a concept that refers to alterations in social phenomena at various levels of human life, from the individual to the global. Vago (1980) further identifies six interrelated analytic components, which he suggests fall on a continuum. These are: level, identity, duration, direction, magnitude, and rate. These elements provide a broad, useful framework for discussing social change in this chapter. We will briefly discuss four of these elements. Firstly, the idea of levels of social change has been used in community psychology (Reiff, 1977) and is useful for specifying the location of social change. Secondly,

identity is broadly defined as a specific social phenomenon undergoing transformation (Vago, 1980). Thirdly, elements such as duration and direction refer to a sense of time or history. While most theorists would agree with this broad definition and the associated elements of change, they would differ considerably on the forms, causes, and consequences of social change. Accordingly, Vago (1980) identifies five main theories of social change. These are the evolutionary, conflict, structural-functional, systems, and social-psychological explanations of social change.

It is argued that the Marxist conflict perspective on social change differs fundamentally from other perspectives on change. One crucial difference between Marxist and most non-Marxist perspectives on social change is that the latter invariably accepts the dominant social formation, i.e. capitalism, implicitly or explicitly. The methodologies, theories, and practices emanating from the non-Marxist perspectives do not sufficiently challenge oppressive and exploitative social relations. The Marxist conflict perspective, by contrast, offers a radical worldview, methodology, and guiding principles for social change. From a Marxist perspective, social change is defined as a struggle to transform oppressive and exploitative social relations, and social change is thus inevitable, desirable, and a necessary process to address inequality. (See Chapter 4 by Hamber, Masilela, and Terre Blanche in this volume for a more detailed discussion of this issue.)

2.1 Psychology and social change

The main differences we have identified above between Marxist and non-Marxist perspectives are also reflected in psychological discourse and practice. Mainstream psychological theory and practice have been criticized for reproducing and maintaining oppressive and exploitative social relations (Ibáñez and Íñiquez, 1997; Moll, 1983; Nicholas and Cooper, 1990; Nicholas, 1993; Serrano-García, López, and Rivera-Medina, 1987). These critiques raise many challenges for mainstream psychological theory and practice, and also represent attempts at developing an alternative psychology.

While there are considerable differences in the approaches grouped together as 'alternative', they share some common ground with the issue of social change. Mainstream approaches wittingly or unwittingly support capitalism as the dominant social formation and maintain traditional systems of knowledge and power. These dominant systems of knowledge and power are oppressive and exploitative, maintain inequalities, and retard rather than facilitate the process of social change. Alternative approaches tend to challenge these traditional systems of knowledge and power. For example, mainstream views that medicalize 'mental illness' or psychological distress implicitly or explicitly locate pathology in the individual and ignore the broader socio-political context. In contrast, alternative approaches might suggest that 'mental illness' is related to political and social inequality, and may also attempt to address these inequalities. For our analysis then, a social change perspective is one that challenges dominant psychological discourses, presents an alternative view of social reality, and suggests alternative modes of intervention. It is within this context that Rappaport's

(1977) claim of a paradigm shift becomes significant. Community psychology can be viewed as an alternative approach because it challenges dominant psychological discourses and tackles a range of issues that relate to social change. Through our review of some of the perspectives in community psychology we will examine the extent to which community psychology meets the criteria of social change that we have enunciated above.

3 Models[2] of community psychology

It is useful to think of community psychology as having several distinct orientations rather than a unified viewpoint (Heller and Monahan, 1977). Mann (1978) identifies four models in community psychology. (The reader is also referred to Heller and Monahan, 1977, as well as Iscoe, Bloom, and Spielberger, 1977, for a more detailed discussion of these models.) We will discuss two of the four models identified by Mann (1978), namely, the mental health model and the social action model. They are chosen because they represent very different perspectives in community psychology and differ considerably in their assumptions about social change. We will also look at the model by Serrano-Garcia et al. (1987), which was developed as a response to some of the criticisms levelled at both mainstream and community psychology. It represents the Latin-American experience (Monterro, 1996) and provides a useful way forward for community psychology.

3.1 The mental health model

The mental health perspective aims to treat and prevent mental disorders within a geographical catchment area, and the role of the psychologist is to give expert, professional advice to individuals and organizations in the community. The model is thus strong on rational and economic considerations, and has the potential to mobilize community structures. Mental health care is integrated with other services and forms part of a broader primary health-care framework. An attempt is made to facilitate greater access to health resources through local clinics. While direct service delivery is part of the model, the main emphasis is on prevention.

One of the primary assumptions of this model is that earlier and larger scale intervention is more cost-effective and helps to reduce the incidence of mental health problems. Primary prevention is aimed at reducing the number of new cases vis-à-vis incidence. Secondary prevention is aimed at reducing the extent and duration of symptoms when they occur. Tertiary prevention aims at minimizing the impact of a disorder on an individual's life and preventing relapse to the acute phase of the disorder (Caplan, 1964). For example, in dealing with a mental health problem like depression, interventions through support groups for depressed patients would reduce chronicity and severity, and intervening with risk factors such as a lack of social support would reduce the incidence of depression.

The mental health model does not explicitly address the issue of social change. However, through its emphasis on prevention and access, it contains assumptions about social change that differ considerably from mainstream approaches. It intervenes at the level of groups within a community rather than the individual level and it recognizes that there are broader environmental forces relating to mental health. Social change is clearly circumscribed in terms of a geographical catchment area (i.e community), problem definition (i.e. mental health), as well as professional roles and expertise. The professional retains his or her expert role and social change occurs as a consequence of the transfer of this expertise. Through this transfer of knowledge and skills new structures of change can be established or older structures can be restructured or reactivated. However, these changes in social systems and structures within a geographical area are usually incidental to the main goal, which aims at a reduction in the incidence and prevalence of mental health problems. The index of social change in this model then is very specific: a change in the distribution of mental health problems in the community.

One of the major problems with this model is that its assumptions remain far too rooted in mainstream medical discourse to be able to adequately deal with issues of social change. Mental illness is understood as a disease that can be treated or prevented. One of the most consistent criticisms against this approach concerns its usefulness or relevance for understanding human subjectivity and distress or pathology (Parker et al., 1995). By retaining this medical or disease metaphor traditional systems of knowledge and power are also retained. Pathology is still viewed as being located in the individual, complex socio-political processes are reduced to environmental variables, and the professional retains his or her role as the source of expertise and power.

While the model broadens its perspective on change to include the environment, the latter is still conceptualized in terms of an individual focus. It does not have a theory of social institutions and socio-political forces, and is unable to link structural inequality and mental health. For example, even though twice as many women as compared to men are diagnosed with a major depressive episode (DSM-IV, 1994), this model is unable to provide a socio-political explanation for this diagnostic tendency. In summary, the mental health model provides a different perspective and mode of intervention to mainstream clinical models. While it identifies and intervenes at many levels, social change is usually incidental rather than central to its modus operandi. Traditional systems of skills, power, and knowledge are retained and there is no explicit commitment to transforming oppressive and exploitative social conditions. The changes in level from individual to community, and the change in emphasis from treatment to prevention are not substantive enough to represent a radical departure from mainstream clinical models. It does not adequately address issues of social change in terms of the criteria we have identified earlier.

3.2 The social action model

The social action model has its roots in the war on poverty during the Kennedy and Johnson administrations of the United States in the 1960s (Mann, 1978). National legislation through the 1964 Economic Opportunity Act was aimed at dealing with social problems by generating community responsibility and participation (Mann, 1978). The broader socio-political context included the civil rights movement campaigning for black rights, and protests against the Vietnam War.

One of the main assumptions of this model is the failure of mainstream approaches to consider the link between behaviour and social systems. Mainstream approaches were considered to be excessively intra-psychic and as Reiff (cited in Mann, 1978, p. 157) argues, 'such tangible social conditions as housing and transportation, or even such non-tangible social conditions as literacy and free speech, play little or no role in the clinician's conceptualisation of individual behaviour'.

The social action perspective emphasizes the structural inequalities in society, and their impact on communities and individuals in these communities. Its main aim is to produce the circumstances that will allow pressure to be put on those in power to bring about the changes necessary to improve the quality of life of these communities. The model challenges the mainstream psychological and dominant ideological view that holds individuals entirely responsible for their own fate. According to this dominant, individualistic view, conditions of poverty could be attributed to personal failings rather than structural inequality. The social action model challenges this view and links conditions of poverty and powerlessness to structural inequality. It suggests that structural inequality results in a range of psychological and social problems.

Interventions that arise from this framework raise different psychological goals and professional roles. Reiff (cited in Mann, 1978) suggests that self-determination rather than self-actualization is more appropriate for community interventions. Self-determination in this context is understood as a collective struggle for freedom and justice in society. The role of a community psychologist in this model is to organize, activate, mobilize, empower, conscientize, and provide resources or make contacts that were not there before. The psychologist is not neutral in this model and the ultimate goal is to empower the disempowered.

The goal of social change is central to this model and there is a clear political and ideological commitment to transforming oppressive social conditions. There is a recognition of the link between people's daily experiences, social structures, and power and resource imbalances in society. The professional takes on the role of an activist who helps the community achieve self-determination. Community in this model is thus defined as a political constituency in conflict with the broader institutions of society. Social change is accordingly measured by individual and community empowerment, an improvement in social conditions that communities face, and the extent to which societal institutions become more responsive to community demands.

While the social action model has utility for people's daily struggles to bring about social change, there are two major problems. First, if social change is viewed as an attempt to make social institutions more responsive to community demands, this limits change to constituencies. The model identifies conditions of inequality but is unable to theorize or address them beyond a constituency level. Second, there is a paradox in the model; it identifies the contradictions of capitalism while at the same time accepting capitalism as the dominant world-view (Seedat, Cloete, and Shochet, 1988). There is an acknowledgement of the power and resource imbalance in society, but the broader economic, political, and ideological parameters that relate to inequality are not sufficiently addressed.

An example may serve to illustrate some of these issues. Crime is a source of concern for many South Africans (*Cape Times*, 1999, March 12). It is both a local community and a national concern. Within a social action model one way of addressing crime is to make local or national authorities more responsive to community concerns. However, many more broader, historical, political, and ideological considerations to the issue need to be considered: Who defines crime? How is crime defined? What is the link between crime, class, race, and gender? Do the affluent and poverty stricken share the same experiences and understanding of crime, and how to address it? How have the discourses on crime changed historically? These are complex questions and they suggest that crime, like other social and psychological problems, is located in broader historical, socio-political processes. The social action model needs to draw on other theoretical formulations that provide a more comprehensive and critical analysis to address these issues.

The social action model is the perspective in community psychology most closely linked to protest politics. Historically, political and social struggles have taken on different forms. Social action in the present context needs to take into account the changed global context and the emergence of contemporary social movements (Melluci, 1985). In the South African context one needs to explore how the nature of protest politics has changed in the post-apartheid era (Carrim and Sayed, 1992). The key question that needs to be addressed is whether the forms of social action envisaged in the model are relevant to the present context.

In summary, the social action model best captures the essence of social change in community psychology. It tackles a range of issues outside of a narrow mental health framework, acknowledges issues of power and inequality, and defines the professional as a politically and ideologically aligned social change agent. The empowerment metaphor is the heart of this model and it is a very powerful metaphor for transforming social conditions through individual and social action. Rappaport's (1981) argument for a policy of empowerment over prevention and the call for a social movement represents a significant departure from mainstream models.

3.3 The social community approach

The model proposed by Serrano-Garcia et al. (1987) attempts to address the problems associated with mainstream psychology and suggests that community psychology as an attempted solution has not been successful. In this model there is an explicit commitment to social change and the professional has the responsibility of finding solutions to social problems. According to Serrano-Garcia (1994, p. 2) 'the main goal of community psychology is to promote social change to alter unjust and oppressive situations by generating knowledge, carrying out research and developing interventions'.

Theoretically, the social community approach is interdisciplinary and draws from different frameworks. There are two key elements to this approach. First, there is an acknowledgement of the historically changing structural determinants of social reality. An understanding of this element is located in a sociological analysis of social formations, such as capitalism, that promote specific social realities. Second, the model incorporates an analysis of human subjectivity and agency that is grounded in social constructivism but acknowledges broader socio-political and ideological factors as well. By referring to modes of production, there is an acknowledgement that subjectivity and social reality are tied to particular social and economic formations at specific historical moments (Serrano-Garcia et al., 1987).

In terms of intervention the professional is seen as a social change agent who can intervene at different levels with different objectives. The professional can use his or her skills and knowledge to facilitate an adaptation to the prevailing values in society. This is referred to as a change in function. The professional can also attempt to change or establish structures that will better respond to prevailing values. This is a longer term intervention and is referred to as a change in forms, i.e. a change in the attitudes and values of social institutions. The professional can work towards an adaptation or a change in social reality (Serrano-Garcia et al., 1987).

From within this model human subjectivity is understood historically and within broader social, economic, and political parameters. By conceptualizing humans as constructing social reality it allows for human agency in social action. There is a legitimization of 'popular' culture and consciousness, and the dissemination of knowledge is considered to be essential for empowerment. The model highlights the need for information and holds that participation is achieved through consciousness. It stresses both individual and community empowerment, and social change is understood as a process that allows people to construct as well as change social reality.

The model can be viewed as developing the social action model within a Marxist framework and it addresses some of the concerns we raised about the social action model. Social change is central to the model and the professional plays a key role as a social change agent. Social change is conceptualized as occurring at different levels and involves both collective action as well as a change in consciousness (i.e. attitudes or values). By referring to changes in function it also suggests that social institutions can be changed to meet human needs.

The strength of the social community model lies in the way it addresses a key issue with regard to social change, namely, human subjectivity or agency. Human subjectivity is located within a broader Marxist, socio-historical framework and the model emphasizes a change in consciousness. In this framework social reality is contained in, but not determined by, broader socio-historical processes. Humans have the ability to construct and engage with social reality. The social constructivist framework suggests that while institutions shape human experience and consciousness, humans also have the ability to shape institutions. For example, the dominant medical discourse on psychological distress reinforces dominant ideological positions and plays a powerful role in shaping people's understanding of psychological distress. However, people are also able to challenge this dominant discourse and their understanding may differ from the mainstream idea that psychological disorders are caused mainly by biological abnormalities.

Unlike the social action model, the social community model uses Marxism in its analysis and intervention. This is a significant development that raises different issues and possibilities for social change. However, there are two areas that need further development. First, in the exposition of the model there seems to be a greater emphasis on human subjectivity. For addressing issues of social change more broadly it would also be useful to more fully engage with other areas of Marxist thought. Second, the level of intervention needs to be established. Serrano-Garcia (1984) raises the difficulty in choosing, in the light of scarce resources, the level of intervention. The author argues that community is an important level of intervention and addresses all levels of intervention besides the macro-social. Below we explore the possibilities for social action at the macro-social level.

4 Taking community psychology forward: silences and issues of change

As our discussion of the models indicates, community psychology offers a different perspective on psychological and social problems. At this stage it would be useful to consider to what extent community psychology measures up in terms of our social change criteria. While social change can be defined in a number of ways, our discussion has centred on two key related aspects. First, dominant systems of knowledge can be constraining, oppressive, and exploitative, and social change involves a process of challenging this through an alternative definition of social reality. Second, social change also involves an attempt to transform oppressive and exploitative conditions. As our review of the models has suggested, community psychology addresses both aspects in terms of its theories, modes of intervention, and its notions of social change. Below we look at possibilities for further engaging with some of the issues, as well as some silences in community psychology.

4.1 Theoretical and methodological issues

Rappaport's (1977) assertion that community psychology represents a paradigm shift can be questioned. While the notion of 'science' can be contested, community psychology has not successfully developed a systematic alternative 'scientific' or methodological framework for viewing social phe-

nomena. There has been little critical examination of positivist frameworks or an engagement with meta-theoretical and epistemological issues. The research produced still predominantly remains rooted in the mainstream approach. In a content analysis of over 700 research articles in the *American Journal of Community Psychology* and the *Journal of Community Psychology* in the period 1973 to 1982, it was found that only 8 per cent of the projects reviewed moved beyond an individual level of analysis and only 12 per cent drew implications at the level of community or society (Lounsbury, in Orford, 1992). The researchers' conclusion is, 'we feel uneasy about the lack of a community perspective in most of the research articles we examined . . . [and] the nearly exclusive focus on individual as the unit of analysis' (Lounsbury, in Orford, 1992, p. 12).

This finding is significant and highlights two important issues. It suggests that if social change is to be measured by the development of an alternative voice, then, in the arena of academic and professional development, community psychology has not been very successful. This is not to suggest that the critical voice of community psychology is or should be confined to this space, however. In fact, the strength of community psychology lies in its dissemination and popularization of academic knowledge best exemplified by the social community model. Part of the challenge for community psychology, like most of psychology, lies in exploring and redefining the boundaries of the discipline, critically examining the nature of the subject, and finding new ways of conducting psychological research (Smith,

Harre, and Van Langenhove, 1995).

Part of the continued growth of community psychology lies in more vigorously challenging dominant systems of knowledge, and providing theoretical and methodological alternatives. While community psychology has drawn from alternative frameworks such as critical psychology, critical social psychology, post-modernism, and Marxism, among others, the challenge lies in more fully integrating contributions from these frameworks into community psychology. In terms of its academic and professional engagement, community psychology needs to provide a viable theoretical alternative to mainstream approaches. In this regard the social community model's attempt at using critical frameworks within community psychology is a useful one.

4.2 Notions of social change within community psychology

Community psychology is characterized by its engagement with issues of social change. While there are differences between the various perspectives in community psychology, social change is clearly seen as an important or desirable goal. Community psychology tackles a range of issues outside of a narrow mental health framework and moves beyond the individual unit in its interventions. Reiff (1977) identifies five different levels of intervention from the individual level to the social level, and Levine and Perkins (1987) suggest that interventions beyond the individual level shade into political action. The goals of intervention are not 'curative' but aim for both personal and community empowerment (Rappaport,

1981; Riesel, 1994) and a striving for a sense of community identity (Sarason, 1976) as a collective value to counteract individualism as a value. Professional roles have been diversified, there is a greater awareness of the professional's ideological and political role, and there is a strong emphasis on the democritization of skills and knowledge. Communities are considered to be important social forces in the process of change, and form the focal point of community psychology interventions.

In terms of the elements of social change that we have highlighted, community psychology moves towards challenging the dominant social reality as well as offering strategies for transforming social conditions. There are, however, some key issues in the area of social change that have not been adequately addressed, as well as some significant 'silences'. Firstly, the ahistorical approach to social change is inadequate. Secondly, the relationship between human subjectivity/agency and social change is complex and requires further analysis. Finally, the relationship between conditions of structural inequality and social change is complex and can also be explored as an issue of political economy. We briefly explore these and look at ways in which a more critical and contextual view could be taken of present notions of social change in community psychology.

5 A socio-historical approach to social change

All definitions of change contain the element of time, and change is measured or analysed by various indices indicating a temporal dimension. While notions of social change contain implicit or explicit references to time or history, critical frameworks highlight the need for adopting a socio-historical approach. The social community approach explores this notion and raises a crucial idea, that social reality is a dynamic, context-specific process tied to different historical periods and different social formations.

Socio-historical approaches suggest that ideas and practices do not develop in a vacuum. They suggest that in different historical periods there are different role players, vested interests, and social forces. Ideas and practices that may have been considered to be 'progressive' initially may have different consequences in later historical periods (Tolman, 1997). It is for this reason that community psychology discourses and practices needed to be located in a socio-historical context. For example, while difficulties in defining the concept of empowerment are highlighted (Perkins and Zimmerman, 1995; Riesel, 1994; Zimmerman, 1995), the location of this concept in a socio-historical framework, as in the social community model, seems to be the exception rather than the trend. Community psychology concepts such as empowerment emerged during the protests against the Vietnam war and the civil rights protests. As a concept and a goal is it still applicable to our present context? How have the discourses relating to empowerment changed historically? Is empowerment a useful concept and goal for the South African context? How does empowerment relate to social formations such as capitalism?

6 Human subjectivity/agency and social change

One of the major limitations of mainstream approaches to psychology is the explicit and implicit assumption that the individual should be the focal point of change. Socio-historical approaches such as Marxism challenge this idea and suggest that social change should be understood as a socio-political process with the focus on changing social structures. Classical Marxism views social change as an inevitable process arising from the contradictions of capitalism. The role of human subjectivity/agency in this process is a complex and thorny issue both within and beyond Marxism, and this debate is beyond the scope of the present text. Thus, rather than enter into the debate, it is perhaps more useful to suggest that human subjectivity/agency remains a crucial area for discussion.

Humans devise social reality and actively participate in the process of change. Symbolic activity and meaning making are therefore crucial areas of engagement for community psychology. The use of social constructivism in the social community model addresses this issue. It suggests that not only do social structures act on humans, but humans also interact with and shape social structures. The processes by which humans construct and change social reality constitute an important area for discussion in community psychology.

Post-modern perspectives differ from Marxist perspectives in their approach to human subjectivity/agency. They highlight the specific and local contexts of knowledge and action (as opposed to grand theories or narratives) and point to the relativity in social reality. These approaches can serve to give voice to issues beyond the major forms of structural inequality, namely, class, race, and gender. They allow space for all marginalized voices and acknowledge the role of human agency in social change. These approaches are also useful for deconstructing and reconstructing accepted notions of social change. It is suggested that the present engagement of community psychology with post-modern discourse is a fruitful one. Griffin, Beardslee, and Holland (cited in Newbrough, 1995) distinguish between a deconstructionist and a constructionist move in post-modern thought. While Newbrough (1995) argues for a constructionist emphasis, both merit further engagement.

While post-modernism remains an important contribution, there is a danger of extreme relativism and an emphasis on the purely subjective psychological domain. Spears (1997) argues against this position and, like the social community model (Serrano-Garcia et al., 1987), points to the constraints of power and social reality. According to Spears (1997) extreme relativism (all truths are equally valid) is unsatisfactory, and he calls for a theory of subject to guide political action. Post-modernism needs to be marked by a call to political action rather than an inability or unwillingness for political action, as has been the case (Spears, 1997). In addition, an understanding of broader political and economic structures should inform an understanding of human subjectivity/agency. The integration of Marxism and social constructivism in

the social community model addresses both these concerns. While the marriage of Marxism and post-modernism has stimulated vigorous debate, it merits further exploration.

7 Structural inequality and social change

As we have highlighted above, there are significant issues relating to social change and structural inequality that community psychology does not sufficiently address. Structural inequality is mainly understood as a power and resource imbalance, without critically analysing the differing forms of inequalities, the reasons for, or causes of, these inequalities, and the many ways of trying to change these inequalities. The three main forms of inequalities that we have identified are class, race, and gender, yet there has not been sufficient engagement in community psychology with some of the critical discourses relating to these forms of oppression. There are many perspectives and theories on these forms (and other forms) of inequality, but we will not be able to engage with them within the scope of the present chapter. Rather than enter into these debates, we will look at Marxist and neo-Marxist approaches to these forms of inequalities. It is suggested that Marxism provides a useful way forward as it is able to theorize and link the different forms of inequality, relate these to an analysis of capitalism, and provide possibilities for engaging in different forms of collective action.

The contribution of Marxism to community psychology is more fully discussed elsewhere (see Chapter 4 by Hamber, Masilela, and Terre Blanche in this volume), so we will confine our discussion to possibilities for engaging in different forms of collective action. According to Marxist thought, capitalism is characterized by an unequal and conflictual relationship between capital and labour (the economic base), from which all other political and ideological structures (the superstructure) arise. The ideological and political structures 'hide' these unequal social relations and serve to maintain the domination of the working class by the ruling class. This oppressive and exploitative relationship between the two classes is antagonistic and irreconcilable and results in a political struggle. The ruling class want to retain the economic resources (mode of production), power, and control, while the working class struggle to transform their subordinate position. Social change then is a process of destroying this exploitative and unequal system and establishing a new, democratic, and just social order - socialism or communism.

A Marxist perspective poses a number of challenges for community psychology in three key areas. First, while there is much voice given to conditions of oppression there is often a silence around economic exploitation and the link between economic exploitation and oppression. Second, while the call to social and political action is a feature of community psychology, Marxist approaches highlight and emphasize possibilities for different sites and forms of collective action. Third, Marxist approaches challenge some of the implicit and explicit assumptions about

society, societal institutions, and individual and citizen participation that underlie much of community psychology.

7.1 Economic exploitation

Marxist approaches emphasize the economic structure (mode of production) of society as the foundation from which all other political and social processes arise. While it is not possible to analyse this crucial statement in detail, it is important to note that this perspective differs fundamentally from other perspectives on social change. For community psychology they raise two crucial implications for social change. First, social change, according to this definition, should include an attempt to change the economic structures of society. Second, it identifies a different set of issues or struggles around which community psychology has been silent, particularly issues relating to economic exploitation and class struggle. Economic exploitation can take different forms at different levels. The unequal economic relationship between capital (owners) and labour (producers of wealth) in countries is also related to the exploitation and underdevelopment of 'Third' World economies by 'First' World economies, and the present trend towards the concentration of wealth in fewer and fewer hands (global economy). It is estimated that the poorest receive 1,4 per cent of the total world income and the richest receive 82,7 per cent of the total world income (UNDP Human Development report cited in the *Cape Times*, 1999, June 25). Apart from the social community model there has been very little acknowledgement of these issues in community psychology, and it is imperative that this silence be addressed.

The thesis that political and social change can be understood by changes in economic structures and processes is a powerful one and challenges community psychologists to expand the definition of social change to include economic structures. For example, as a community psychologist you may be confronted by the scarcity of and inequality in the distribution of resources in the local community context. Nationally this local situation is also related to the vast discrepancy between the rich and the poor (capital vs. labour). At the international level South Africa as an 'underdeveloped' country has a tremendous debt to the World Bank (which includes the debt accrued during the apartheid era). To repay this debt it has to exercise fiscal discipline, which means that less money is available for state expenditure and services like health. While there is no simple relationship between the local, national, and international context, it does suggest that the local community context is strongly influenced by the global economy.

For the community psychologist this raises possibilities for a different range of social change strategies. Most community psychologists address inequality at the local community level. While this is important, it may exclude other social change strategies. One could at the national level attempt to address the unequal distribution of resources as a national problem (for example, campaigns that call for greater state expenditure on social services, or organized labour campaigns), or even as an international problem (for example, the campaign to write off the debts of 'developing' countries, which place

an enormous burden on their already scarce resources). While there is a strong acknowledgement of the power and resource imbalances in community psychology, Marxist approaches contribute greatly to our understanding of these imbalances by suggesting they are linked to economic exploitation and global economic trends.

7.2 Collective action, the state, and civil society

Collective action is a distinctive feature of community psychology. Community psychology interventions are often based on an advocacy model aimed at influencing decision making. The assumption is that if issues are clearly and loudly articulated they will be heard. This occurs mostly at the local authority level and at the national level with a view to making social institutions more responsive to constituency demands. While Rappaport (1981) argues strongly that advocacy involves both a struggle for rights as well as resources, most advocacy frameworks draw from a liberal-democratic ideology (Sayed, 1995), which does not sufficiently analyse or challenge capitalism. Marxism, on the other hand, locates inequality in the context of social formations like capitalism, and analyses the different social forces in society, how and why certain voices (rather than all) are heard, and the complex relationship between state, citizenship, and social formations.

Advocacy frameworks that draw from a liberal-democratic ideology hold the implicit assumption that the state is a neutral force for distributing resources for which differing groups compete. Marxist approaches, by contrast, question the notion of a neutral state. These approaches emphasize the link between the state and capitalism, and some theorists view the state as a powerful agent of control. Althusser (1971) views the state as an instrument of capital (the ruling class), which, through its institutions, reproduces and maintains oppressive and exploitative social relations. While this assumption has been vigorously contested, and there are alternative conceptions of the state (Dale, 1989), the neutrality of the state remains in question. The state represents particular group interests, which, according to Althusser (1971), are the interests of capital.

An understanding of the state can also be expanded to include the notion of civil society as a space that falls outside of the state and party political structures. The notion of civil society is itself vigorously debated (Narsoo, 1991), but we will define it as all private organizations that fall outside the public apparatuses of the state (Simon, 1982). While the ruling classes maintain power through the control of state apparatuses, they also want to assert political and ideological dominance in all places (churches, civic and community organizations) that fall outside of the state's public apparatuses. This dominance, however, is challenged by these social forces, resulting in a struggle for control or hegemony (Simon, 1982). In summary, the struggle to end economic and political domination occurs at the level of state structures as well as civil society, and involves a struggle for economic, political, and ideological control.

Civil society is also the space in which social movements operate and form part of the struggle. Social movements, as used in the present context, refer to any grouping outside of the public apparatuses of the state. They are distinct from political parties that have or seek representation in formal parliamentary structures through elections. Social movements may develop into political parties but often arise from collective action around specific issues (Melluci, 1985), either nationally or internationally. Social movements develop organically and, like other sectors of civil society, challenge the dominant ideology or cultural code (Melluci, 1985).

This has been a highly simplified examination of complex theoretical areas and the accounts presented have been vigorously contested. We can, however, identify useful areas of engagement for community psychology. Apart from the social community model, most community psychology frameworks draw, implicitly or explicitly, from a liberal-democratic framework, which Marxism would argue does not sufficiently challenge capitalism. From a Marxist perspective we have raised two key ideas that need further engagement. The first is the idea that power and resource imbalances are not accidental, but a result of the attempts of the ruling classes (those in power) to maintain power and control. The second is the idea that community struggles form part of a bigger economic, political, and ideological struggle that occurs in all sectors of society. Marxism identifies more clearly the levels and forms of citizen participation (local, national, international, party politics, civil society), the divisions along class, race, and gender lines, as well as the contexts and constraints of power.

The Marxist approach raises a number of key challenges for notions of collective action and social change in community psychology. It suggests that social reality and social change are historically specific sociopolitical processes rooted in a particular social formation, i.e. capitalism. The key issues that community psychology needs to deal with from this perspective are issues of class conflict and economic exploitation, 'development' and 'underdevelopment' in the changing global economy, and the role that the state and social structures play in maintaining and reproducing oppressive and exploitative social relations. Marxist perspectives generate a much wider range of social change strategies. National and international politics, the politics of class, race and gender, and national and international social movements considerably expand the boundaries and possibilities for social change.

The use of Marxism to examine the above issues is not to suggest that its usage is unproblematic. There are vigorous debates within Marxism about some of the areas we have covered. Furthermore, changing global conditions and post-modern approaches are two significant challenges to Marxism. Three issues which we have raised but which we have not fully discussed are critical. These are Marxism's economic reductionism, the view that social change is inevitable, and the structure/agency debate. Marxism has and should continue its engagement with these issues.

8 Conclusion

Through a review of some of the models in community psychology we have explored notions of social change in community psychology. It has been argued that community psychology differs considerably from mainstream perspectives and is marked by its commitment to social change. However, its conceptualization of and commitment to social change are still largely evolutionary rather than revolutionary. It has been suggested that the use of a Marxist framework in community psychology, as attempted by the social community model, provides a useful way forward. Marxist perspectives on social change differ from other perspectives and they also address some key silences in community psychology that need to be addressed. This is an important intellectual task, but the real challenge is perhaps one of 'practical adequacy', that is, the extent to which theories resonate with the real and potential struggles of ordinary people (Spears, 1997). To paraphrase Marx, philosophers interpret the world, our duty is to change it.

Exercises

1 What are some of the main criticisms that have been levelled at mainstream discourses in psychology?

2 Adopting the role of a social change agent, as proposed in community psychology, challenges traditional professional roles, values, and boundaries. Consider how the adoption of this role relates to your personal value system. As a group, did you reach consensus that the psychologist needs to adapt the role of a social change agent? What were the points of agreement/disagreement?

3 Write an essay on your understanding of human subjectivity. Which approaches do you find the most useful for this topic?

4 How does the Marxist approach differ from most community psychology approaches in its understanding of macro-social processes?

5 As a group, discuss more fully some of the criticisms levelled at mainstream discourses in psychology. Choose a journal article or reading that you consider to be part of mainstream discourse as the basis for your discussions.

6 One of the silences in community psychology has been around the issue of racism. Review some recent texts and journal articles, and analyse how the issue of racism is addressed. Do you agree that there is a silence around this issue? How is the issue of racism discussed?

7 As a group consider what contribution community psychologists make at the macro-social level. Should community psychology interventions be confined to the community level? What interventions are possible at the macro-social level?

8 Community psychology perspectives differ from mainstream perspectives in a number of ways. We have not covered all these differences and you might want to explore the basic principles and underlying assumptions in community psychology by examining some of the key concepts in community psychology. Besides the important concepts we have covered, such as community, advocacy, and empowerment, it will also be useful to look at deprofessionalization, blaming the victim, causal attribution, and deficit and resiliency perspectives. Do these concepts more directly address issues of social change as compared with mainstream approaches? How do these concepts measure up in terms of our social change criteria?

9 Events like the fall of communism and post-modern approaches call to question Marxism. As a group you can consider whether a Marxist analysis is still useful or relevant for the South African context. Refer to Callinicos (1987) for a Marxist critique of post-modernism.

10 Two models we have not covered are the ecological and the organizational models (Mann, 1978). The ecological model is an influential model in community psychology and uses a systems metaphor for understanding human behaviour. Trickett (1984) defines it as a metaphor for the understanding of the 'community embeddedness of persons and the nature of communities'. The study of organizations and organizational dynamics has its roots in industrial psychology and is very useful for working with a range of service organizations in communities. Study these models and try to identify their assumptions about social change. Do these assumptions differ from the models we cover? In what way?

Notes

1 We would like to thank Mohamed Seedat whose patience, many reviews, and constructive comments helped shape this piece. Thanks to Sandy Lazarus and Norman Duncan for their reviews and constructive comments. A final thank you to all our colleagues, friends, and family members who helped in various ways.

2 While the term model is retained and used for consistency there is a debate around the use of the term and 'perspective' is perhaps more accurate.

References

ALTHUSSER, L. (1971). *Essays on ideology.* London: Verso.

CALLINICOS, A. (1987). *Making history.* Oxford: Polity/Blackwell.

CAPE TIMES. (1999, March 12). *Crime is SA's major concern.* Gill Gifford.

CAPE TIMES. (1999). *Cracks start to show in global free markets.* Melanie Gosling. 25 June.

CAPLAN, G. (1964). *Principles of preventive psychiatry.* New York: Basic Books.

CARRIM, N. and SAYED, Y. (1992). Civil society, social movements and the National Education Co-ordinating Committee (NECC). *Perspectives in Education,* 14(1), 21–34.

DALE, R. (1989). *The state and education policy.* Great Britain: Open University Press.

DSM-IV (1994). *Diagnostic and statistical manual of mental disorders.* Washington, DC: American Psychiatric Association.

HELLER, K. and MONAHAN, J. (1977). *Psychology and community change.* Homewood, IL: Dorsey.

IBÁÑEZ, T. and ÍÑIQUEZ, L. (Eds.). (1997). *Critical social psychology.* London: Sage.

ISCOE, I., BLOOM, B.L., and SPIELBERGER, C. (Eds.). (1977). *Proceedings of the national conference on training in community psychology.* Washington, DC: Hemisphere.

LAUER, R. H. (1982). *Perspectives on social change.* (3d ed.). Boston: Allyn and Bacon.

LEVINE, M. and PERKINS, D. N. (1987). *Principles of community psychology: Perspectives and applications.* New York: Oxford University Press.

MANN, P. A. (1978). *Community psychology: Concepts and applications.* New York: Free Press.

MOLL, I. (1983). Answering the question: What is psychology? *Psychology in Society,* 1, 59–77.

MELLUCI, A. (1985). The symbolic challenge of contemporary movements. *Social Research,* 52(4), 789–817.

MONTERRO, M. (1996). Parallel lives: Community psychology in Latin America and the United States. *American Journal of Community Psychology,* 24(4), 589–605.

NARSOO, M. (1991). Civil society: A contested terrain. *Work in Progress,* 76, 24–27.

NEWBROUGH, J. R. (1995). Toward community: A third position. *American Journal of Community Psychology,* 23(1), 9–31.

NICHOLAS, L. J. (Ed.). (1993). *Psychology and oppression: Critiques and proposals.* Johannesburg: Skotaville.

NICHOLAS, L. J. and COOPER, S. (Eds.). (1990). *Psychology and apartheid.* Cape Town: Vision.

NISBET, R. (1972). *Social change.* New York: Harper & Row.

ORFORD, J. (1992). *Community psychology theory and practice.* England: John Wiley and Sons.

PARKER, I., GEORGACA, E., HARPER, D., MCLAUGLIN, T., and STOWELL-SMITH, M. (1995). *Deconstructing pathology.* London: Sage.

PERKINS, D. D. and ZIMMERMAN, M. A. (1995). Empowerment theory, research and application. *American Journal of Psychology,* 23(5), 569–57.

RAPPAPORT, J. (1977). *Community psychology: Values, research and action.* New York: Holt, Rhinehart and Winston.

RAPPAPORT, J. (1981). In praise of paradox: A social policy of empowerment over prevention. *American Journal of Community Psychology,* 9(1), 1–21.

REIFF, R. (1977). Ya gotta believe. In I. Iscoe, B. L. Bloom, and C. D. Spielberger (Eds.), *Proceedings of the national conference on training in community psychology.* Washington, DC: Hemisphere.

RIESEL, C. (1994). Empowerment: The holy grail

of health promotion. *Health Promotion International,* 9(1), 39–45.

SARASON, S. B. (1976). *The psychological sense of community: Prospects for a community psychology.* San Francisco: Jossey-Bass.

SAYED, Y. (1995). *Educational policy developments in South Africa, 1990–1994: A critical examination of the policy of educational decentralisation.* Unpublished doctoral dissertation, University of Bristol.

SCHNEIDERMAN, L. (1988). *The psychology of social change.* New York: Human Sciences Press.

SEEDAT, M. A., CLOETE, N., and SHOCHET, I. (1988). Community psychology: Panic or panacea. *Psychology in Society,* 11, 39–54.

SERRANO-GARCIA, I. (1984). The illusion of empowerment: Community development within a colonial context. In J. Rappaport, C. I. A. Swift, and R. Hess (Eds.), *Studies in empowerment: Steps towards understanding and action.* New York: Hawthorn.

SERRANO-GARCIA, I. (1994). The ethics of the powerful and the power of ethics. *American Journal of Community Psychology,* 22(1), 1–20.

SERRANO-GARCIA, I., LÓPEZ, M. M., and RIVERA-

MEDINA, E. (1987). Toward a social-community psychology. *Journal of Community Psychology,* 15, 431–446.

SIMON, R. (1982). *Gramsci's political thought: An introduction.* London: Lawrence and Wishart.

SMITH, J. A., HARRÉ, R., and VAN LANGHOVE, L. (1995). *Rethinking methods in psychology.* London: Sage.

SPEARS, R. (1997). Introduction. In T. Ibáñez and L. Íñiquez (Eds.), *Critical social psychology.* London: Sage.

TOLMAN, C. W. (1997). *Psychology, society and subjectivity: An introduction to German critical psychology.* London: Routledge.

TRICKETT, E. J. (1984). Toward a distinctive community psychology: An ecological metaphor for the conduct of community research and the nature of training. *American Journal of Community Psychology,* 12(3), 261–280.

VAGO, S. (1980). *Social change.* New York: Holt, Rinehart and Winston.

ZIMMERMAN, M. A. (1995). Psychological empowerment: Issues and illustrations. *American Journal of Community Psychology,* 23(5), 581–599.

6 Models of community mental health services for children

Anthony Pillay
Rafiq Lockhat

Study objectives

After a study of this chapter you should be able to:

- understand the extent of childhood mental health problems and the need to vigorously formulate methods of addressing the problems;
- obtain some insight into a few of the mental health problems affecting children in South Africa;
- understand the economic issues involved in child mental health; and
- examine a few of the available models of mental health service delivery.

1 Introduction and historical background

Mental health services for children are underprovided in most countries around the world, and not only in low-income coun-tries. Furthermore, at the level of national health policies, mental health for people under nineteen years is not receiving the priority rating it deserves. In general, chil-dren from poorer families are more disad-vantaged in terms of access to services, with the result that underlying and manifest problems are left untreated, only to develop into more chronic or complicated conditions that are sometimes treatment-resistant.

It is widely acknowledged that an ade-quate number of mental health specialists, such as psychologists and psychiatrists, will probably never be available to meet the needs of children in low- to middle-income coun-tries such as South Africa, and even in high-income countries such as the United States (Kelleher and Long, 1994). Of course, this issue relates to the failure of the tradi-tional mental health model to provide ade-quate and equitable care to those in need. Despite its rather lengthy existence, there has been a distinct failure over the years to appropriately transform the traditional model to suit the times and needs. The profession of clinical psychology, which celebrated its 100th anniversary in the United States of America in 1996, has, for example, only recently begun to seriously recognize the deficiencies of the traditional practice model. Although this discipline is much younger in South Africa, local psychologists have not waited as long as their American counterparts to criticize the traditional mental health model.

There is certainly a need to replace or substantially modify the traditional mental health model, which has a history of passively waiting for people who have the necessary insight and economic resources to seek consultations from mental health specialists. This approach is not applicable to the majority of South Africans, and certainly not to disadvantaged children whose parents are not able to afford mental health consultations or even identify problems as being psychological in nature. It is, therefore, imperative that we take a fresh look into alternative models of providing mental health care to children across the spectrum of the South African population.

Planning an efficient child mental health service requires a clear perspective of the rates of psychological and psychiatric morbidity, nationally and even regionally. However, the absence of adequate health-management information systems means that high-quality epidemiological data is lacking in South Africa, with the result that information on service needs is sketchy and inadequate. Using projections from international prevalence studies, and notwithstanding the cultural and political variables, it is reasonable to expect that at least 15 per cent of the country's children are affected by mental health problems of one form or another. This means that in excess of 3 million South African children could benefit from psychological or psychiatric intervention in order to improve their quality of life. Considering the discriminatory and hostile policies of apartheid to which the majority of the nation's children have been subjected, it would be understandable for them to show a much higher rate of psychological morbidity than children in other industrialized countries (Pillay and Lockhat, 1997). Dawes (1985) described the apartheid policies as 'psychopathogenic', with the government jeopardizing the mental health of its people.

To date, child mental health services have been concentrated in the metropolitan areas, including the large cities of Cape Town, Johannesburg, and Durban, and based mainly in state psychiatric hospitals and their satellite clinics, a few general hospitals, university child guidance centres, social welfare organizations, and non-governmental organizations (NGOs). A survey by Duncan and Rock (1994) found that 85 000 children were attended to by non-government welfare services during 1990, suggestive of the role played by this sector in child mental health. The country has less than five specialized in-patient child mental health centres, despite the relatively large number of such facilities and in-patient beds for adults. This must be viewed against the fact that, at the time of writing this chapter, almost 20 million (46,8 per cent) of South Africa's population was under nineteen years of age (Central Statistical Services, 1996). The only in-patient specialist facility for this age group in the province of KwaZulu-Natal, which has almost 4 million children and adolescents, was closed in 1996. Most of the country's nine provinces had no such specialized units. An investigation in the Western Cape region found that the outpatient mental health services were overwhelmed by adult patients, with children and adolescents constituting only 18 per cent of the attendees (Ensink, Leger, and Robertson, 1994).

The current ratio of child psychiatrists to children in South Africa is approximately 1:1 million, compared with the World Health Organization (WHO) recommended ratio of 1:35 000 (Dawes et al., 1997). The ratio of psychologists to children is difficult to calculate since many psychologists see children and adults. Some urban areas have relatively large numbers of psychologists and a few psychiatrists in private practice. A smattering of educational psychological services is available, but these are clearly remnant of the apartheid education system, favouring the historically white schools with virtually no such services in most black schools.

At the level of community mental health services for children there is really no infrastructure in South Africa. Apart from a few isolated, but well-intentioned endeavours, mental health services for children in communities outside the metropolitan boundaries are virtually non-existent. Many of the services developed to date are informal and have evolved in reactive circumstances such as violence and other social problems affecting children. The need, therefore, for carefully constructed, pro-actively oriented community services is evident. Certainly, this type of approach is likely to achieve more widespread success in the long term than the 'band-aid' approach we have been forced to use during the 1980s and 1990s.

2 Types of childhood mental health problems in disadvantaged communities

In discussing childhood problems presenting in community mental health contexts, the socio-economically disadvantaged child inevitably takes precedence. However, there is little reason to believe that the psychological disorders affecting children in different social-class contexts is likely to differ significantly, although conditions like poverty do bring additional stresses and mental health sequelae, since children from advantaged backgrounds generally have access to private or other urban-based health services. Private practitioners are usually located in urban areas and are only accessible to affluent families or those who are members of medical aid societies. Also, specialized state-funded facilities are almost always urban-based and out of reach of rural communities. To date, literature and research on childhood mental health problems in this country have been skewed and have been more concerned with advantaged and urban children, with the result that little is known about the problems of children from poorer, rural, and peri-urban communities. Perusal of the psychological and psychiatric literature published in and about South Africa in the past few decades bears testimony to this.

2.1 Poverty and its mental health effects

It is well known that sustained periods of poverty can have marked effects on children's cognitive development (Illback, 1994). Poverty is also known to affect and inhibit the quality of parenting that these children receive (McAdoo, 1988). Considering the high levels of unemployment and general deprivation in rural areas of South Africa, exceedingly high numbers of children in these communities are malnourished. Recent research indicates that 10 per cent of pre-school-aged children are underweight, and 25 per cent show growth stunting due to nutritional deficiency (Health Systems Trust, 1996). This means that over 1,5 million children are stunted due to long-term malnutrition. Many of these children manifest either mental retardation or specific learning disabilities but are usually not appropriately diagnosed or managed. Recent research in the KwaZulu-Natal Midlands region showed that 15 per cent of rural and peri-urban children with mental health problems presented with mental retardation, while a further 11 per cent manifested specific scholastic difficulties in the absence of mental retardation (Pillay and Lockhat, 1997). This means that over one-quarter of the children exhibited cognitive problems that affected their schooling. Unfortunately, these children tend to remain in the same grade for several years due to a lack of progress, without any assessment or remediation attempts. Cases of children held in the same grade (e.g., Grade 1 or 2) for as long as five years have come to the authors' attention on numerous occasions. Considering the emphasis on

children's education since the inception of the country's first democratic government in 1994, the impact of poverty on children's cognitive development will certainly require much attention in the next few years.

2.2 Post-traumatic stress disorder

A significant problem requiring psychological intervention among rural children is post-traumatic stress disorder (PTSD). The political violence that became a part of the South African landscape during the past two decades has taken a severe toll on children and adolescents in conflict-ridden communities. Several mental health effects have been identified in children exposed to violence (Dawes, 1994). These include symptoms of hyper-arousal, re-experiencing the traumatic events through intrusive thoughts, dreams, and even re-enactment of the event through play. Research on affected children in KwaZulu-Natal found higher levels of distress among boys than girls, possibly due to the greater involvement of males in the combat situations (Pillay, Magwaza, and Peterson, 1992). Widespread intervention programmes are needed to address this problem. While there are several efforts in progress, mainly from NGOs, there is a distinct need for these to be formalized and collaborative in order to facilitate the required networking process. Also, in view of the extent of this problem, specific government support and initiatives through its Department of Health would be beneficial and unifying in the long term. It must be borne in mind that many other children are affected at sub-clinical levels. These affected children's drawings and play behaviour tend to be more aggressive and often mimic armed combat situations (Killian, 1993).

2.3 Sexual abuse

Sexual abuse is a related problem, especially in the sense of its violence and PTSD sequelae. While there is no real evidence to suggest that the sexual abuse of children is more common in rural than urban communities, the lack of after-care and support facilities for abused children in the rural areas is a crucial distinguishing factor. A recent investigation noted a much lower proportion of sexual abuse cases in an urban clinic in Durban than in a rural/peri-urban context in the KwaZulu-Natal Midlands periodically visited by clinical psychologists (Pillay and Naidoo, 1997). However, this difference was ascribed to the fact that urban sexual abuse cases presented at any one of the numerous available facilities, while the rural children had to wait for the monthly visiting psychological services catering to children within a 100 km radius. As an indication of reported crimes, police department statistics in South Africa revealed that over 16 000 cases of sexual offences against children were reported to their Child Protection Units during the year 1995 (*Daily News*, 1996, July 11).

2.4 Attention-deficit/hyperactivity disorder

The condition of attention-deficit/hyperactivity disorder (ADHD) is one that is certainly underidentified in rural children. According to the American Psychiatric Association (1994) 3 to 5 per cent of school-aged

children are affected with this disorder, which has a marked impact on their attention and concentration abilities, and inevitably their learning potential, with excessive activity levels also hindering their adaptive functioning. Interestingly, the urban/rural comparative study cited earlier noted that the proportion of ADHD cases seen at the urban clinic was almost three times as high as that seen among rural children referred with mental health problems (Pillay and Naidoo, 1997). This variance, however, is really related to the problems associated with identifying and referring affected children for mental health assistance. Since ADHD is a condition that is, in most cases, identified by school teachers, including pre-school teachers, the education system in rural areas does not facilitate this process. With extremely large classes and the structural disadvantages in these schools, teachers are not identifying psychological problems in individual pupils as easily as is the case in urban schools (Pillay, Naidoo, and Lockhat, 1998).

2.5 Self-destructive behaviours

All over the world research has come to recognize the presence of depressive disorders and associated self-destructive behaviours among children and adolescents (Kovacs, 1996). In South Africa there is a similar increasing identification of self-destructive behaviours among black children (Mkize, 1992).

A recent study conducted by Mayekiso (1995) in the Eastern Cape showed that over one-third of high-school pupils considered suicidal behaviour as an option in the face of stressful life events. In an earlier study, Mkize and Mayekiso (1993) also identified high levels of depression in school-aged adolescents in the Eastern Cape area. Preventive programmes, aimed at family dynamics and stressful life events, are therefore important community outreach programmes that could markedly decrease self-destructive responses in adolescents (Pillay and Wassenaar, 1997a; 1997b).

The mental health problems outlined above are just a few of those affecting children and adolescents in peri-urban and rural communities that desperately require psychological intervention. Community psychologists have a pivotal role to play in managing and preventing these problems. Apart from the traditional case-consultation approach, the importance of intersectoral collaboration and training must be emphasized. For example, liaison with the Department of Education is necessary to help school teachers to identify and appropriately refer children with mental health problems. In a similar manner, collaborative work with the Departments of Safety and Security, and Justice, can be instrumental in developing prevention programmes and encouraging timeous intervention in the case of sexual violence against children.

3 Economic considerations

Ascertaining the financial costs of children's mental health problems is no simple task. These costs are made up of (1) direct costs relating to diagnostic, treatment, and rehabilitative procedures, and (2) projected costs

to the nation as measured by the loss of healthy life years due to disability or premature death.

Direct treatment costs for mental health problems are likely to be higher than is commonly envisaged, since individuals with mental disorders are more frequent users of primary health care services than those without psychological problems (Hansson and Sandlund, 1992). Children and adolescents with somatoform or suicidal conditions, for example, are also known to make extensive use of general hospital services where the treatment is largely medical, unless mental health personnel are immediately available (Pillay and Lalloo, 1989; Pillay and Wassenaar, 1995). Mental health care costs for children are also high due to the breadth of treatment that is usually initiated. Very seldom is a psychologically disturbed child treated in isolation from family members. Unlike the physically ill child, the one with mental health problems often receives treatment in conjunction with his or her family. Parent training programmes and family therapy techniques constitute adjunctive treatments, which, despite their necessity and appropriateness, inevitably escalate the overall treatment costs. However, the use of appropriately trained mental health workers at the primary health care (PHC) level can substantially reduce costs by virtue of early diagnosis and management. Many mental health problems presenting at PHC points are often treated with multiple drugs, including anxiolytics and analgesics, as well as unnecessary hospitalizations and medical procedures (Ustun and Gater, 1994).

The devolution of mental health care from psychiatric hospitals, reduced in-patient care and the consequent emphasis on out-patient, community-based mental health care could also have positive economic repercussions. This is because most of the direct costs of managing mental health problems are attributed to specialist in-patient care with very little funding devoted to community-based care relative to the high proportion of mental health problems presenting at the PHC level (National Advisory Mental Health Council, USA, 1993). The South African situation is similar. In the Western Cape region, for example, 93 per cent of the mental health funds are allocated to psychiatric hospitals (Ensink, Leger, and Robertson, 1994). This form of mental health spending does not inspire confidence in the prevailing mental health policy, especially since psychiatric hospital in-patients represent between 0,2 per cent and 0,5 per cent of the general population (Goldberg and Huxley, 1992). Assuming a psychological morbidity rate of around 15 per cent, it follows that 93 per cent of mental health funds are spent on 3 to 4 per cent of the mentally ill. While this analysis is obviously an over-simplification, since many psychiatric hospitals also pro-vide some community care out of their allotted budgets, the unfavourable skewing against community mental health is evi-dent.

Research has demonstrated that im-proved community mental health services for children reduces the need for psychiatric hospitalization and decreases the duration of in-patient treatment when required (Rosenblatt and Attkisson, 1992). American child mental health programmes have shown average annual cost-savings per child

of between 25 per cent and 50 per cent by increasing and improving community-based care (Bickman, 1993; Illback, 1993). These and many other studies provide evi-dence of the cost-efficiency of managing childhood mental health problems outside resource-intensive specialist psychiatric hospitals. It is important that decisions regarding the choice of model for the deliv-ery of care not be made purely on the basis of financial costs but, more importantly, also on the efficacy of the model, especially its accessibility.

The second type of economic cost burden resulting from mental health problems relates to disability or premature death and the healthy life years lost to the nation. The Disability Adjusted Life Years (DALY) Index, which reflects this cost, is obviously more severe in the case of children – compared with adults – with mental health problems in view of their developmental level and the greater loss of productive years. Research literature over the years has suggested that psychological problems in children have a high probability of persisting for several years with the odds of persistence increasing according to the length or frequency of pre-vious morbidity (Costello et al., 1988). Certainly the need to minimize periods of illness through early intervention tech-niques is evident. The improvement of mental health service provision, especially at the level of community care and, very importantly, the integration of services in collaborative efforts, could substantially reduce problems such as chronicity and incomplete recovery, thereby decreasing the overall economic burden of childhood mental health problems.

4 Models of child mental health service delivery

Given the failure of the traditional mental health model to provide the required level of care to people in most parts of the world, the search for alternative models of service provision has resulted in vigorous local and international debate over which is the ideal model. In the section that follows we discuss a few of these models in the context of child mental health, taking into consideration South African and international developments. We discuss the community mental health model; the primary health care model; the comprehensive help and guidance centre model; the psychiatric hospital model; and the private practice model in turn, below. In addition, the practice of non-governmental organizations will be discussed, even though the NGO approach is not based on any one of the models reviewed below. Thereafter, the authors' own proposed model is outlined.

4.1 The community mental health model

This model has its roots in the 1960s and is linked to the lobby favouring the de-institutionalization of the mentally ill in the United States. However, history has shown that the intention of this endeavour was more forceful in attempts to empty psychiatric hospitals than to provide the necessary support and after-care that was required to sustain affected individuals in the community (Barham, 1992). Nevertheless, there are strong arguments in the United States, South Africa, and elsewhere supporting the evolution and development of a more insightfully contemplated version of this model to provide mental health care at a grass-roots level.

The community mental health centres (CMHCs) as described in the box below are not currently in existence in South Africa, but are quite prevalent in some of the countries in Europe and North America. Children are brought to the CMHC on the accord of their parents, or may be referred by school teachers, the family physician, or primary health care clinics. Older children and adolescents may even be self-referred. The simple referral process is valuable in that fewer children are 'lost' in the system as is often apparent in large health care bureaucracies. Also, easier access to the mental health service is likely to influence the motivation to seek help.

Central features of the community mental health model

The central features of the community mental health model, as distinct from the traditional mental health model, may be summarised as follows:

1. Mental health care is available where people live and within the social context of the community. It is not restricted to remote institutions far removed from communities.
2. Community mental health centres (CMHCs) are relatively smaller service organizations located in the heart of residential areas, resulting in easier access. Only out-patient care is provided at this level.

3 These centres are staffed by mental health professionals such as psychologists, psychiatrists, psychiatric nurses, and social workers, in full or part-time capacities, depending on the needs and size of the community being served. The staff structure is not intensive but appropriately skilled.

4 These centres are directed solely at mental health care and adopt a generalist approach, providing care to all age groups and servicing all mental health problems.

5 The community is actively involved in supporting its mental health centre and participates in its control. Very importantly, the CMHC is perceived as belonging to the community, quite unlike the large psychiatric institutions where consumers feel like intruders.

6 The CMHCs have the function of treating mental health problems, preventing mental illness, and promoting mental health in their respective communities. Liaison with schools in the area serves not only to identify early childhood problems, but also to promote positive mental health development among the young.

7 These centres have links with, and access to, secondary and tertiary mental health care facilities and specialized units (e.g., child abuse units, eating disorder units) at regional and provincial level, so as to accommodate those cases that cannot be dealt with at the generalist out-patient level.

The CMHC should be a state-funded service and consequently fees would be levied in a similar manner to current state health services or compensated by a national health insurance. There are many advantages to including mental health in a national health insurance, which are discussed in detail elsewhere (Freeman, 1992; De Beer and Broomberg, 1990). Again the minimal cost implication for individual families will also serve to encourage the use of this resource.

Virtually all types of childhood mental health problems can be dealt with at the CMHC, where patients are initially assessed and screened by a community psychiatric nurse. If necessary, referrals are then made to the centre's psychologist, psychiatrist, or social worker for further assessment and management. The psychiatric nurses at the CMHC are specifically trained for independent work in the community context and are able to assess and intervene in uncomplicated mental health problems as and when necessary. They do not feel totally reliant on the psychologist or psychiatrist.

4.1.1 Advantages and disadvantages

In essence the CMHC functions as a composite mental health service located in the community and accessible to all socio-economic groups. Referrals to higher levels of mental health care should not occur frequently and, therefore, reduce cost burdens on tertiary care centres. However, in view of the infrastructure and specialized staff requirements in the establishment of CMHCs, these are likely to be relatively expensive projects, especially if attempts are made to have them evenly spread and within easy reach of all communities. Nevertheless, the benefits, especially in the context of early detection and management of childhood problems, and those of adults, far outweigh the immediate concerns regarding financial implications. Of course, another negative factor relating to CMHCs is the attention paid solely to mental health problems and the consequent neglect of physical problems. In other words, this model does not offer a truly holistic approach. (See Chapter 19 for a further critique of this model.)

3 Tertiary level care occurs at a provincial level and is very often provided at academic hospitals with super-specialist staff and facilities. Referral to this level is mainly from the secondary level and the emphasis is on a consultative, highly specialized approach that keeps in-patient care to a minimum. Follow-up treatment and rehabilitative care is usually re-routed back to the secondary or PHC levels.

4.2 The primary health care model

Primary health care (PHC), by definition, refers to first or front-line health care that can be accessed in the case of any health problem. The three different levels of health care, namely, primary, secondary, and tertiary health care, are detailed in the box below.

Levels of health care

1 Primary health care (PHC) refers to first-contact health care, traditionally concerned with physical health problems. PHC also targets children at risk. In South Africa PHC sites include district hospitals, primary health clinics, general medical practitioners, traditional healers, and adolescent health services.
2 Secondary level care refers to the care generally provided by relatively more specialized providers or facilities to those cases that cannot be managed at the PHC level. These are usually regional general hospitals, child guidance clinics, specialist welfare services, or private practices.

Having been formalized internationally as a specific model in the past two decades or so, the PHC approach can be traced much further back, especially in its applications in low-income countries. The approach was conceived as a non-specialist approach essentially in contexts where specialized services were not affordable. The aim has been to make general health care accessible to all citizens regardless of their income levels or socio-economic status. One of the key assumptions of this model, as outlined by the World Health Organization (WHO) (1978), is that quality health care should be made accessible to all members of the community at an affordable cost, and that it should include their full participation. In addition, the model emphasizes intersectorial collaboration, empowerment of the communities being served, and cost-effective services that are community oriented. Despite being developed to meet the needs of low-income countries, this model is also being contemplated and introduced in some high-income countries of Europe. While PHC has been in existence for many years in

South Africa, operating through various delivery structures and levels of complexity, the PHC system in this country is yet to include mental health in its services. However, the national health policy guidelines of the African National Congress (1994) advocated the incorporation of mental health care into the PHC infrastructure.

Although traditionally conceived within the dichotomous mind-body model as aimed solely at physical health problems, there is no plausible reason to exclude mental health problems from being attended to in this setting. Facilities providing primary health care include general hospital out-patient departments, general practitioners, and, of course, the various state PHC clinics that are being established with the aim of providing basic, first-line health care mainly to people of low socio-economic backgrounds. With the national health policy suggesting a strong emphasis on PHC services in South Africa, it is clear that this is the resource structure that will reach and be accessed by more inhabitants than any other health system. Each PHC clinic is staffed by nurses specifically trained in primary care vis-à-vis the identification and treatment of physical ailments of an uncomplicated nature. Medical practitioners also staff these clinics, not necessarily in a full-time capacity. The need to train PHC nurses in the area of mental health has been emphasized and even introduced in certain areas (Pillay and Lockhat, 1997). The PHC personnel can be trained to deal with all types of childhood mental health problems. More complicated or pervasive conditions can be referred to the secondary care level for assessment and intervention.

A recent epidemiological study of children in Nigeria showed that approximately one out of five, i.e. 20 per cent, child attenders at PHC centres exhibited psychiatric problems, with conduct disorder and major depression having the highest prevalence, namely 6,1 per cent and 6,0 per cent, respectively (Gureje et al., 1994). A British investigation noted an even higher prevalence rate of 28 per cent for mental health problems among children attending general paediatric clinics with 'emotional' disorders present in two-thirds of the affected children (Garralda and Bailey, 1989). Similarly, an American study of paediatric primary care patients at a health maintenance organization noted a psychiatric morbidity rate of almost 25 per cent (Costello et al., 1988). Research findings such as those cited above led the WHO, in its Declaration of Alma Ata, to call for the integration of mental health care into the PHC system (World Health Organization, 1978).

4.2.1 Advantages and disadvantages

Among the advantages of incorporating mental health care into PHC are the grass-roots level service structure, the broadly holistic approach, and the relative lack of stigma attached to receiving mental health care in a general facility. Also, childhood mental health problems (e.g., mental retardation, attention-deficit/hyperactivity disorder) can be easily identified during visits for common physical complaints. Furthermore, each PHC centre has access to a district community psychiatric nurse (CPN) to advise, consult, and provide the vital link between PHC and the mental health specialists at secondary (regional hospital) and tertiary (specialist and super-specialist units) levels.

Unfortunately, the detection rate of psychological problems at the PHC level is exceedingly low (Reeler and Todd, 1994). Research has shown that patients with mental health problems presenting at PHC centres more often receive medication for physical symptoms than appropriate treatment for their psychological conditions (Simon et al., 1995). Another major concern is that PHC personnel are finding themselves heavily burdened by the large numbers of cases presenting (with physical problems) at their clinics. The possibility that this situation could result in mental health care being given a back seat to physical health is worrying. Of course, this issue could be addressed by increasing the human resource provision at PHC centres and also educating PHC personnel against giving priority to physical health over mental health. A further criticism of this model is that it tends to be mainly service oriented and will not be able to address the broader issues of mental health, which could be undertaken by the CMHCs. Also, there is a concern that the powerful medical model within which the PHC operates could engulf mental health to the point where truly holistic care is not achieved (Freeman, 1992). (See Swartz and Gibson, Chapter 3, for additional limitations associated with this model.)

4.3 Comprehensive help and guidance centre model

This model, which has been put forward by Nell (1994), relates to attempts to de-medicalize the health-care system through the establishment of a Department of Human Services and the establishment of a network of comprehensive help and guidance centres. Such centres are to be located within the community with the proposal that each be resourced to serve up to 500 000 people. Typically the staffing component would comprise a wide range of professionals to include psychologists, social workers, vocational guidance and rehabilitation specialists, counsellors skilled in parenting issues and abuse, occupational therapists, injury prevention specialists, paralegal workers, and networkers to access agencies and service components.

According to Nell's (1994) proposed model, these centres would target individuals of all ages with non-psychiatric conditions but who are experiencing life problems or crises. People with somatic symptoms related to psychological distress will form part of the attender population and primary health care nurses will do the initial screening. A centre worker thereafter decides on the intervention direction and plan, which would usually involve group therapeutic formats in favour of individual approaches, thus effecting better use of resources.

4.3.1 Advantages and disadvantages

An advantage of this proposed model lies in its ability to offer a range of services, including to abused women and children, adolescent groups aimed at prevention of mental health problems, and related programmes that interface health and social services. However, the targeting of non-psychiatric consumers could cause difficulties and confusion, especially in terms of defining and distinguishing this group from those having psychiatric problems. Also, educating families and the general public about who should and should not attend these centres could prove difficult, especially considering the general public's understanding of psychiatric, psychological, and social problems. The cost factor in establishing such centres could be prohibitive in view of the specialized staff required, as compared with the PHC model, for example.

4.4 Psychiatric hospital model

Having its roots in the traditional mental health model, psychiatric hospital care has unfortunately over the years tended to become synonymous with institutional care and even institutionalization. Clearly this type of care does not render itself to positive sentiments when considering child mental health. However, the psychiatric hospital model should not be operative purely at the institutional care level.

It is evident that in-patient psychiatric care, where there is the advantage of a wider range of specialist treatments, for example, occupational and rehabilitation facilities, will always be required (Gelder, Gath, and Mayou, 1994). Of course, substantial work needs to be done to reduce the social stigma of these specialist hospitals. The formulation of adequate admission and discharge practices could contribute to changing

community perceptions of these highly resourced facilities. Very importantly, the practice of lengthy periods of admission needs to be modified.

At the level of tertiary care, such specialist facilities provide valuable teaching opportunities, especially in cases of treatment-resistant conditions, diagnostic problems, and the less common conditions that require highly intensive attention. Ideally, this model needs to be implemented in a manner that takes specific cognizance of the tertiary care function of psychiatric hospitals. The model is best understood when seen as analogous to the specialist tertiary care hospitals providing high-tech cardiothoracic or neurosurgical care, for example. Psychiatric hospitals should be functioning in a similar manner, providing specialist services for complex or treatment-resistant cases, which, for reasons of expertise or facilities, could not be effectively managed at the primary or secondary care level.

In practice, this model functions in a supportive and consultative role to PHC personnel and regional general hospitals dealing with childhood mental health problems. The latter levels of care have access to the psychiatric hospitals when specialist care is required. Again, this is a state-funded facility that provides care at a nominal cost to parents and should be linked to a national health insurance. Of course, specialist hospitals such as these are extremely expensive to maintain in view of their extensive resources and facilities, but they are certainly required at a provincial level. It is envisaged that each province should have at least one such hospital.

This model provides for the establishment of super-specialist units, such as adolescent units and eating disorder units, staffed by mental health workers specifically trained in these areas of child mental health care. Units such as these should be few in number across the country in view of their cost, but also because only the very severe cases should be dealt with at this level.

The psychiatric hospital largely functions as an in-patient facility, which is why the cost of running this facility is higher than that of the CMHC, for example. However, these costs could be substantially trimmed by keeping admission time to a minimum, with the children's maintenance and follow-up treatments conducted by regional general hospitals or PHC centres. This approach entrenches the consultative nature of the psychiatric hospital and serves to deviate from the traditional mental health model where psychiatric hospitals were asylums that institutionalized the mentally ill in order to separate them from society.

4.4.1 Advantages and disadvantages

The psychiatric hospital has several benefits when perceived as part of a collaborative effort in the treatment of mental health problems. Its ability to provide multidisciplinary care, containment for acute mental disorders, respite for families of severely ill individuals, specialist units, and training facilities are some of the positive features of psychiatric hospitals. However, one disadvantage remains: the social stigma that is still attached to treatment in this type of facility. The need for community awareness and education programmes must be em-

phasized if we are to address this issue. A further problem affecting this model is the vulnerability to abuse. Examples of abuse include the involuntary admission procedures, maltreatment in the name of 'restraint' of acutely ill individuals, and the length of admission. Of course, these can be addressed through appropriate legislation entrenching the rights of the mentally ill. The exorbitant costs of in-patient care is another negative feature of this model.

4.5 Private practice model

This model of mental health care for children is applicable to those from more affluent families or whose health care is covered by medical aid insurance. In view of prevailing tariffs, children from families outside of these two groups will be unlikely to afford this type of mental health care. Typically, the private practice model operates in urban areas with a few psychologists, psychiatrists, social workers, and occupational therapists specializing in child mental health. Referrals to these practitioners are made either by medical practitioners, other health workers, or parents. All types of mental health problems can be dealt with in the context of this model, with the option for specialist or super-specialist referral in the larger urban settings.

Unlike in the CMHC or PHC clinics where less emphasis is given to psychometric evaluations, psychological testing does constitute a small proportion of the consultation time in private practice contexts. Psychological testing, by its very nature, is rather costly and time-consuming, but can produce very useful findings. In private practice settings children experiencing difficulty with scholastic performance, for example, may be intensively assessed through cognitive testing in order to identify the specific problem area(s) and institute management. However, such an approach is not always possible through state-funded health or education departments.

Therapeutic work with children in private practice situations tends to involve more medium- to long-term therapy, unlike the PHC and CMHC facilities where crisis intervention and short-term work is undertaken. Similarly, the private practice model concentrates on individual therapy while the tendency towards group therapy programmes is increasing in state-funded facilities in order to make better use of scarce resources (Nell, 1994).

4.5.1 Advantages and disadvantages

The choice of the private practice model is largely determined by socio-economic status. A high standard of care is available through this model for those who can afford this type of care. Another advantage is that with the more affluent using private health care, the burden on state-funded health care is decreased. This also increases the availability of state-funded health care to low-income groups. Among the disadvantages of this model is the élitism that it generates. Also, the quality of care, or access to certain forms of specialist care available to private practice patients, may differ from that available to patients of state-funded services (e.g., in the case of low birth weight neonates who are not provided with survival assistance in state-funded hospitals).

4.6 Non-governmental organizations

Non-governmental organizations (NGOs) in South Africa involved in the upliftment of children's mental health include the child welfare societies, mental health societies, and organizations dealing with specific problems such as violence, trauma, and abuse, among others. Essentially, these organizations are funded through various sources, including the private sector, business, and overseas development aid programmes. Some also receive government subsidies.

The philosophical and theoretical underpinnings of the NGO delivery system are different to those of the formal models discussed. NGOs have evolved essentially within a needs-driven context, rather than a theoretical one. Most NGOs, especially the non-state-subsidized organizations during the apartheid era, worked within a framework of empowerment, seeking to provide skills, training, and networking systems to bring relief and resources to oppressed and disadvantaged communities (Parekh, McKay, and Petersen, 1997). As such, the work of these organizations has been in direct response to the needs of specific geographically or sociologically defined communities. Examples include: (1) the Project for the Survivors of Violence established to assist individuals, families, and communities affected by political violence, and (2) Childline, developed in response to the large numbers of children suffering abuse of a physical or sexual nature.

NGOs providing mental health and related services to children have generally been highly valued for their contributions to the field. Services provided include actual case management as well as numerous support and rehabilitative services. The service infrastructures that have been developed over the years by these organizations have complemented those of government departments, with the result that liaison between these two types of structures does occur, but can also be substantially improved. Ideally, government departments and NGOs need to work co-operatively in a manner that is neither duplicative nor competitive, and essentially in the interest of the community.

There are several areas of child mental health where NGOs play a crucial role. The large population of 'street children' in this country, for example, which is currently being addressed to some degree by NGOs, requires much more attention. Until their involvement it appeared as if these children were falling through the 'cracks', since the government departments, especially in the pre-democracy era, did not seem to see themselves responsible for these youths. The fact that the mental health and social development of these children are being jeopardized by their life on the streets has been blatantly overlooked. The role of apartheid policies in the evolution of the black 'street child' was also not acknowledged by the previous apartheid government. South African research has also emphasized the serious problem of sexually transmitted diseases among children living on the streets, bearing in mind that they are easy prey for situations of sexual abuse (Naidoo, 1997). The NGOs that have initiated work with affected children have concerned themselves with organizing, re-socializing, educating, and rehabilitating them in a structured format. Unfortunately this work occurs on a relatively small scale, obviously largely due to financial constraints. The need for greater investment from all sectors in such NGO programmes must certainly be seen as a priority if we are to effectively address this problem.

Similarly, NGO programmes for children with substance abuse problems are an area that requires attention. While organizations such as the South African National Council on Alcoholism and Drug Dependence (SANCA) undertake much work in the general area of substance abuse, the need for increased services aimed specifically at curative and preventive aspects of childhood and adolescent substance abuse is enormous. Education programmes aimed at increasing awareness of this problem need to be intensified, highly focused, and, most importantly, sustained. Occasional talks to school children are unlikely to have the desired effects in the long term. NGOs have a vital role in terms of liaison functions with schools and health departments. There are numerous other areas where NGOs can and do play a significant role in children's mental health.

4.6.1 Advantages and disadvantages

Clearly one of the advantages of NGO services is the lack of bureaucracy and 'red-tape', which allows these services to be implemented wherever and whenever they are required. They are neither geographically nor sectorially bound. In addition, most NGOs related to child mental health are able to pay attention to specific risk groups, such as survivors of violence and child abuse, allowing for in-depth work in these areas, unlike most government departments, which have to adopt a generalist approach. Unfortunately, funding difficulties can cause uncertainty in the planning of specific mental health programmes for children. Therefore, the financing of NGOs needs attention if we are going to incorporate these valuable resources into child mental health policy and structures in South Africa.

5 Proposed hybrid model

Considering the advantages and disadvantages of all the models discussed above, the authors propose a hybrid model amalgamating concepts of the community mental health model and the PHC model. This proposal is based on the view that neither of these models is exclusively capable of meeting the country's mental health needs within the context of current financial constraints. Very simply, the delivery of mental health care through the PHC infrastructure is advocated, but should be supported by a dedicated community mental health service. It is proposed that the front-line PHC workers, mainly nurses but also including medical practitioners where possible, be trained to deal with mental health problems in all age groups, using a generalist approach. However, each district, as demarcated in the national Health Department's District Health System, should have at least one community psychiatric nurse (CPN) who co-ordinates, oversees, and renders specialized mental health care for the dis-

trict. The CPN provides the specialist support to the PHC staff and, very importantly, is the link between PHC and secondary level care, including the general hospital mental health units.

This proposed model assures a dedicated mental health service either at or close to the PHC level, thereby ensuring that mental health care cannot be side-lined or pushed into obscurity by the overwhelming physical health needs, as is possible when using the PHC model in its traditional form. Another advantage is that the role of the CPN will also include training, advocacy, and community empowerment in the area of mental health. The rest of his or her functions should include enhancing mental health services, developing community awareness, networking with relevant organizations, and reinforcing the liaison between primary, secondary, and tertiary levels of care. This model is, therefore, not exclusively service-oriented as is the PHC model. It is expected to be considerably less expensive to finance than the community mental health model, since the CPN would be the only specialist personnel at the district level, with all other mental health specialists operating at the secondary and tertiary care level. While not ideal, this model could provide affordable mental health care to all at grass-roots level, as well as specialist care upon referral to secondary or tertiary facilities. (See Chapter 3 for a more critical view on these proposals.)

6 **Conclusion**

Mental health services for children are in short supply in most parts of the world, including many high-income countries. However, the situation in South Africa is of even greater concern, since the prevalence of childhood mental health problems is expected to be higher than in other countries due to the apartheid history that disadvantaged the black majority.

The widely recognized failure of the traditional mental health model has resulted in a search for alternative, community-oriented models that could provide basic mental health care to all citizens, regardless of their socio-economic status. Models currently being considered include community mental health, primary health care, comprehensive help and guidance centres, private practice, and NGOs. A hybrid model integrating the community mental health and PHC models was also proposed. The economic costs of child mental health problems must also be taken into consideration. These include direct treatment costs as well as long-term costs to the nation in terms of healthy, productive life years lost.

Exercises

1 Consider and discuss childhood mental health problems, other than those mentioned in this chapter. Review those that may be unusual or unique because of South Africa's history.
2 Detail other models of child mental health service delivery that you consider applicable in geographical areas with which you are familiar.

3 Try to calculate the approximate economic cost to the nation of a debilitating, untreated mental illness afflicting an eight-year-old girl, rendering her unable to secure formal employment in later life.

References

AFRICAN NATIONAL CONGRESS. (1994). *A national health plan for South Africa.* Johannesburg: African National Congress.

AMERICAN PSYCHIATRIC ASSOCIATION. (1994). *Diagnostic and statistical manual of mental disorders.* Washington, DC: American Psychiatric Association.

ARAYA, R., WYNN, R., LEONARD, R., and LEWIS, G. (1994). Psychiatric morbidity in primary health care in Santiago, Chile. *British Journal of Psychiatry,* **165**, 530–533.

BARHAM, P. (1992). *Closing the asylum.* London: Penguin.

BICKMAN, L. (1993). *The evaluation of the Fort Bragg demonstration project.* Nashville: Vanderbilt University, Centre for Mental Health Policy.

CENTRAL STATISTICAL SERVICES. (1996). *Statistical release PO 317.* Pretoria: Central Statistical Services.

COSTELLO, E. J., COSTELLO, A. J., EDELBROCK, C., BURNS, B. J., DULCAN, M. K., BRENT, D., and JANISZWESKI, S. (1988). Psychiatric disorders in paediatric primary care. *Archives of General Psychiatry,* **45**, 1107–1116.

DAILY NEWS. (Durban). (1996, July 11). *Incidence of child abuse rockets.* p. 15.

DAWES, A. (1985). Politics and mental health. *South African Journal of Psychology,* **15**, 55–61.

DAWES, A. (1994). The emotional impact of political violence. In A. Dawes and D. Donald (Eds.), *Childhood and adversity* (pp. 177–199). Cape Town: David Philip.

DAWES, A., ROBERTSON, B., DUNCAN, N., ENSINK, K., JACKSON, A., REYNOLDS, P.,

PILLAY, S., and RICHTER, L. (1997). Child and adolescent mental health policy. In D. Foster, M. Freeman, and Y. Pillay (Eds.), *Mental health policy issues for South Africa* (pp. 193–215). Cape Town: MASA Multimedia.

DE BEER, C. and BROOMBERG, J. (1990). Financing health care for all: Is national health insurance the first step? *South African Medical Journal, 78*, 144–148.

DUNCAN, N. and ROCK, B. (1994). *Inquiry into the effects of public violence on children.* Johannesburg: Goldstone Commission of inquiry regarding the prevention of public violence and intimidation.

ENSINK, K., LEGER, P., and ROBERTSON, B. (1994). *Public sector mental health services in the Western Cape.* Paper presented at the Primary Mental Health Care Workshop, Durban.

FREEMAN, M. (1992*). Providing mental health care for all in South Africa: Structure and strategy.* Paper No. 24. Johannesburg: Centre for Health Policy, University of the Witwatersrand.

GARRALDA, M. E. and BAILEY, D. (1989). Psychiatric disorders in general paediatric referrals. *Archives of Disease in Childhood, 64*, 1727–1733.

GELDER, M., GATH, D., and MAYOU, R. (1994). *Concise Oxford textbook of psychiatry.* Oxford: Oxford University Press.

GOLDBERG, D. and HUXLEY, P. (1992). *Common mental disorders.* London: Routledge.

GUREJE, O., OMIGBODUN, O. O., GATER, R., ACHA, R. A., IKUESAN, B. A., and MORRIS, J. (1994). Psychiatric disorders in a paediatric primary care clinic. *British Journal of Psychiatry, 165*, 527–530.

HANSSON, L. and SANDLUND, M. (1992). Utilisation and patterns of care in comprehensive psychiatric care organisations. *Acta Psychiatrical Scandinavica, 86*, 255–261.

HEALTH SYSTEMS TRUST (1996). *South African health review.* Durban: Author.

ILLBACK, R. J.(1994). Poverty and the crisis in children's services: The need for services integration. *Journal of Clinical Child Psychology, 23*, 413–424.

KELLEHER, K. and LONG, N. (1994). Barriers and new directions in mental health services research in the primary care setting. *Journal of Clinical Child Psychology, 23*, 133–142.

KILLIAN, B. (1993). *The disintegration of family life of black people in South Africa.* Paper presented at the Family and Child Symposium (South African Association for Child and Adolescent Psychiatry and Allied Professions: KZN Branch), Pietermaritzburg.

KOVACS, M. (1996). Presentation and course of major depressive disorder during childhood and later years of the lifespan. *Journal of the American Academy of Child & Adolescent Psychiatry, 35*, 705–715.

MAYEKISO, T. V. (1995). Attitudes of black adolescents towards suicide. In L. Schlebusch (Ed.), *Suicidal behaviour, 3* (pp. 46–53). Durban: University of Natal.

MCADOO, H. P. (1988). *Black families.* Newbury Park, CA: Sage.

MKIZE, D. L. (1992). Suicide rate in Umtata: 1971–1990. In L. Schlebusch (Ed.), *Suicidal behaviour, 2* (pp. 9-22). Durban: University of Natal.

MKIZE, D. L. and MAYEKISO, T. V. (1993). *The prevalence of depression amongst adolescents in the Transkei.* Paper presented at the 9th National Congress of the South African Association for Child and Adolescent Psychiatry, Cape Town.

NAIDOO, S. (1997). *The development, implementation and evaluation of an AIDS health education programme for youth on the street in the greater Durban area.* Unpublished doctoral thesis, University of Fort Hare.

NATIONAL ADVISORY MENTAL HEALTH COUNCIL – USA. (1993). Health care reform for Americans with severe mental illness. *American Journal of Psychiatry, 150*, 1447–1465.

NELL, V. (1994). Critical psychology and the problems of mental health. *Psychology in Society, 19*, 31–44.

PAREKH, A., MCKAY, A., and PETERSEN, I. (1997). Non-governmental organizations. In D. Foster, M. Freeman, and Y. Pillay (Eds.), *Mental health policy issues for South Africa* (pp. 122–131). Cape Town: MASA Multimedia.

PILLAY, A. L. and LALLOO, M. (1989). Psychogenic pain disorder in children. *South African Medical Journal, 76*, 195–196.

PILLAY, A. L. and LOCKHAT, M. R. (1997). Developing community mental health services for children in South Africa. *Social Science & Medicine* (in press).

PILLAY, A. L. and NAIDOO, P. (1997). The need for an alternative model of mental health service delivery for children in South Africa. In D. R. Trent (Ed.), *Promotion of mental health: Volume 6* (in press).

PILLAY, A. L., NAIDOO, P., and LOCKHAT M. R. (1998). *Mental health problems in urban and rural/peri-urban children.* Paper presented at the 4th annual congress of the Psychological Society of South Africa, Cape Town.

PILLAY, A. L. and WASSENAAR, D. R. (1995). Psychological intervention, spontaneous remission, hopelessness, and psychiatric disturbance in adolescent parasuicides. *Suicide & Life Threatening Behaviour,* 25, 386–392.

PILLAY, A. L. and WASSENAAR, D. R. (1997a). Recent stressors and family satisfaction in suicidal adolescents in South Africa. *Journal of Adolescence,* 20, 155–162.

PILLAY, A. L. and WASSENAAR, D. R. (1997b). Family dynamics, hopelessness and psychiatric disturbance in parasuicidal adolescents. *Australian & New Zealand Journal of Psychiatry,* 31, 227–231.

PILLAY, Y., MAGWAZA, A., and PETERSEN, I. (1992). Civil conflict in Mpumalanga: Some mental health sequelae in a sample of children and primary caregivers. *Southern African Journal of Child and Adolescent Psychiatry,* 4, 42–45.

REELER, A. P. and TODD, C. H. (1994). *An overview of psychological disorders and psychiatric services in Zimbabwe.* Paper presented at the Primary Mental Health Care Workshop, Durban.

REELER, A. P., WILLIAMS, H., and TODD, C. H. (1993). Psycho-pathology in primary care. *Central African Journal of Medicine,* 39, 1–8.

REGIER, D. A., NARROW, W. E., RAE, D. S., MANDERSCHEID, R. W., LOCKE, B. Z., and GOODWIN, F. K. (1993). The *de facto* US Mental and Addictive Disorder Service System: Epidemiologic catchment area prospective 1 year prevalence rates of disorders and services. *Archives of General Psychiatry,* 50, 85–94.

ROSENBLATT, A. and ATTKISSON, C. (1992). Integrating systems of care in California for youth with severe emotional disturbance. *Journal of Child & Family Studies,* 2, 119–141.

SARTORIUS, N., USTUN, T. B., COSTA, E., SILVA, J. A., GOLDBERG, D., LECRUBIER, Y., ORMEL, J., VON KORFF, M., and WITTCHEN, H. U. (1993). An international study of psychological problems in primary care. *Archives of General Psychiatry,* 50, 819–823.

SEEDAT, M., BUTCHART, A., and NELL, V. (1991). Family therapy in primary health care: Skills training and outcome evaluation. *Contemporary Family Therapy,* 13, 143–163.

SIMON, G., ORMEL, J., VON KORFF, M., and BARLOW, W. (1995). Health care costs associated with depressive and anxiety disorders in primary care. *American Journal of Psychiatry,* 152, 352–357.

USTUN, T. B. and GATER, R. (1994). Integrating mental health into primary care. *Current Opinion in Psychiatry,* 7, 173–180.

WORLD HEALTH ORGANIZATION (1978). *Alma Ata: Primary health care report.* Geneva: WHO.

7 Discovering Agape: forming and re-forming a healing community

Stanley Lifschitz
Corinne Oosthuizen

Study objectives

In telling the story about the process of formation and re-formation of the Agape Healing Community, we form a window for the reader to view the practice of community psychology. Our intention in doing this is to provoke you, the reader, into thinking about what the community psychologist needs to know in the performance of this healing profession.

1 Introduction

Any book on community psychology would be incomplete without a section exploring the pragmatics of the profession. This chapter, different to those that precede and follow, provides a window onto the personal and practical worlds of community psychologists. From these accounts we can gain appreciation for what is generally referred to as the praxis of the profession.

While theories, research methodologies, and policies all have instructive value by giving expression to ways of thinking and being accountable, they are all meta-considerations, that is, considerations about the practice of community psychology rather than the activity itself. They might enhance or limit the dance of the practitioner in forming relationships within communities or in achieving goals, but they always remain one step removed from the practical situations and circumstances in which the community psychologist works.

No theory, paradigm, methodology, or policy can in itself bring about the commitment and involvement called for in the practice of community psychology. Without the often presumed preparedness of the practitioner to be dedicated and to become an integral member of the community with whom she or he works, even the best of meta-consideration will do no more than sound good. In this vein, in a comprehensive study to try and pinpoint the essential characteristics of effective community projects, the World Health Organization (WHO) could only identify one common denominator: the passion of the people involved (WHO Study Group, 1984).

Our effort in this chapter is to tell the story of forming and re-forming a healing community; a story of the struggles and passions of people committed to staying within often difficult situations, which are not always responsive to the community psychologist's preferred position or expectations.

Staying with the confusion and discomfort is an essential pragmatic of community work that allows interpersonal processes to evolve. In this way a community is a continuously co-created set of relationships in which sufficient trust forms between its participants to deal with issues of mistrust.

Neatly packaged community programmes and time-limited research projects are too often executed without regard for the bigger and more subtle impact on the ecology of people involved. They can provoke and escalate processes such as the forming of an even stronger sense of helplessness in their reconfirmation of the need for external input, or the building of mistrust and anger around unfulfilled expectations raised by interventions, as well as by people appearing and disappearing.

Community psychologists need to be accountable not only to their employers, funders, or scientific collectives, but also above all to the community of people who are touched by, and form around the ideas and issues that emerge in the process of doing this work. It is in staying in the process, in ongoing face-to-face encounters,

that an accountability emerges that ensures an ethic of practice no theory or paradigm can generate.

The aim of this chapter is to share with the reader the trials and tribulations of a few psychologists working in community psychology. This story is intended to convey how the process of struggle not only creates community, but also generates ideas that shape the way a community psychologist plies his or her profession among people.

Whether a theory, a policy, or an intervention is healing or hurtful is ultimately declared and demonstrated by those involved. No a priori theory or paradigm can predict this or substitute for the experiences of those involved.

We invite you now into our story to share with us something that brought us and others together in the declaration and continual re-formation of a healing community.

2 A story about Agape

2.1 One version of Agape

In keeping with our idea that healing happens when the crisis of our living finds safe places to occur, a community called Agape formed. This story tells of the struggle in forming and re-forming this healing community. When we began to work in the township of Mamelodi[1] some ten years ago, we sought out places to practise psychotherapy that would be safest for us, the therapists. We were given sanctuary in a wing of the offices of the local SOS Children's Village. From inside this building, guarded by our diary, we waited for the needy to avail themselves of our services.

In those days our intention was, and it still is, to practise psychotherapy in the townships. So we began by duplicating our ways of working as if all places are the same. Our assumption then, we see now, was that psychotherapy can be applied in any place without regard for context.

When we began in Mamelodi we announced our presence and initiated a struggle to declare what it is that we do. This struggle brought questions about why we were here and what it is that the therapist does. These were difficult and different questions from those we confronted before we began to work in Mamelodi.

Wanting to do something for those who had been deprived of the services of clinical psychologists[2] was a good-sounding purpose in other domains like that of the university or other contexts of ideological debate. However, in the township the differences between charity and healing, between being a patron and belonging, were the issues that confronted us continually in the work we were trying to do.

The year was 1987. Few whites were to be seen in the townships then. Those who did venture there were noticed and often announced with calls of *lekoa* (white people). It was not unusual then for a white person to become the target of aggression as this single person became the symbol of an oppressive regime. Apartheid was almost forty years old. By then it was increasingly driven by the tyranny of fear and hidden anger that produced processes of suspicion and oppression as it folded in on itself.

It was in these initial moments that the very idea of psychotherapy as the talking cure was brought into our conversations, as we struggled to convey what it is that we do.

Few people in Mamelodi had heard of psychologists or psychotherapy, so we spoke of healing. Finding words to describe the work of a psychotherapist beyond a professional vocabulary and assumed shared meanings, which we had come to accept, brought us to profound points of questioning. We sometimes wondered whether we could do anything at all, or whether we were just frauds.

At this early stage, our uncertainty and sometimes our fear were disguised and translated into sophisticated psychologies, which invariably placed the problem with the clients, the system, the environment, or with the country and its history, anywhere but with ourselves. In this we found comfort and protection from what sometimes felt like an unwelcoming community.

Some people said that they would not come to our clinic because there were whites there. Others came to our clinic because there were whites there. Some came asking politely what it is that we do, and others brought their sick babies swaddled in blankets. Each brought questions, which were also about ourselves and what we were doing.

The idea that healing is also for the healer arose from our living across the borderlines of our own safety. It announced a way of bringing ourselves into what we were doing through an acknowledgement and appreciation of our own struggle.

We began to note that our own sense of disconnectedness and lostness was echoed and reflected in the struggle of those who we sought to help. Confessing this first to one another, we began to use our own experiences of lostness as the source of being informed about those who came to see us. In giving voice to our own struggle, we found words to guide us in the hidden worlds of those who had come. And so we found ways of proceeding in the realization that therapists are informed not by the theories they purport to subscribe to, but by their experiences in the domain of relationships.

By giving words to these experiences in particular situations we found languages of connection and understanding – beyond culture and race – with those who had come. Voices declaring the unspeakable within, in the safety of connection, brought healing to all those involved. In this realization we rediscovered an age-old wisdom: that healing is also for the healer.

With this expression of faith, which is now part of our credo, we began to form a community with a larger body of healers, some of whom were sangomas and shamans and prophets of the world.[3]

By then many people from different places were coming to talk. Our meetings became a mix of apparent differences, finding commonality in our mutual lostness. The acknowledgement of this allowed for the naming of Agape. The naming arose from a meeting in a room filled with people who had come together to give substance to their meanings of being located in lostness. Someone called out Agape as a name for us through the din of the crowd. Then he left, only to appear four years later, calling our names from the voting lines in the informal settlements where we stood to cast our ballot, then for the first time as one nation.

And so it was in people's continued connection that Agape took form. Every Wednesday we would meet, year after year, talking and talking to those who came to our clinic. Sometimes we would huddle together for hours, acting in ways that revealed our struggle. On other days we would weave through the township, attending ceremonies and rituals, and going into homes. In this way, along unexpected ways, we wove webs of connection.

We once met a drama group called Lazar at a community meeting and developed a play with them about psychotherapy. We thought it would help us to spread the idea and availability of psychotherapy through the township of Mamelodi. Doing what we thought right took us to an altar upon which we continued our struggle to create meaning out of what we, the psychologists, do.

Once the play with Lazar was formed, we went from the Old Beer Hall, where we would meet every week, to perform at schools, churches, and trade union meetings. One memorable occasion was at Broederstroom[4], where the play was performed in place of a plenary session at an international conference of family and marital therapy.[5]

Year after year we spread in this network, performing and talking about what we do. And what we did kept shifting and re-forming, forming community for those who connected with this struggle.

2.1.1 From the building to the tree

It was in the early nineties now, in the last hours before the dawn. Talk on the street was about with whom you belonged. From the pavements people shouted. We were told to join up. The young folk were organizing for the day of deliverance. They danced and sang, giving flame to their fears.

It was in the confrontation of all this that we were put out onto the street. The place in which we once found sanctuary told us and everybody else using their space to keep projects in the township going, to leave. Homeless, with nowhere to go, we stood on the pavement with new questions about staying and leaving, and about beginnings and endings. We were lost once again.

Then someone offered us the use of three zozos, prefabricated huts, just inside the yard of the Young Men's Christian Association (YMCA) next door. So on Wednesdays we sat under the huge bluegum tree in front of the zozos, which were either too hot in summer or too cold in winter. And people kept coming; some limping, some drowning, to sit in the shade with the others who were there.

Little huddles would form, pulled slightly away from the group by the tree. They would struggle together to find ways of being in the eye of their storm. Others would sit in the shifting shade of the tree, talking and dancing and drawing together, mapping and showing the ecology that was forming.

Agape shifted from being only a clinic to being a healing community when we began to acknowledge the different ways in which people come. We recognized that sometimes people came defining themselves as patients or ill simply because this was the only option we allowed for within our community. We began to realize that people also come in search of belonging or looking for a place where lostness can be shared. In this we also heard echoes of ourselves and of many therapists who came to the tree for reasons other than giving or receiving psychotherapy or treatment.

So we began projects that allowed people to come to Agape in various ways. People like teachers or social workers would arrive, with a variety of ideas, to talk of their work difficulties. We would form groups, composed of those who came and those who were interested or connected to these issues in some way through the details of their own circumstances, and encourage these people to meet for as long as they wanted.

From our weekly Agape meetings under the tree, we would pick up on the issues that were echoing through our various activities. Often waves of difficulty around school problems or sexual abuse would besiege Agape. By collecting those who were touched, we would collectively initiate projects that would take us to the places from where the people reporting these problems had come. For the kids who appeared during school holidays or just through the day, we would form groups to play football or dance, before we sat in a rough circle to talk of their living. Some people who came struggling with meaninglessness and loss would also be connected to existing projects or groups. In this way they would find healing by discovering alternative definitions of themselves as care-givers or parents beyond the definition of patient or victim.

We would urge all of Agape to use their talents and skills in all that they do. One member used her love of movement and music, and so dancing became one of the ways in which a healing context was formed for children who were abused. Others would be trained by remedial teachers to give after-hours help to children with learning difficulties.

We would also answer calls for advice, like the one from the retired nurses who had volunteered their services at the home for the elderly. One idea that emerged out of collective talking was to connect these forgotten old men with a local youth drama group who was searching to find life stories that they could make into plays. In these forming and re-forming webs, discarded people could become valuable again as they transformed from being patients to emerge as the storytellers and the keepers of wisdom.

All through this time, local and overseas people came to look at our work. We would insist that they participate rather than sit on the sidelines. In doing this we wanted to be true to our idea that community is built in the participation of everyone who is there. We would include these visitors in groups, in therapies, in supervisions, or conversations with those who were there, depending where they fitted or wanted to be.

Within all this, our ideas of who were the ones doing therapy drastically changed. We, the official therapists, were being trained by artists, social workers, and many others who had been honed through the difficult circumstances of their lives. And our thinking about the official categories that separate clinical psychology, counselling psychology, community psychology, social work, and community workers from each other began to blur.

We noticed how some psychologists appeared and re-appeared in different ways. Sometimes they would be recognizable as social workers, then as community psychologists. Then these same people would re-appear at different times as charity givers or researchers, sometimes as individuals in crisis, and then again as psychologists. It was in acknowledging the shifts between different forms of involvement that we came to appreciate the usefulness of psychologists practising in various ways within the unofficial communities each one finds.

Then the almost forgotten owner of the big zozo appeared to claim his hut and the other two we gave to a self-help group making bricks. By then we had repeatedly confirmed our reasons for staying, and letting the zozos go brought with it a feeling of being part of a community.

Then, in a misguided effort to clean up the surrounds, a bulldozer levelled the yard, leaving a dust bowl around the bluegum tree. And still we continued, week after week, then to sit in the dust under the tree, shifting with the shade to find shelter from the sun, making spaces to practise, now in various ways.

2.1.2 Between shelter and exposure

In this process of sitting under the tree, our ways of doing therapy were also falteringly being transformed. Rituals of conservation and those of transformation were the words we would then use to describe our practices of healing. There were times when we would be acutely aware of doing nothing more than perpetuating the problems of the people we worked with. Our reluctance and fear would keep us from connecting with their pain and aloneness. And then there were moments when we would find connection and trust in the shaded spaces that would transform into holy temples and sacred sanctuaries for all.

Supervision would happen while walking on the pavements or in the mealie patch, or sitting on the low wall under the eaves of the big YMCA building. In the breaks between the long two- or three-hour sessions, our trainees came to talk of their 'stuckness' and we would struggle together, finding ways to give voice to the void. Being 'outside' and 'inside', and 'using place to find space', became regular ways of talking about the work we were doing. 'In the eye of the storm' and 'finding safe spaces for crises' are ways in which we still talk of our practices today.

We would entreat the therapists to go out to the homes and places of living of those who came. They would follow these trails, discovering hidden 'family' in the places they visited. And so we all came to know of poverty in disconnection, of the wealth of connectedness, and the metaphorical meanings of 'family' and 'home' beyond biology and place.

Then the question re-appeared about having a building or not. The idea had come up before. At those times we had gotten into all sorts of 'stuckness' around issues of funds and ownership, and of being 'inside' and 'outside'. We had no budget. We preferred not to be sponsored as we did not want to be tied to the dictates of the givers, nor did we want to become a welfare organization with a formal constitution and an executive body removed from the grass-roots functioning of the community itself.

We wanted to be visible and also protected from the wind and the rain. So,

sometimes, we drew in the dust while talking of a structure. From this came a design for a shelter that is based on a spiral. It has low, undulating, circling walls, spiralling into an open thatched-roof hut in the centre. The structure allows us to be inside and still remain connected to the flow on the street.

Our shelter was built from the gifts brought by the people who are of Agape. Some brought bricks and cement, some building know-how, others gave money or brought voices of encouragement or confirmation, all of which were now mixed into the substance of this shelter.

The shelter exposed us to new questions about how we are 'here'. Are we a 'cult of the new-age movement', as somebody once said? Or are we the 'New South Africa', as Andrew, a long-standing Agape member, repeatedly says; and what does this mean? Are we a community or organization now that we have located in structure? And are we still a healing community, searching for 'home'? In this we face yet another difficulty in which we are strung between becoming too safe in the place where we built our shelter, and still believing our ideas about healing and crisis and re-forming communities.

Agape began as an idea that creates place. It opened a talking space for some, and a place to meet or do activities for others. It is a context for the ritual of psychotherapy and the beginning point for projects that spiral out to the schools and into the informal settlements beyond. It is the place that brings forth sounds and songs from the silence of cold wars and from the tyranny of violence. It is the reservoir from which 'family' can arise beyond blood lines or oppression. It is the cauldron of crisis. It is a confluence and an altar. It is a shifting idea that finds life in connection. It is the creation of many and the possession of none.

2.2 Other versions of Agape

Many written (Blokland, 1993; Joffe, 1993; Lifschitz, Van Niekerk and Kgoadi, 1991; Magodielo, 1994; Migerode, 1992) and drawn documents, videos, banners, and photographs are continually being collected, which record impressions and versions of Agape. These are important in forming our history and mapping contexts to think about our doing. They are the artefacts of Agape. This process reflects Agape as a living community, growing and working in the ever-moving spaces between people. In this section extracts and examples of some of these artefacts are brought together to tell more stories about Agape.

2.2.1 Thinking about the tree

Lieven, a Belgian psychotherapy trainer, writes an article in the Belgian *Tijdschrift voor Familietherapie* after visiting Agape, titled 'Mamelodi – Verhaal van een ontmoeting in Afrika' (Migerode, 1992)[6]. An extract from this article, translated from Flemish, reads:

> Imagine the following: each Wednesday the trainers and their students sit in a circle of rickety chairs in the African shade of a tree. In the middle of the township talking to each other. Almost unnoticed people filter into the 'waiting room': a young man and

his companion, a woman with a baby on her arm, her family. Some had been here before and immediately made contact with their therapists from a previous conversation. Others approached the group hesitantly. Their hesitation is a signal for the students to go and ask them whether they are looking for the clinic. Through a short discussion the group decides which of the students is to see the person. In the course of the morning the most remarkable landscape develops around the tree. At different distances from the tree small circles of helpers and clients are talking.

2.2.2 Re-forming versions of community

Agape offers a place to people to form community in various ways. Here Dyke and Michael, who participated in an Agape project at their school, write a letter to find connection:

> Dear Agape
> Our names are Dyke and Michael.[7] We are 12 years old. We are asking what can we do when we want to be a member of 'Agape' or join 'Agape'.
> We are the children of confidence. Since 'Agape' came to our school we began to change our life. Things that we do are very very important. We like to learn more from you. Dyke and Michael.

'I did meet many people at Agape and it's no longer just a place where I spent time', wrote Clifford, one of the therapists who trained at Agape.

The community of Agape, like any community, is made up of people and what happens between them. The form that Agape takes shifts as people go through processes of giving substance(s) to their personal meanings of being together. All account for the community as they co-create its ever-shifting form. It is in the encounters between people that profound human experiences become part of the fabric of this healing community. For example, when Johannes Mnisi, a regular at Agape, was killed on the road, our mourning for him redefined the community at Agape. Betty then said: 'Now that we have lost a member, we have truly become a "family".'

In this participation of community, people's understanding of 'community' transforms. Magodielo (1994) records how the meaning of 'community' shifts for many trainees spending time in Agape, beyond only a geographical focus or a political definition. Tabea, a clinical psychology student who did her training at Agape, for example, says that she initially thought that 'the concept of community in my mind was applicable to black people only. White people could in no way be a community' (p.72).

Magodielo (1994) refers to Renei, an Agape member who has come to view the process of forming or belonging to a community as important because, as she expresses it, 'it gives one a psychological sense of causality' (p.78). Renei adds:

After a while [community] became a word that almost expressed emotion to me. I stopped defining community

in terms of boundaries and in terms of race. It has become an emotive expression for me. What stayed the same was that it was a place where people are well connected in a special way. For me, Mamelodi became more of a pursuit for community, to find that in people. So I moved from an academic, abstract way of thinking about it, to an emotional way of thinking about it. (Magodielo, 1994, p.79)

2.2.3 Connecting through self in community

A masters student who did his training at Agape writes a poem of his world, giving us a glimpse into his experience of forming community at Agape:

A HEALING CIRCLE CLOSED

I see it from a distance
through the dusty glow
of this different world.
A world of
hopelessness and hope,
ecstasy and despair,
The tree provides protection;
Its roots firmly in the soil,
Its canopy of branches;
caring shade.

I open and open
unto this foreign world,
A world of dust and heat
and sun and cold,
A world of being unsure,
what to do?
where to head?
I cannot stand on this shifting sand,

I sweep away without a hold.
What to do? what to say?
to this despair and pain
and hope and joy.
And then by letting go,
by not holding on to what I know,
or to who I think I am;
It comes unknown from deep within.

With him I connect to myself;
A healing circle closed.

The emphasis on what emerges of self in community is a thread that runs through all of the activities in Agape. Sam, an artist, who has been part of Agape from its beginning, says:

From my side, I find Agape as a home, a different home. I've learned that in a home a father can be a child and a child can be a father too. A father can be a child in that he finds that he has a crisis, or falls into a situation, whereby he needs to be understood.

I too have brothers and sisters who come and go. This house is a bridge that tries to build a sense of community between different people, to show them that they as people can learn from one another and feel what the other's inner part is like.

Agape forms a confluence in which some people find connection beyond the boundaries of their own comfort. In this, people keep re-forming and informing themselves in their relationships with others. Lieven, a visiting Belgian psychotherapist, recalls how one trainee therapist, Mark, carried a gun in his bag for the first three months after coming to Mamelodi.

Stan, the programme co-ordinator, never directly confronted this. He simply maintained an air of awareness of the gun, by playing with the bag in which the gun was kept from time to time. When I asked the student now, almost two years later what had changed in his thinking, he said that he came with his theories and ideas that led him to expect to encounter in this context mainly social problems around work and food at the clinic. Now he experiences that, no matter what their social situation, in spite of hunger, in spite of the racial circumstances, people still attach a moving amount of importance to their personal relationships, that love and emotional hunger exist everywhere and that people can move no matter what.

One day, soon after joining Agape, Mark met Paul, a released ex-death row prisoner who was convicted for his bystander involvement in a witchburning. The student, who once worked for the police, connects with this ex-accused and helps Paul to write his story. Paul, in turn, helps Mark to write his dissertation, as they link to find connection and healing for both themselves and each other. Mark writes in the epilogue to Paul's story, called *In my suffering times,* which is included in his dissertation (Joffe, 1993):

Paul, my friend, you have taught me so much. I have learned about politics, family history, the struggle, the justice system, and your life. Above all you have taught me about courage, sacrifice, bravery and strength. All these qualities you mix with the modesty, humility and softness that drew me to you the very first time we met.

Paul and Mark's encounter contains an experience that many of us have in moving through Agape. It entails finding yourself in connection in ways that push you beyond singular or safe identities. Individuals find themselves confronting their own issues of life.

Being in the fray of relationships often challenges a person's ways of thinking and categories of classification. John, an academic and behaviour therapist from the United States of America, recalls some incidents of coming up against his own categories of classification during a visit to Agape:

I'm in a small group when a young active apparently psychotic man, that I hear shouting nonsense from the other side of the fence, appears, and watch as Stan assigns Jean, a masters student doing his clinical training at Agape, to go and connect with him in some effective way. I question why linear, anti-psychotic treatment would not be in order and am somewhat confused but intrigued by Stan's comeback, connecting him to some relational community context. I recognise the systems conceptualisation. Interesting and lots of face validity, but I question its utility, especially

in the light of what I see as the pressing need for quick action and clear functional results. I shut up and watch, sceptical, but open to be proved wrong. Jean comes back from visiting his house and proves me wrong. He has been greeted by the whole family and community who are no doubt an extremely important and healing resource. I begin to connect this approach with chaos theory, dynamic healing factors which may be uncontrollable yet may be trustworthy. I become more convinced of the value of this oblique but patient approach to establishing meaning and focus on family problems as I see the smile and physical closeness of the aunt and the sister and her troubled daughter walking away with Kevin in tow, sheepish smile of humble but apparent victory on their faces.

Connecting beyond reified categories can provoke the formation of spaces in which voice is given to the unspoken or even the long-held hurtful secrets we keep.

Thabangile, at the time a client who has since become an Agape member, describes how she found a space at Agape to voice her silent, inner pain:

Now I see myself as different, as I've discovered another Beauty here. Agape has taught me to talk and use my voice and not keep more and more secrets.

Re-forming self in community is not always a comfortable circumstance. It often takes time and sometimes only becomes apparent when one has shifted to another complex of community involvement. Clifford reflects back on his experiences in Agape from another place where he was working:

> I'm not sure whether I did good work in Mamelodi. I'm not sure whether I dared enough. I do trust myself more than I used to, but this is simply because I now believe that what I experienced is valid, and this allows me to explore rather than simply to deny and react in a destructive manner.
>
> How to work in Agape is only now becoming clear to me. My interventions throughout the year had been very linear in their conceptualisation and I often lapsed into a nasty cycle of advice-giving. Chief amongst my failures was Kagiso and her mother. I don't think I ever broke through to them.

3 A credimus

The ideas and notions noted here have arisen from our living in the flow of our work. They simultaneously describe the ways we work and what we believe. Together they provide a lexicon of our language and also a vocabulary for our practice. The relevance of this credo for the reader is in providing and provoking ideas for the practice and training of clinical and community psychologists.

For the authors there is also relevance to be found, through writing this piece, in creating a place to report to the fraternity. In this we are attending to the important issue concerned with the ethics of practice where all practitioners need to account for themselves to their community.

What is said here is not new or original. Many people know of these ideas and some have written of them from within different disciplines and practices like religion, art, and physics. Within the fraternity of contemporary psychologists, Bateson (1972), Jung (1963), Mutwa (1964, 1986), and Sullivan (1953) are a few who have written eloquently about these ideas. As practising ecological psychologists, we also believe that the ideas and notions stated here will shift as we continue to re-form and inform our work.[8]

- Healers are informed and re-formed through their experiences in living rather than by the theories they subscribe to.
- Healing happens in the languages that bring the unspoken into conversation.
- Every conversation in healing can be usefully viewed as cross-cultural and every person as multicultural.
- Training and healing happen when we find safe spaces to connect within crisis.
- Healing is also for the healer.
- When community forms in crisis, the possibility of transformation is opened.
- Crisis is the cauldron of transformation.

4 An epilogue

The ongoing journey of re-forming what we have come to know as the Agape Healing Community has also led to our continual forming and re-forming of ideas about essences of the work. This process has made us respectful of grass-roots experience as teachers and transformers, realizing that theoretical instruction alone is not sufficient preparation to be able to perform work usefully. Indeed, it too often serves as a shield to keep psychologists, teachers, supervisors, policy makers, and so on from having to get their hands dirty and thereby to encounter the struggle entailed in what is often spoken about too easily.

On the other hand, the continual struggle to formulate and also share those ideas that are forming through and recursively guiding the work is an important part of an effort to be accountable for what we are doing. Much of the difficulty we encounter in trying to convey in writing the essence of a process that emanates from the unpredictable encounters between people, lies in having to use a mechological medium and metaphor for something that is most profoundly ecological.

The premises underlying this profound difference can be summarized as follows. The rules of mechologic include the assumption of a fixed, absolute reality; the use of a machine metaphor for the person and for living; a breaking up of the whole into fragments, which are regarded separately; a reverence for a set hierarchy of knowers and knowledge; an assumption of linear causality; and a belief that something is only scientific and therefore valuable if it is observable and measurable (Auerswald, 1969).

On the other hand, the rules of ecology include a belief in a multiverse of realities, rather than in master codes; a move towards seeing knowledge as a product of social negotiation and a consideration of its social

function; an acknowledgement of the interrelatedness of everything, and the importance of context; a focus on perspective and pattern rather than discrete facts; and a challenge to the so-called knower's position as an expert and a demagogue (Auerswald, 1969).

The dialectic between the certainty and limitations of the world of formal theory and teaching, and the uncertainty and vagueness of encountering not-knowing at grass-roots level have profound reverberations. Often the more essential human processes are omitted in our formal accounts of our work. The discomfort of this dialectic is also, however, precisely what informs and reforms our work and life. It can move us beyond the restrictions of worn-out prescriptions.

4.1 A crisis of fragmentation

Coping, on the one hand, with the extreme fragmentation of our worlds, and on the other hand, with feeling overwhelmed by sensing the interrelatedness of everything, is detectable at all levels of our living. It echoes through the issues about psychology in South Africa, and as a profession or body of knowledge in general; through the different facets of crisis that this country has been experiencing for many decades now; and through the struggling of all people in all times to find useful ways to be themselves in the presence of others.

The processes in this country[9], while passing through the rigidities of an oppressive system and the redefinition of societal transformation, have produced contexts of intense crisis and uncertainty. It was and is a context marked by the intense struggle between separateness and togetherness, between authority and equality, between certainty and uncertainty, and between desperation and hope.

This struggle is often echoed in the crisis in psychology: Who can or should the psychologist be? With whom, what, and where should or shouldn't we work? How do we know which set of beliefs or language is the right/best/politically correct one? In which categories, for example, clinical or counselling, should we organize ourselves, and how rigidly should we keep these categories apart? Is it answers that are needed now, or could it in any way be useful to admit our many questions?

Perhaps one can say that it is our experience of smallness and helplessness in the immense interconnectedness of living and dying that pushes us to construct fragmentation as a means of finding control over ourselves and our worlds. The growth of Newtonian science's legitimation of the mechanistic fragmentation of the person and her or his world – as a way of attaining clarity and predictability – is one echo of this.

Institutionalized fragmentation, like apartheid, that is too singular, lasting, and absolute interferes with the necessary evolution of patterns in the domains of living and work. Our options become reduced, and in our ensuing alienation and helplessness is a profound sense of crisis. This crisis of too much mechanistic fragmentation can also be described as energizing the movement towards postmodernism (Kvale, 1992; Rosenau, 1992), the growing open search for spirituality, and the need for new and more languages of relating – both personally and professionally (Rorty, 1982).

However, it is neither fragmentation nor wholeness that can in itself be good or bad. What is called for is that the evolution that emerges from the tension between these counterparts can proceed. Thus, natural shifts and movement are frozen when this rhythm is interfered with. In South Africa we face the particular crisis of having blocked natural social evolution through the stultification of specific separations. The institutionalization of a mechological epistemology has pushed a one-sided approach, in which individuality and specific group identities are revered.

The word 'crisis' derives from the Greek word '*krinein*', which means 'to separate' (McNamee, 1992). It is often rigid patterns or unexpected events of separation that precipitates a sense of crisis. Conversely, the experience of crisis also brings separation. Not only are we removed from the intimate and seemingly safe interactional spaces we know. We are also removed from previous meanings – from the sense that the world, as we knew it before, used to make.

Often people's dealing with such a crisis entails mainly conservational processes. In this we curb the crisis in some overt or covert way, while still ensuring the status quo – still maintaining old identities, meanings, and ways of relating. However, it is when we find ways of entering and sharing the uncertainty, of being together in crisis, that possibilities for transformation evolve. It is in this that crisis can also be seen as a resource.[10] It is the circumstance that can mobilize us to move beyond the safety and familiarity of old set ways of compartmentalizing and fractionalizing our selves and our work.

This is in keeping with Auerswald's (1969) comment that what he calls the systems thinker cannot work in a context of safety. Rather, our fuller participation can only land us in a crisis of uncertainty and not knowing. Acknowledging the notion of context-bound knowledge challenges not only our cognitive styles and professional ways of living, but also our total life styles. It means a turbulent period of disintegration and reintegration, of being willing and able to tolerate the fragmentation of identity boundaries. This is in contrast with trying to maintain the stance of the clinical scientist that is the product of the specialized fragmentation of the modern world of science. Being this kind of scientist can get you caught up in the sequences prescribed by the content-based training of a highly specialized and circumscribed discipline upon which you can also eventually depend for the very definition of your personal identity. This safety of seeming truths can enable one not to have to face oneself, or the crisis of not knowing, or the demand of personal transformation. It enables one to maintain a sense of clear self-esteem, values, and of status in the vertical hierarchies of society. Auerswald (1969) describes this kind of construction of a world that is sufficiently fragmented to deny one's participation in what emerges and can emerge, as the abdication of responsibility.

Our work in Agape, which has been organized by this very crisis of fragmentation, has brought us to an increasing respect for the need, at this time, to be part of processes within which traditional prescribed boundaries, political, professional, and personal, can be bridged or at least straddled. It is for this that the idea of the Agape Healing Community currently provides a context (Lifschitz, 1996).

4.2 The relevance debate

We have seen the fragmentation in psychology and also in this country take form in the growing debate over the past few decades about the development of contextually relevant applications for psychology in South African settings (Berger and Lazarus, 1987; Biesheuvel, 1991; Butchart, 1995; Dawes, 1985, 1986; Gilbert, 1989; Nell, 1989; Seedat and Nell, 1992). The question that arose was whether, and how, to cross the great divide between the selective consulting room and the needy masses.

It is in this that the dialectic between effectively fragmented, yet undeniably interrelated worlds is again encountered. In psychology we are stuck in apartheid. Through the traditions of our profession, we also face the rigid and narrow prescription of togetherness and separateness, all through the rigid prescription of singular, formalized, and fragmented professional identities. This rigid and problematic prescription of boundaries within the profession can be detected at many levels. Consider, for example, traditional ideas, which have often been linked to socio-economic constructions, about who can benefit from psychology; the highly contentious strict and arbitrary previous delineation of categories of psychologists (often echoing the self-preservation issues of professionals more than it reflects the nuances of living and needs at grass-roots level); and also the prescription of which parts of the psychologist and her or his repertoire of relating are irrelevant or even noxious in her or his work (positing her or his personhood as either a non-issue or problematic to her or him as a professional).

Many responses to the crisis of fragmentation seem to perpetuate the delineation of rigid boundaries. Most typically, our personal and professional efforts at dealing with this crisis entail trying to remove the crisis, or sense thereof, as quickly as possible. In this we often seem to achieve some relief, but simultaneously subtly perpetuate the singular prescription of boundaries and limits.

Consider two typical and opposite responses to the relevance debate. On the one hand, many mainstream positivistic voices, described by Biesheuvel (1991), expressed their concern that traditional psychology will be limited and deprofessionalized if it is politicized. These voices fit within a traditional medical model orientation in the field and thus rest on a set of beliefs that perpetuate hierarchy and separateness (Kvale, 1992). The academically trained professional is seen as a problem-free expert who gives one-way help to the helpless and needy person. The emphasis is on eradicating problems that are always recognizable in the form of formal diagnoses. This approach rests on an absolute belief in reified categories that are seen to be true across time and setting, regardless of context.

The responses from these voices to the relevance debate typically take the form of actions that seem to shift the geographical and some pragmatic parameters of psychological practices, but which still perpetuate hierarchy and separateness. This is often called the mental health model in community psychology (Mann, 1978). From this

stance, most typically, hierarchically based services would be replicated in other 'under-privileged' areas, making more experts available to the needy masses. This approach implies a geographical understanding of what community means and a non-regard for the recursive impact of context. The input is one-directional, keeping professionals safe from having to shift away from the clarity of their beliefs or the safety of their unquestionable expertise.

On the other hand, another position that psychologists took within the crisis of this country was to advocate an emphasis on the mental health effects of political repression, pointing out that traditional mental health services have helped to legitimize and perpetuate the patterns of apartheid in South Africa (Berger and Lazarus, 1987; Dawes, 1986; Seedat and Nell, 1992). These voices call for us to position ourselves, almost exclusively, as social activists, contributing to a bottom-up process of mobilizing people against an unjust system. This is often referred to as the social action model in community psychology (Glidewell (1984); Mann (1978); McCulloch (1995); Sonnleitner (1987); and Wolff (1986).

In this approach the definition of community is constructed along the societal patterns of power distribution, distinguishing the have's and have-not's of power. Again, this effort at changing the playing fields of psychology can be seen as perpetuating separateness in a non-useful way. Although psychologists can shift from their position as the only experts and the acknowledgement of their role as change agents is undeniably important, they can still be seen as essentially keeping themselves safe while others put themselves on the line for the struggle. Furthermore, the issue narrowed to socio-political identity can limit the co-evolution of richer ways of relating. The singular prescription of either separateness or togetherness patterns is a typical answer to the relevance debate. But what responses within the relevance debate often seem to neglect is a process in which both similarities and differences, separateness and togetherness, can become part of a complex and naturally evolving process.

The categories and descriptions of models in this section can seem effortlessly clear, and that calls for a moment's reflection. What is ignored in such a theoretical description is that our ideas and theories, which are so rational in the academic domain, also emerge from those parts of ourselves that are very personal or hidden. The models we choose or discard do not reflect only our intellectual efforts. They are also the clues as to where our greatest struggles are as people. The different paradigmatic and epistemological choices we describe in this writing always profoundly echo what we need, are scared of, or are trying to conserve for ourselves as people. Such a perspective implies that one should not only judge any thinking or doing on its first appearance. Rather, they are also useful as subtle indications of the particular rings of crisis circling in the webs of our lives.

4.3 Understanding 'community' within psychology beyond geography and politics

The idea of community psychology in its contemporary definition (Levine and Per-

kins, 1987; Mann, 1978; Orford, 1992) has been limited by the way in which it has been used as an answer to the problem of psychology and unreached peoples. A field called 'community psychology' came to be seen as a pragmatic reaction against the limitations of a problem-oriented and individual-centred traditional psychology. In South Africa, given the context of the struggle against apartheid and its concomitant skewing of services, 'community psychology' came to be understood as working with underprivileged black people, and 'community' as mostly signifying, through a combination of political and geographical lenses, black townships.

This way of posing community psychology as the answer to psychology's apartheid problems once again perpetuates a system of separateness by simply inventing another too absolute and too singular a category. By simply seeing community psychology as yet another separate speciality field in psychology, different, for example, from clinical psychology, the urgent challenge to the ways in which psychology is informed and practised is uselessly averted.

While the injustices of an oppressive apartheid system certainly necessitate explicit and far-reaching attention, we also need to acknowledge that the crisis of fragmentation with its petrified patterns of group identity are detectable at all levels of existence. It is not simply a localized practical problem. It emanates from the formal and informal epistemologies that inform most of our work and living. This perspective calls for a process in which all of the nuances of our relating can be addressed and challenged – also in unpredictable ways and places.

This ecological focus rests on an appreciation that it is from an acknowledgement of interrelation that a way of being emerges that can allow opportunity for healing and transformation. From this position, 'community' can be understood not as an irreversible given but as process, something that evolves, that is interactively created (Biggers, 1996; Bozzoli, 1987; Dunham, 1984; Oosthuizen, 1995, 1997). It is the space where the crisis and possibilities of the interrelatedness of people, ideas, and issues can be encountered. From this encounter, a profound transformation of previous stultified identities, meanings, and patterns can evolve. New options for who we are in our togetherness and separateness emerge.

Such a process demands of us as psychologists to enter into places and processes where we are unsure of ourselves. It means that we have to put ourselves on the line without the guarantees of set theories, pre-planned programmes, or contexts that continually confirm our expertise. It calls for us not to endeavour to simply posit ourselves as neutral professionals or conveyors of information, but rather to openly take a position, to, in Price's (1989) words, 'bear witness'. It entails us having to work without the boundaries that usually serve the purpose of effectively hiding when we fall flat on our faces. It also means that we allow for the possibility to be profoundly, not just seemingly, transformed in this process. Through stepping into our own uncertainty, within the crises of ourselves and our profession, we allow ourselves to be unpredictably pushed by circumstances and by people, regardless of the labels we can give them: student, client, organizer, or disadvantaged community.

Similarly, people's helplessness transforms in a co-evolution of community that does not simply hide the so-called professional's uncertainty and exposure, or the unpredictability of the outcome (Anderson and Goolishian, 1992; Byrne and McCarthy, 1988; Lifschitz, 1988; Lifschitz et al., 1991). No theory, model, life-skills programme, or questionnaire can convey or replace the importance of being in the unpredictable process of forming increasingly personal webs of connection. However much theoretical ideas can be useful guiding principles, many people will attest to how they soon lose their impact when they are confronted with the harshness of putting themselves to work at grass-roots level. Thus, a question that theory can be measured against is whether it gives one a language to voice one's own issues, or to divert one from it.

Furthermore, while a theoretical model is tempting in the sense of the predictability it brings, it can simply get one to carry reductionistic preconceptions into the context. This can prevent one from going through one's own process in order to evolve a way of thinking and being that can make possible personal connections and disconnections within the never-ending process of evolving community.

From this perspective, 'relevance' can be redefined in terms of people and professionals in the field, working at their own edges between certainty and uncertainty, and not only in terms of prescriptions of how and where they need to work. Such a redefinition can contribute to a profound transformation of ourselves and our work. It also enables us to note and attend to the many spaces (not just the current politically correct ones) where people are stuck, no matter who or where they are.

Thus, 'community psychology' indicates an appreciation of the processes that emerge when people come together in crisis. It is in crisis where people become most compelled to move beyond what is known, stultified, and stuck. In this crisis, community psychology indicates attention to the mobilization of the hidden and of unexplored possibilities. This happens in a process within which people can explore and re-form their ideas of self and others in continuously forming, and re-forming, a safe space to find new identities, express hidden stories, and explore more ways of being together and separate.

In this vein, Gadamer (in Anderson and Goolishian, 1988) sees a therapeutic process as one of 'expanding the unsaid' (p. 381), and describes the immensity of the domain of hidden stories as 'the infinity of the unsaid' (p. 3890). Making space for an exploration of the stories people live, hide, and tell forms an important part of the co-creation of a healing space. It opens up a domain within which to work against the paralyzing silence evolving in people's lives, so that people's voices can be heard again or anew. Additionally, the process of storying our experiences also provides a useful epistemological template for exploring the processes we are part of in our work (Lyotard, 1984; Parry, 1991).

Another important essence of what can be called the pragmatics of community psychology entails the co-creation of networks through which everyone's resourcefulness

can be explored (Glidewell, 1984; Kelly, 1986; Oosthuizen, 1997; Trickett, 1984; Wolff, 1986). This refers on the one hand to participation by all in planning and doing the work. On the other hand, it also calls for participation by all in reflecting on the work, ourselves, and the inequalities we and our relationships inherit from the systems we are part of. Such a process of continual shared investigation, and the creative intelligence elicited from everyone through this ongoing dialoguing, also serves to work against the even subtle perpetuation of oppressive helping regimes and cultures of silence. It also continually reconfirms the right of each person to, as Freire (1972), puts it, 'say his own word, to name the world' (p. 12).

In essence, it is in connecting in struggling, and in trying to find new ways through uncertainty, that people's most profound resourcefulness is uncovered.

4.4 Seeing every interaction as cross-cultural and multilingual

Calling, in the particular context of South Africa, for a process that builds the moreness of our selves and our relationships, also demands of us to question the singular meanings we attach to people and their ways. Very often these emerge in the guise of talk about culture.

Considerations around the concept 'culture' often elicit content-bound prescriptions of how we should understand or deal with people, or how psychology or healing should be practised. However, such prescriptions are highly problematic themselves. The notion that we need a special Third World psychology for certain settings is one example of such a prescription. We agree with Nell's (1989) idea that this ethnopsychological trap can be avoided by acknowledging that our ideas about healing can be sufficiently sophisticated and ecological to deal with the so-called intercultural differences between people as different manifestations of the one and the same humanity that we all share.

It is of more use to consider the dilemmas inherent in the way the word 'culture' is typically used. These problematic uses include: viewing a person's culture as an absolute ontological reality; the historical South African euphemism of using the word 'culture' to denote race; and an ignorance of how the specific way we choose to use this term in itself organizes a social world. The issue is not to ignore the existence and political ramifications of differences between groups (Gobodo, 1990), or to do away with this term. Rather, the issue is for us to mainly consider the usually ignored functions and restrictions inherent in the way the term is being used. Most typically, using this term gets people stuck in a sense of absolute knowledge, that is, reified content knowledge about reified categories of people, absolute ideas about which differences between people are noteworthy, and seemingly clear understandings of where culture is and is not to be found. Such a sense of absolute truth also precludes a consideration of the way specific chosen understandings of culture serve strong political and economic power patterns.

Categorizing people in terms of reified 'cultural' identities, and enhancing the 'importance' of such categories by using the label 'cross-cultural' to denote seemingly irreconcilable differences between people, often become reductionistic and immobilizing (Oosthuizen, 1995). Introducing such cultural talk into relationships often brings about a circumstance in which people become objects or artefacts of reified concepts and in which the possibilities for human connection and understanding then become radically reduced.

This idea takes our consideration of the concept onto an epistemological level: a thinking about our thinking. Constructing culture as collective ways of punctuating and understanding similarity and difference between people enables us to see how we organize social interaction through the way in which we use the word. It also reminds us to ask the question: why does the term culture and the usual accompanying issues come up at some times and not at others? Such a constructionist exploration of the concept 'culture' and its use can be aided by texts such as those by Geertz (1973, 1986), Van Gennep (1960), and Wetherell and Potter (1992).

Our notion is not that so-called cultural differences are irrelevant, but that our arbitrary use of the term serves an organizing epistemological function, and does not have much use at an ontological explanatory level. Through confrontation with our senses of self and our own beliefs – some of which were described earlier in the story of Agape – we have come to believe that the richness of similarity and difference at play in all human contact necessitates the view that all human interaction is simultaneously cross-cultural and not. Thus culture is co-created in each and every conversation. This does not assume similarity and equal positions, and does not negate the organizing role of power structures. It does, however, assert that our understanding(s) of 'culture' is always simultaneously and recursively a function of the relationships we are in, and also an organizer of the way we perpetuate our social worlds. We can all be seen as multi-cultural creatures; it is just that we prefer some ways of relating to others.

Similarly, the possibilities for dealing with what is seen as a multilingual context are reduced when we only understand language to be an ontological given. It certainly is necessary to be open to learning more official languages in the South African context. But if we only ask the question whether we can speak Tswana, English, Zulu, and so forth, we limit the possibilities of connection between the narrow denotative boundaries of formally punctuated languages.

In this narrow focus we ignore that there are in the processes of interaction many different kinds of English, Zulu, and so forth. Language can be understood as only ever subjective and frequently re-created if we take the connotative domains of the spoken word into account.

Even more importantly, we lose, in this narrow focus, the opportunities for connection inherent in other languages of sharing that can emerge between people. In moving beyond the constraints of the traditional consultation room, we can and need to develop more than just the language of the talking cure. Also important are the languages of ritual, of art, of movement, of distance, or of physically working or being together.

Through Agape we have learned to respect, show, and use the language of cele-

bration, of mourning, of joking, and of giving up. We have discovered the difficulty and the space of silence. Even more essentially, we have come to an understanding that a language grows each time anew between people, that there always are some levels of understanding to be found through personal connection, that we always build in translation, and that we need to be most cautious of those instances where we assume that we do speak the same language.[11]

4.5 Ethics through mutuality

Acknowledging the multiplicity of ourselves moves the emphasis from visiting to constantly trying to co-create communities, and onto the multisidedness of the therapist as well. This brings forth the idea that everybody involved in the process both needs to and can give healing – in many different forms – and that our healing potential is mobilized through an encounter with our own pain and difficulty. This notion ties in with the age-old maxim to be found in most healing traditions: that the healer can only heal through her or his own woundedness, and that she or he creates contexts that are also, but not exclusively, for her or his own healing (Keeney, 1994; Kreinheder, 1989o; Meyerhoff, 1976; Somé, 1993).

This idea is captured in *The fall* by Camus (1957), in which the character of the fallen judge who becomes the barman at the frontier of existence can be likened to the therapist who learns to heal through his or her own failings or woundedness, and also in the legend of the wounded healer. According to this legend, Chiron, the healer centaur, suffers from an incurable wound originally caused by a poisoned arrow of Hercules. Thus, he is a healer who needs healing himself. It is also to him that Asclepius is given to raise. Under Chiron's tutelage, Asclepius becomes the Greek god of healing (Graves, 1955).

The idea of the healer also needing help brings a recognition of the possibility that psychologists can also have a calling to their helping professions as part of their own journey of seeking healing. It is only in professional communities that are mainly informed by mechanistic Newtonian science that treatment or practice is exclusively reserved for the patient. Here a reverence for clarity, as conceptualized by mechological thinking, leads to warnings against the mystification of the science, and interpretations of the ethics of dealing with people only along the lines of technical expertise and a reduction of the encounter to something clearly delineated as professional. In this traditional approach the perpetuation of boundaries (for example, between expert and patient, between thinking and sensing, between knowing and believing) again works against the transformation possible through richer encounters between people. Perhaps the Newtonian psychological maxim, 'If it moves, measure it', most poignantly demonstrates how the richness of humanness is effectively ruled out by a too singular reverence for the mechanical and demonstrable.

Believing in the ancient wisdom that healing is also for the healer evokes an ethic of practice that flows from the humility brought about by the healer her- or himself having been recruited through the struggles of her or his own living.

5 Conclusion

The processes described above in the bifurcating languages of experience and of ideas continually bring us back to a re-encounter with essential meanings inherent in the journey of co-creating community – meanings also embodied in possible meanings of 'Agape', the name given to this healing community. On the one hand, it carries the meaning of the Greek word for brotherly and sisterly love (*agapé*). On the other hand, it also contains the Sotho word '*gape*', which means 'again'. This reflects what we have continually, even sometimes unwillingly, been reminded of: that we have to come again, stay in the process, face what comes after what had gone before, and that it is in this, most essentially, that a living and healing community can grow and transform – both itself and those who participate in it.

In conclusion we want to acknowledge and thank all those whose words have been placed in this text. These people, together with the many others who have created the confluence called Agape: without you all, there would not be a story to tell, and with you we can move beyond the ideas we have come to here.

Reflecting back over the text now it seems to us, just as it did to Clifford when he wrote in another piece about Agape:

> [We] did not set out to write a comprehensive piece. At most [we] want to give an idea of what Agape is for [us]. It doesn't [only] involve well-structured paragraphs and eloquent deep passages, but a variety of

stories and ideas that connect [our] memories of Agape. It is the connections that make this place special. There are many people who [we] are fond of, and who [we] hope will have long and happy lives. Whenever writing about Agape it was often with tiredness. It is better to be there than to write about it.

The writing and reading of this chapter brings another opportunity to co-create community. So in the spirit of Agape we invite you to join with us in a process of forming and re-forming our healing community.

Exercises

In the flow of telling the Agape story, certain ideas, concepts, and issues were raised, which may challenge you to ponder about what you think a community psychologist needs to know. We pose a few questions that could provoke you to continue actively in enquiring about this question.

1 Does a community psychologist serve or co-create a community?
2 What do you understand a community to be?
3 How personally involved should a community psychologist be with the community members with whom she or he works?
4 How is success measured in community psychology?
5 Does healing mean the same as curing?

6 When and by whom does a community project get planned?
7 Which languages should a community psychologist speak?
8 When does a community psychologist work cross-culturally and when not?
9 How does the practice of community psychology account for ethics?
10 Does a community psychologist do psychotherapy?

Notes

1 Mamelodi is situated east of Pretoria. Agape forms every Wednesday on the grounds of the Young Men's Christian Association (YMCA).
2 The way an oppressive social system has contributed to the serious skewing of the availability and nature of psychological services in South Africa is taken as a basic assumption and will not be discussed here. Suffice it here to refer to examples of numerous useful texts on this matter, such as Dawes (1985, 1986), Dawes and Donald (1994), Mholi (1987), and Berger and Lazarus (1987), who write about the South African context. Furthermore, colonial mental health science as a system of knowledge and power is discussed and analysed in depth in seminal publications by writers such as McCulloch (1995), Sonnleiter (1987), and Foucault (1973).
3 The useful and instructive dialogue possible between the domain of the psychotherapist and the domain of the sangoma or the shaman can be explored further through readings by authors such as Cheetam and Griffiths (1982), Mutwa (1964), Hammond-Tooke (1989), Mankazana (1979), Katz and Kimani (1982), and Meyerhoff (1976). In this chapter the concept 'healer' is used interchangeably with clinical and community psychologist.

4 This was a conference location for the SA Association of Family and Marital Psychology during 1990.

5 Auerswald (1992) refers to this event, which he was part of, as one that brought the audience at the conference to a creative mode of ecological thinking.

6 One account of such a visit can be found in Migerode (1992).

7 Two school children from Mamelodi who were involved in an Agape project dealing with violence at their school.

8 While respectful of the official categories, we use the designation 'healer' to include people from both the categories of clinical and community psychology.

9 Some useful interpretations of these processes can be found in Leatt, Kneifel, and Nurmberger (1986), the OASSSA publication on apartheid and mental health, and Dawes and Donald's (1994) text on childhood and adversity in South Africa.

10 See in this regard also McNamee (1992). Prigogine and Stengers's (1984) ideas about bifurcation in evolutionary systems can be useful in further explorations of this point.

11 The constructionist notion of language as constantly intersubjectively created rests strongly on Wittgenstein's (1958) ideas and is explored in depth in many texts. Some that can be useful are: Bruner (1991), Derrida (1982), Goolishian and Anderson (1987), Harré (1990), Mair (1990), Parker (1990), Parry (1991), Ricoeur (1991), and Zimmerman and Dickerson (1994).

References

ANDERSON, H. and GOOLISHIAN, H. A. (1988). Human systems as linguistic systems: Preliminary and evolving ideas about the implications for clinical theory. *Family Process*, 27, 371–393.

ANDERSON, H. and GOOLISHIAN, H. A. (1992). The client is the expert: A not-knowing approach to therapy. In S. McNamee and K. J. Gergen (Eds.), *Therapy as social construction* (pp. 25–39). London: Sage.

AUERSWALD, E. H. (1969). Interdisciplinary versus ecological approach. In W. Gray, F.J. Duhl, and N. D. Rizzo (Eds.), *General systems theory and psychiatry* (pp. 373–386). Boston: Little, Brown.

AUERSWALD, E. (1992). The roots of dissonance in human affairs. In J. Mason, J. Rubenstein, and S. Shuda (Eds.), *From diversity to healing* (pp. 1–35). Durban: SAIMFT.

BATESON, G. (1972). *Steps to an ecology of mind.* New York: Ballantine.

BERGER, S. and LAZARUS, S. (1987). The views of community organizers on the relevance of psychological practice in South Africa. *Psychology in Society*, 7, 6–23.

BIESHEUVEL, S. (1991). Neutrality, relevance and accountability in psychological research and practice in South Africa. *South African Journal of Psychology*, 21, 34–47.

BIGGERS, J. (1996). *From the dusty soil: The story of Mitraniketan community education and development in rural India.* Kerala, India: Mitraniketan Publishers and Printers.

BLOKLAND, L. M. (1993). *Psychotherapy training: The Mamelodi experience.* Unpublished MA dissertation, UNISA, Pretoria.

BOZZOLI, B. (1987). Class, community and ideology in the evolution of South African society. In B. Bozzoli (Ed.), *Class, community and conflict in the South African perspective* (pp. 1–43). Johannesburg: Ravan.

BRUNER, J. (1991). The narrative construction of reality. *Critical Inquiry*, 18, 1–21

BUTCHART, R. A. (1995). *On the anatomy of power: Bodies of knowledge in South African socio-medical discourse.* Unpublished doctoral thesis, UNISA, Pretoria.

BYRNE, N. O. and MCCARTHY, I. C. (1988). Moving statutes: Requesting ambivalence through ambiguous discourse. *The Irish Journal of Psychology*, 9, 173–182.

CAMUS, A. (1957). *The fall.* Middlesex: Penguin.

CHEETHAM, R. W. S. and GRIFFITHS, J. A. (1982). The traditional healer/diviner as psychotherapist. *South African Medical Journal*, 52, 957–958.

DAWES, A. (1985). Politics and mental health: The position of clinical psychology in South Africa.

South African Journal of Psychology,
15, 55–61.

DAWES, A. (1986). The notion of relevant psychology with particular reference to Africanist pragmatic initiatives. *Psychology in Society,* 5, 28–48.

DAWES, A. and DONALD, S. (1994). *Childhood and adversity.* Cape Town: David Philip.

DERRIDA, J. (1982). *Writing and difference.* Chicago: University of Chicago Press.

DUNHAM, M. (1984). Community as process: Maintaining the delicate balance. *American Journal of Community Psychology,* 5, 257–268.

FOUCAULT, M. (1973). *Madness and civilization.* New York: Vintage.

FREIRE, P. (1972). *Pedagogy of the oppressed.* London: Penguin.

GADAMER, H. G. (1975). *Truth and method.* New York: Continuum.

GEERTZ, C. (1973). *The interpretation of cultures.* New York: Basic Books.

GEERTZ, C. (1986). Making experiences, authoring selves. In P. Rabinow and W. M. Sullivan (Eds.), *The anthropology of experience.* Chicago: University of Illinois Press.

GILBERT, A. (1989). Things fall apart? Psychological theory in the face of rapid social change. *South African Journal of Psychology,* 19, 91–100.

GLIDEWELL, J. C. (1984). Training for the role of advocate. *American Journal of Community Psychology,* 12, 193–197.

GOBODO, P. (1990). Notions about culture in understanding black psychopathology: Are we trying to raise the dead? *South African Journal of Psychology,* 20, 93–98.

GOOLISHIAN, H. A. and ANDERSON, H. (1987, Fall). Language systems and therapy: An evolving idea. *Psychotherapy,* 24, 529–538.

GRAVES, R. (1955). *The Greek myths: Volume 1.* New York: Penguin.

HAMMOND-TOOKE, D. (1989). *Rituals and medicines.* Johannesburg: Paper Books.

HARRÉ, R. (1990). Language games and the texts of identity. In J. Shotter and K. J. Gergen (Eds.), *Texts of identity* (pp. 20–35). London: Sage.

JOFFE, M. G. (1993). *Stories about stories about stories from death row: Post-traumatic stress disorder*

revisited. Unpublished MA dissertation, UNISA, Pretoria.

JUNG, C. G. (1963). *Memories, dreams, reflections.* London: Collins and Routledge & Kegan.

KATZ, S. H. and KIMANI, V. N. (1982). Why patients go to traditional healers. *East African Medical Journal,* 59, 170–174.

KEENEY, B. (1994). *Shaking out the spirits: A psychotherapist's entry into the healing mysteries of global shamanism.* New York: Station Hill Press.

KELLY, J. G. (1986). Context and process: An ecological view of the interdependence of practice and research. *American Journal of Community Psychology,* 14, 573–589.

KREINHEDER, A. (1980, Spring). The healing power of illness. *Psychological Perspectives,* 11, 9–18.

KVALE, S. (1992). *Psychology and postmodernism.* London: Sage.

LEATT, J., KNEIFEL, T., and NURNBERGER, K. (1986). *Contending ideologies in South Africa.* Cape Town: David Philip.

LEVINE, M. and PERKINS, J. (1987). *Principles of community psychology: Perspectives and applications.* New York: Oxford University Press.

LIFSCHITZ, S. (1988). The story of the cave. In G. Mason and J. Rubenstein (Eds.), *Family therapy in South Africa today.* Pinetown: Robprint.

LIFSCHITZ, S., VAN NIEKERK, S., and KGOADI, B. (1991). Three views of psychotherapy. In G. Mason, J. Rubenstein, and S. Shuda (Eds.), *From diversity to healing.* Pinetown: Robprint.

LIFSCHITZ, S. (1996). *Agape Healing Community video: Crisis, culture and transformation.* Pretoria: UNISA.

LYOTARD, J. F. (1984). *The postmodern condition: A report on knowledge.* Manchester: Manchester University Press.

MAIR, M. (1990). Telling psychological tales. *International Journal of Personal Construct Psychology,* 3, 121–135.

MANN, P. A. (1978). *Community psychology: Theories and applications.* New York: The Free Press.

MAGODIELO, T. D. H. (1994). *A psychotherapy clinic in the township: Exploring the concept of community.* Unpublished MA dissertation, UNISA, Pretoria.

MANKAZANA, E. M. (1979). A case for the traditional healer in South Africa. *South African Medical Journal*, 1003–1007.

MCCULLOCH, J. (1995). *Colonial psychiatry and 'the African mind'*. New York: Cambridge University Press.

MCNAMEE, S. (1992). Reconstructing identity: The communal construction of crisis. In S. McNamee and K.J. Gergen (Eds.), *Therapy as social construction* (pp. 186–199). London: Sage.

MEYERHOFF, B. G. (1976). Balancing between worlds: The shaman's calling. *Parabola*, 1, 6–13.

MIGERODE, L. (1992). Mamelodi: Verhaal van een ontmoeting in Afrika. *Tijdschrift voor Familietherapie*, 2.

MJOLI, Q. T. (1987). The role of the psychologist in culturally diverse South Africa. *Development Southern Africa*, 4, 7–19.

MUTWA, C. V. (1964). *Indaba, my children*. Johannesburg: Blue Crane Books.

MUTWA, C. V. (1986). *Let not my country die*. Pretoria: United Publishers International.

NELL, V. (1989). One world, one psychology: 'Relevance' and ethnopsychology. *South African Journal of Psychology*, 20, 129–140.

OOSTHUIZEN, C. J. (1995). From visiting to co-creating communities: I. A conceptual map. *The Social Work Practioner Researcher*, 8(4), 279–288.

OOSTHUIZEN, C. J. (1997). From visiting to co-creating communities: II. A case report. *The Social Work Practioner Researcher*, 10(1), 70–79.

ORFORD, J. (1992). *Community psychology: Theory and practice*. New York: Wiley.

PARKER, I. (1990). Discourse and power. In J. Shotter and K. J. Gergen (Eds.), *Texts of identity* (pp. 56–69). London: Sage.

PARRY, A. (1991). A universe of stories. *Family Process*, 30, 37–54.

PRICE, R. H. (1989). Bearing witness. *American Journal of Community Psychology*, 9, 1–26.

PRIGOGINE, I and STENGERS, I. (1984). *Order out of chaos: Man's new dialogue with nature*. London: Heinemann.

RICOEUR, P. (1991). Life in quest of narrative. In D. Wood (Ed.), *On Paul Ricoeur: Narrative and interpretation* (pp. 20–33). London: Routledge.

RORTY, R. (1982). *Consequences of pragmatism*. Minneapolis: University of Minnesota Press.

ROSENAU, P. M. (1992). *Post-modernism and the social sciences: Insights, inroads and intrusions*. Princeton: Princeton University Press.

SEEDAT, M. and NELL, V. (1992). Authoritarianism and autonomy. I. Conflicting value systems in the introduction of psychological services in a South African Primary Health Care System. *South African Journal of Psychology*, 22, 53–75.

SOMÉ, M. P. (1993). *Ritual: Power healing and community*. Portland: Swan/Raven.

SONNLEITNER, M. W. (1987). Of logic and liberation: Frantz Fanon on terrorism. *Journal of Black Studies*, 17, 287–304.

SULLIVAN, H. S. (1953). *The interpersonal theory of psychiatry*. New York: Norton.

TRICKETT, E. J. (1984). Toward a distinctive community psychology: An ecological metaphor for the conduct of community research and the nature of training. *American Journal of Community Psychology*, 12, 261–279.

VAN GENNEP, A. (1960). *The rites of passage*. Chicago: University of Chicago Press.

WETHERELL, M. and POTTER, J. (1992). *Mapping the language of racism: Discourse and the legitimation of exploitation*. New York: Harvester Wheatsheaf.

WHO STUDY GROUP. (1984). *Mental health care in developing countries: A critical appraisal of research findings*. Geneva: World Health Organization.

WITTGENSTEIN, L. (1958). *Philosophical investigations*. New York: MacMillan.

WOLFF, T. (1986). Community psychology and empowerment: An activist's insights. *American Journal of Community Psychology*, 14, 595–599.

ZIMMERMAN, J. L. and DICKERSON, V. C. (1994, Sept.). Using a narrative metaphor: Implications for theory and clinical practice. *Family Process*, 33, 233–245.

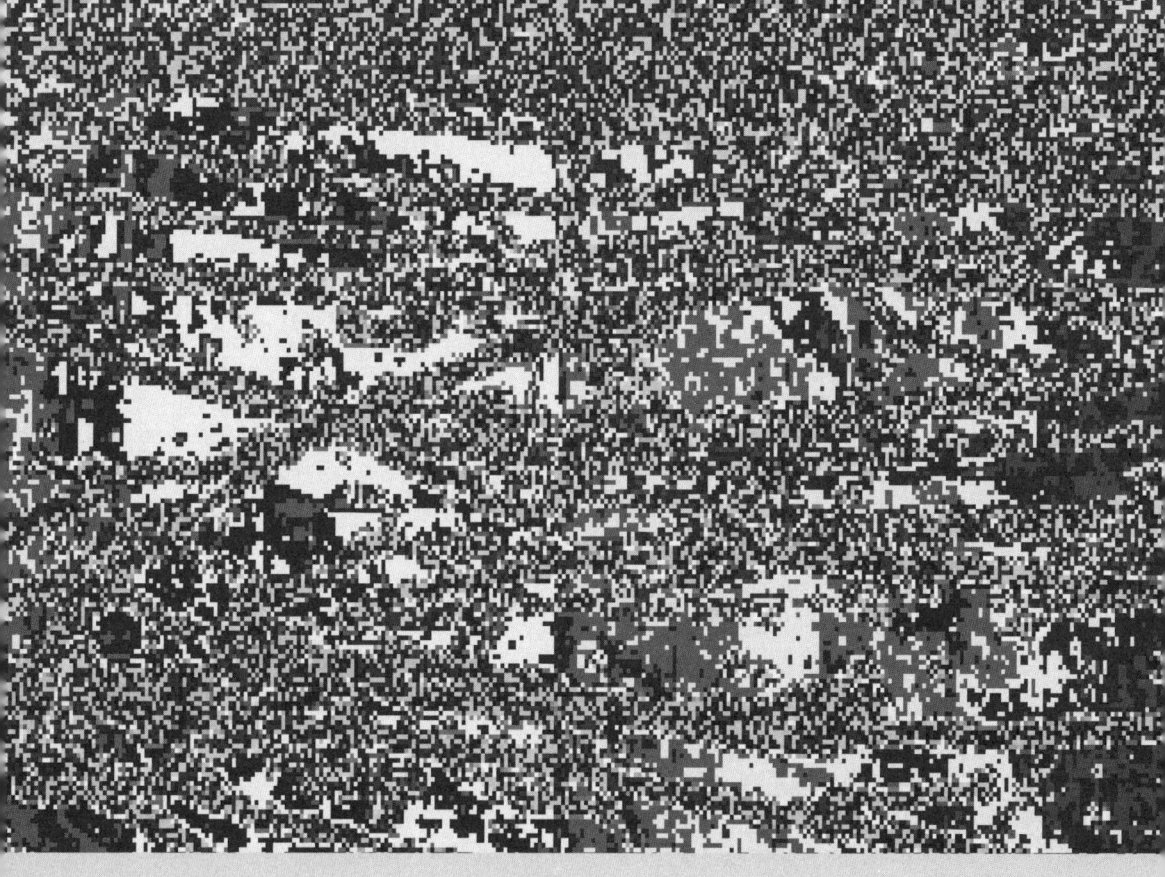

SECTION II

Methodological
considerations

8 Epistemological and methodological issues in community psychology

Arvin Bhana
Anil Kanjee

Study objectives

After reading and studying this chapter you should:
- be familiar with the concepts of science, research, methodology, and epistemology;
- be able to distinguish between the empiricist/positivist, hermeneutics/ interpretive, critical theory, and feminist epistemological positions;
- be able to identify the relationship between the various epistemological positions and qualitative and quantitative methodology;
- understand the relationship between community psychology and the various epistemological positions;
- be familiar with the research methods used in community psychology; and
- be able to apply and use relevant methodology for conducting community psychology research in South Africa.

1 Introduction

Community psychology as a discipline does not have a long history in South Africa. The methodological and research issues in community psychology that preoccupy researchers elsewhere, however, are no less salient in South Africa, as many of the methods used in psychology in South Africa derive from Western Europe and North America. Methods of conducting research in community psychology are influenced by the prevailing methods found in psychology in general, as well as more recent advances in this relatively new field.

Community psychology can trace its earliest roots to the group dynamics and decision-making processes of Kurt Lewin (1948) and the ecological theory of Roger Barker (1968). The ecological approach regards the relationship between the observer and the participant as the source for the construction of meaning about the phenomena being studied. Persons and systems, therefore, become understandable when they are examined as part of a multi-level, multi-structured, multi-determined social context.

Most often the research approach that is adopted is closely allied to the way in which the researcher chooses to understand communities and the way they function. For example, studying individuals in isolation from events or from the setting of the community is not the same as studying individuals from a holistic perspective. It is for this reason that approaches attempting to understand communities from a perspective based on systems and ecological thinking, and that integrates health, human resources, education, social interventions, citizen empowerment, and cultural values into one strategy, are favoured over a piecemeal approach to understanding communities. This integration recognizes the mutual adaptation and interdependence of individuals and social structures so that both individual and collective needs, as well as value orientations may be synergized (Holtzman, 1997, p.382).

This chapter examines the epistemological issues underlying research methodology and their relevance to community psychology. The assumptions underlying various perspectives are examined, including the research methodology associated with each of these. We believe that both qualitative and quantitative methods are important to community research endeavours, and so we argue for methodological eclecticism in community psychology research. The relationship between epistemology, methodology, and specific methods for conducting community psychology research in South Africa is also examined.

2 Epistemology and methodology

The primary purpose of conducting community psychology research is to obtain information in order to address and solve social problems. This central purpose begs the question: how does one do this? That is, what is the most relevant and applicable approach, method, or technique that a researcher should use to obtain relevant information to address specific social problems? Does the researcher merely collect information to highlight what the problems are and let the community find the solutions? Or does the researcher identify specific problems in the community and work towards developing and implementing solutions to these problems?

In addressing these questions we note two critical aspects. First, the information obtained, vis-à-vis the epistemology, and second, the specific processes used for obtaining such information, namely, the methodology. Critical to understanding both of the above aspects is making explicit: (1) the effect of the specific epistemological position, namely, the philosophy of how we know what we know; (2) the consequent methodology, which refers to the principles and procedures of enquiry; (3) the position of the researcher in the research process; and (4) the subsequent knowledge claims. This view is clearly articulated by Usher (1996b), who argues that:

any research, whether in the natural or social sciences, makes knowledge claims and for that reason alone is implicated in epistemological questions.

It could be argued that all research is based on an epistemology even though this is not always made explicit – in fact most of the time the epistemology that underlies a particular piece of research is taken for granted (p. 11).

Prilleltensky (1997) presents a useful overview of the values, assumptions, practices, and potential benefits and risks of some of the major epistemological positions in social science research (See Table 1 overleaf). Underlying each position is a fundamental question: 'Does (the) psychological approach promote the peaceful, respectful, and democratic process whereby citizens have meaningful input into decisions that affect their lives?' (Prilleltensky, 1997, p. 520). For example, the values that traditional approaches would promote are directed at individual needs, and not on making society more equal or fair (distributive justice), as is the case with emancipatory communitarian approaches to research.

3 Definition and purpose of research

The definition of research in the social sciences and the reason for conducting research differs among various researchers (Breakwell, 1995; Dane, 1990; Leedy, 1993; Vogt, 1993). This is evident in the many different conceptions of what constitutes social science research. Common to all these conceptions of research is the notion of research as a process that is (a) systematic and (b) obtains (new) information or knowledge.

In this chapter, research is defined as a systematic process used for collecting data and constructing new knowledge to impact on praxis towards community change. In this definition, three aspects need further clarification. First, there is the systematic process, which refers to the different methods and designs used for identifying and collecting data. The systematic process is what distinguishes social science research from other forms of 'conducting research' or knowledge creation, for example, experience, authority, deductive reasoning, inductive reasoning, tradition, common sense, and myth (Ary et al., 1990; Neuman, 1997). This process refers to the methodological aspects of conducting research (Harding, 1987; Guba and Lincoln, 1991).

Second, the construction of new knowledge, vis-à-vis the epistemological aspects, refers to the use of data collected to identify new information for the development of new knowledge and testing theory (Breakwell, 1995). According to Dane (1990) any information collected in any research process is generally used to: (1) identify the existence of any phenomena (exploration); (2) examine phenomena and more fully define them or differentiate them from other phenomena (description); (3) identify relationships between different phenomena to enable speculation about one thing by knowing about some other thing (prediction); (4) examine cause-effect relationship between two or more phenomena (explanation); and (5) address or solve social problems (action).

The third process is impacting community change, which suggests that the role of research in community psychology should

Table 1 Summary of values, assumptions, and practices
in four psychological approaches

DOMAIN	TRADITIONAL APPROACHES	EMPOWERING APPROACHES	POSTMODERN APPROACHES	EMANCIPATORY APPROACHES
VALUES	Promote caring and self-determination of individuals but neglect distributive justice. Major emphasis on helping individuals, not communities.	Promote human diversity and self-determination of individuals and of marginalized groups.	Promote human diversity and self-determination of individuals. Also concerned with collaboration and participation but has equivocal stance with respect to distributive justice.	Promote balance between self-determination and distributive justice. High degree of concern for well-being of individuals and communities.
ASSUMPTIONS	Based on scientific assumptions about knowledge. Good life and good society are based on value-free liberalism, individualism, and meritocracy.	View knowledge as tool for action research. Good life is based on ideas of personal control. Good society is based on rights and entitlements.	Emphasizes epistemological relativism and moral scepticism. Good life is associated with pursuit of identity. Assumptions informed by social constructionism.	Promote grounded knowledge in the service of moral values. Good life and good society are based on mutuality, obligations, and the removal of oppression.
PRACTICE	Problems defined in asocial- and deficit-oriented terms. Interventions are reactive.	Problems defined in terms of risk and disempowering conditions. Interventions are reactive and proactive.	Problems defined in terms of clients' constructions of their own circumstances. Clients encouraged to pursue their own identity.	Problems defined primarily in terms of interpersonal and social oppression. Interventions seek to change individuals as well as social systems.
POTENTIAL BENEFITS	Preserve values of individuality and freedom.	Address sources of personal and collective disempowerment.	Value the importance of identity, context, and diversity and challenges dogmatic discourses.	Promote a sense of community and emancipation of every member of society.
POTENTIAL RISKS	Victim-blaming and tacit support for unjust social structures.	Social fragmentation through pursuit of own empowerment at expense of others.	Social and political retreatism. Scepticism and lack of moral vision.	Denial of individuality and sacrifice of personal uniqueness for good of the community.

SOURCE: Prilleltensky, 1997, p.525

138

be to address real world problems that affect the community and to serve as an avenue for social action. Tolan et al. (1990) concur with this view and argue for research endeavours in community psychology to be grounded in applying sound methodology to wrestle with real world problems in order to develop alternative solutions for those problems.

All three aspects of this definition are dialectically linked and inevitably determine the outcome of the other. For example, the process by which information is collected impacts on the specific method/s used to collect information, which in turn determines the type of information collected, and the subsequent use made of this information. Similarly, the specific social action necessary to bring about some change will determine the specific knowledge required, which in turn will impact on the research process and methods that can be used to collect the required information.

The immediate question that the above discussion raises, especially within the context of community psychology, is: what should research in community psychology strive towards? Shadish (1990) argues that in order to carry out research directed at social problems in a practical and coherent way, community psychologists must address the following questions:

1   How does social change occur?
2   How is scientific knowledge used in social change?
3   What do we do about values and valuing?
4   What is going to count as knowledge?

There can be no single answer to any of these questions. One possible approach to addressing these questions in a pragmatic

way is to employ what Cook and Shadish (1986) refer to as theories of research practice. These theories provide practical advice about which questions to ask, which methods to use, and what roles the researcher should strive to fulfil. As an example, a useful theory might be one that states explicitly what its target group is and what specifically it claims to be able to change. It may be a theory that advises how to lower the incidence of cigarette smoking among adolescents through innovative educational material that discusses the harmful effects of tobacco. These questions may be addressed by examining the relationship between the research process, knowledge building, and knowledge use. However, in order to understand this relationship, it is important first to understand the various epistemological positions that underlie and guide the research process, and that impact on the outlook and world view of the researcher.

4 Relationship between epistemology and the research process

There are many assumptions that guide psychologists in their research. These assumptions are critical in shaping what we study since they determine how we study it, the questions we ask, and what value or importance we assign to the many elements that we discover in our research. It is therefore always important to know what assumptions we are making before we embark on any research. Making our philosophical assumptions explicit encourages a better understanding of multifaceted phenomena in community psychology. By neglecting to make these assumptions explicit, researchers run the risk of endorsing assumptions that they may not consider to be valid or appropriate to research in community psychology.

4.1 The research process

Two fundamental aspects of the research process are the specific techniques used and the specific procedure/s followed to investigate some subject or phenomenon. Harding (1987) notes the former as method, defined as the techniques for gathering evidence, and the latter as methodology, defined as the theory and analysis of how research should proceed. Guba and Lincoln (1991), and Williams and May (1996) also regard methodology as the more practical branch of the philosophy of science that deals with the methods, systems, and rules for the conduct of enquiry.

4.2 Epistemology

Epistemology is the branch of philosophy that is concerned with the structure and function of knowledge. Thus, epistemologists are concerned with how we know what we know, and how the perceptions, ideas, and knowledge that they have constructed are related to the reality to which they refer. Harding (1987) notes that epistemology also answers questions about who can be a 'knower', what kinds of things can be known, and what constitutes legitimate knowledge.

5 Major epistemological positions

In this section, four epistemological positions relevant to social science research are discussed. These are the empiricist/positivist, hermeneutic/interpretative, critical theory, and feminist positions. Of necessity, discussion of each of these positions can only deal with the broad principles that characterize them. In discussing the various epistemological positions, the following format is used: first, a brief discussion outlining the basic propositions of each position is presented; next, the specific method applied within each position is noted, and finally, the specific problems associated with each of the positions are presented.

5.1 Empiricist/positivist position

The oldest and most dominant epistemological approach within the field of social science research is the positivist position, generally referred to as positivism (Castells and De Ipola, 1976; Neuman, 1997; Robinson, 1993; Usher, 1996b). The positivist position argues that all knowledge is based on observation and measurement that is systematically and methodically applied. In this process, the researcher is seen as an objective, unbiased, value-neutral individual who ensures that personal consideration does not intrude on the research process. Thus, the researcher's subjectivity is supposedly eliminated as a factor in claiming knowledge. The methods and designs of the natural sciences are regarded as the only way of collecting and analysing information and thus constructing new knowledge. Therefore, a clear separation between science and 'non-science' knowledge is possible, and scientific knowledge is regarded as truth. Thus:

> knowledge of observable reality obtained using our senses is superior to other knowledge (e.g. intuition, emotional feelings); it allows us to separate true from false ideas about social life (Neuman, 1997, p. 66).

To qualify as true knowledge, all explanations and new information must meet three criteria: (1) it must be new or logical and without contradiction; (2) it must be consistent with observable facts; and (3) it must be replicable or reproducible. Constituted in this manner, positivistic research ignores the role of context in understanding phenomena. The traditional model of scientific knowledge in its search for 'facts' tends to reduce explanations of human behaviour to elementary phenomena rather than to more complex processes. Positivism tends to assume that these elementary phenomena are universal and can be used to understand similar phenomena in other contexts. The goal of positivistic science, then, is to isolate singular causes of events or phenomena (Mitroff, 1983; Popper, 1968). Within current practice of social science research in general, and psychology in particular, the positivist position is the most dominant position (Neuman, 1997). According to Usher (1996b), this dominance has had two main consequences. First, in the social sciences and in social research a pre-eminent place has been accorded to the production of knowledge based on discovering facts and formulating theory in terms of generalizations. Second, the language, methods, and quantification of the natural sciences has simply been adopted in social and educational research and used as the 'only' model for all research. However, this aspect is being seriously challenged by other emerging epistemological positions, as outlined below.

5.1.1 Methods applied by positivist researchers

In terms of practice, the positivist position is firmly entrenched within the quantitative paradigm. The specific research methods employed thus include surveys and experiments. The quantitative paradigm is regarded as:

> an inquiry into a social or human problem based on testing a theory composed of variables, measured with numbers, and analysed with statistical procedures in order to determine whether the predictive generalisations of the theory hold true (Cresswell, 1994, p. 2).

In the experimental method, the basic aim is to identify causal relationships between the variables under investigation. The researcher is usually able to manipulate at least one variable to study its effect on the other variable. Data is generally selected through some sampling procedure to ensure randomization, and analysis usually involves the use of one or more statistical techniques. Theoretically, all or most of the variable/s between the manipulated variables and the outcome/s are controlled. These studies are conducted either in a laboratory or a natural setting, and usually involve small samples. In the survey method, the basic aim is to describe the population under investigation using information obtained from asking people questions. Information is collected using questionnaires, telephone interviews, and different types of tests, or a combination of these. Typically, this method involves a large number of people who are identified using various sampling techniques. The data collected is in the form of numbers, and analysis usually involves the use of one or more statistical techniques to make sense of the data. Key concepts used in the quantitative paradigm include reliability, which refers to consistency of measurement; validity, which indicates appropriateness of measures; and replication, which outlines the ability to repeat the process.

5.1.2 Shortcomings of the positivist position

Some of the main shortcomings associated with the positivist position include the following:

1 The natural sciences model is viewed as the sole model of knowledge generation.
2 People are reduced to numbers, as the main emphasis of the positivist position lies with abstract laws and formulas that are not relevant to the actual lives of people. The experiences of people and the meanings that they attach to phenomena are completely overlooked. This is especially problematic in multicultural and multilingual communities

that are common throughout South African society.

3 The claim of researcher neutrality in the research process ignores the reality that all humans, including researchers, are socially constructed and that all knowledge produced is always influenced by the social interest of the researcher. Thus in South Africa it was virtually impossible for psychologists to work in oppressed communities without questioning the atrocities of the apartheid regime.

4 The positivist position is unreflexive, because it concentrates exclusively on methods and outcomes, and fails to ask any questions about the research process itself.

5 In the South African context the positivist position tends to promote a disempowering relationship between researcher and participant in all research interactions with or within communities, since, in practice, the academic emphasis on the scientific model as the basis of all knowledge generated typically excludes a significant number of the community from participating in any project as equals.

5.2 Hermeneutic/interpretive position

The hermeneutic position is based on the assumption that all human action is meaningful and has to be interpreted and understood in the context of social practice. Thus, human action can only acquire meaning among people who share the same meaning system that permits them to understand any interaction as socially meaningful and relevant (Neuman, 1997; Robinson 1993; Usher, 1996b). For example, the action of a teenager standing in the street with his or her hand raised and clutching a stone can only acquire a significant meaning if interpreted in the context that it occurs. A raised hand clutching a stone would be interpreted very differently when aimed at a row of tin cans than if it would be aimed at a group of people wearing military uniforms. In order to explain the social world, the researcher has to understand the meanings that construct and are constructed by interactive human behaviour. Thus, the researcher has to interact with the participants to get to know the particular social setting, share in the feelings and interpretations of the people being studied, and see things through their eyes.

Knowledge is concerned not with generalizations, prediction, and control but with interpretation, meaning, and illumination (Usher, 1996b). Unlike positivism, which assumes that everyone shares the same meaning system, the hermeneutic position acknowledges that people experience social and physical reality differently. In this context, facts are regarded as fluid and embedded within a meaning system of people; they are not impartial, objective, and neutral (Neuman, 1997). This, however, causes a major problem for researchers, especially in relation to the idea of objectivity. To address this problem researchers make use of the concept of 'bracketing', which requires them to reflect on, re-examine, and analyse their personal views and feelings, and to identify how this would impact on the research process. Researchers are thus able to set aside personal views and feelings that may affect the research process. Usher (1996a), however, argues that personal feelings and views should not merely be acknowledged but should be used as a starting point for acquiring additional knowledge. The applicability of this approach in a complex community environment, however, is open to debate.

5.2.1 Methods applied by hermeneutic researchers

The methods used within the context of the hermeneutic position are strongly associated with a qualitative paradigm of research (Brannen, 1992; Bryman, 1984). The primary assumptions of the qualitative paradigm (Crabtree and Miller, 1992; Cresswell, 1994; Guba and Lincoln, 1991; Neuman, 1997) include three key components:

First, researchers are concerned primarily with the process rather than the outcomes or products. Thus, research is more descriptive in adequately conveying meaning and understanding of the data. Second, the focus of the research is on the meaning that people attach to their lives and experiences. Third, the researcher is the analytical instrument. Thus data is mediated through human instruments instead of questionnaires or tests.

The methods used typically include interviews and fieldwork, or both, field notes from participant observation studies, discourse analysis, or archival material (Henwood and Pidgeon, 1993). These methods are typical of research approaches such as participatory action research, discourse analysis, ethnography, content analysis, and narrative analysis.

5.2.2 Shortcomings of the hermeneutic position

Some of the shortcomings associated with the hermeneutic position include:

1   An over-emphasis on the interpretation and understanding of people's lives and not enough on changing oppressive social conditions (Usher 1996b). This is especially problematic for communities where the need for social action is greater than that for obtaining additional information or understanding issues.

2   The lack of generalization of findings, since, typically, the methods used apply to specific individuals or groups; thus questions of whether findings apply to other groups or communities are not addressed.

3   The high level of subjectivity leaves serious doubts as to whether research outcomes actually reflect 'reality' or the researcher's perception of reality. This is a complex issue that is extremely difficult to address in the South African context for two main reasons. First, the complex composition of most communities in terms of race, language, culture, and socio-economic status; and second, most researchers typically come from backgrounds different from the socio-economic, racial, and cultural background of the communities that are in most need.

4   The methods used typically alter the behaviour of the group under study, and thus it is not known whether the researcher can ever record information as it naturally occurs. This issue is further complicated by the complexities within communities, and between communities and researchers.

5   The assumption that everything is relative and that nothing is absolute, and that any viewpoint is true for all those who believe in it (Neuman, 1997) can be problematic since it allows for the justification of many different perceptions, which can retard positive social action in the interests of communities.

5.3   The critical theory position

A key aspect of the critical theory position is its emphasis on detecting and unmasking beliefs and practices that limit human freedom, justice, and democracy in order to enable people and communities to change their lives. This is clearly articulated by one writer who defines critical theory as:

> a critical process of inquiry that goes beyond surface illusions to uncover the real structures in the material world in order to help people change conditions and build a better world for themselves (Neuman, 1997, p.74).

The goal of research in critical theory is the empowerment of individuals so that the causes of powerlessness are understood, the oppressive forces acting on individuals and communities are recognized, and the ability of people to change the conditions of their lives is enhanced. For Usher (1996a) this implies that the knowledge claims made by researchers should be emancipatory, should involve the unmasking of ideologies that maintain the status quo, and should promote the raising of consciousness or awareness about the material conditions that oppress or restrict people. By definition, critical theory has to involve praxis, which in this context implies informed and committed action. Unlike the positivist and the hermeneutic positions, both of which are regarded as being detached and only concerned with studying the world instead of acting on it, in critical theory there is no neutral or disinterested perspective. Everyone is socially located, and therefore any new knowledge produced will always be influenced by social interests. As Usher (1996a) argues, knowledge is always socially constructed and therefore always related to either a technicist interest, a communicative 'practical' interest, or a critical 'emancipatory' interest.

Contrary to the hermeneutic position, the issue of objectivity is not a dilemma since the goal of research is to address social problems of the community. In their work, researchers are thus expected to promote specific positions so as to achieve these goals. Objectivity is not regarded as a matter of having the 'right' methods but of having the 'right' arguments and of being prepared and able to subject them to the scrutiny of critical dialogue (Usher, 1996a).

5.3.1 Methods applied by critical theory researchers

Critical theory researchers regard the dichotomy between the qualitative and quantitative paradigms as false (Morrow, 1994), and thus use methods associated with both paradigms. The specific methods used are determined not only by the particulars of the research problem at hand but also by the needs articulated by the community. To this end, an eclectic approach, discussed in the next section, seems most appropriate. However, action research and the historical-comparative method tend to be the favoured methods (Neuman, 1997; Robinson,1993).

5.3.2 Shortcomings of the critical theory position

1 One of the major shortcomings of the critical theory position is its self-proclaimed commitment to the emancipation of people. As Usher (1996b) argues, conducting research in and for communities does not necessarily translate into communities wanting to 'emancipate' themselves. This is an especially sensitive issue in South Africa where communities have been denied the basic right to determine the direction of their own lives. When viewed in the context of the complex interactions of race, language, and socio-economic status in the research process and their impact on communities, the potential for marginalizing the very persons intended to benefit from the research intervention is very likely.

2 An additional shortcoming is that researchers require a thorough understanding of the social, economic, and political realities of communities in which research is conducted, since the outcomes of the research process can have significant negative consequences. Ideally, researchers who themselves are members of the specific community would possess the level of understanding required for adopting a critical theory

position. At this point in the South African context, however, this is highly unlikely owing primarily to the lack of adequately trained and experienced researchers from communities that stand to benefit most from such interventions, namely poor, rural, black communities.

5.4 Feminist position

While many differences exist among feminist researchers, four common themes are identified in the literature (Alcoff and Potter, 1993; Bozalek and Sunde, 1994; Harding, 1987; Hammersley, 1992; Jayaratne, 1993; Mies, 1993; Neuman, 1997; Usher, 1996a).

First, since gender is regarded as a crucial issue in all aspects of life, feminist researchers argue that it has to be taken into account in any research that is conducted. Bozalek and Sunde (1994) note that a common theme of feminist research is the social construction of gender as a central focus of social enquiry. The emphasis here is also on the correction of the male-oriented perspective that has dominated the development of social science.

A second theme is the emphasis on the subjective experiences of women. Neuman (1997) notes that feminist research is based on a heightened awareness that the subjective experience of women differs from an ordinary interpretative perspective. Harding (1987) strongly supports this view and notes that a distinctive feature of feminist research is that it generates its problems from the perspective of women's experiences. In this context, it is the personal experiences of women that are taken as an indicator of the reality against which hypotheses are tested.

The rejection of the hierarchical relationship between researcher and researched person is the third common theme of feminist research. The research relationship is viewed as a reciprocal one in which the views of both the researcher and the researched are open to interrogation. To achieve a shared or collective response to research with those that they study, Usher (1996a) notes that researchers need to form relationships that allow for those who are researched to express for themselves what is significant in their everyday lives. At the same time, researchers are included in the research process, as it is recognised that the beliefs and behaviours of the researcher also significantly affect the research process. As one researcher explains:

> the class, race, culture and gender assumptions, beliefs, and behaviours of the researcher her/himself must be placed within the frame of the picture that s/he attempts to paint (Harding, 1987, p.9).

The fourth theme relates to the goal of research. The central goal for many feminist researchers is not only the production of knowledge but also action towards the emancipation of women. As Mies argues:

> the contemplative, uninvolved 'spectator knowledge' must be replaced by active participation in actions, movements and struggles for women's emancipation (Mies, 1993, p.69).

5.4.1 Methods applied by feminist researchers

Similar to critical theory researchers, feminist researchers also use all methods and reach into various disciplines. Jayaratne (1993) argues that when used appropriately, both qualitative and quantitative methods in the social sciences can prove effective in achieving the goals of feminist researchers. In this respect, an eclectic approach seems highly applicable.

not follow one style or set of ideas

5.4.2 Shortcomings of the feminist position

Some of the main shortcomings associated with the feminist position are:

1 Priority is given to gender over other, sometimes more relevant variables such as race, ethnicity, and language. In the context of South African communities, especially, the issue of race and socio-economic status are critical factors that must be taken into account in any research process, since these factors not only define but may also determine the existence of many communities.
2 An overemphasis on the experiences of women over method. This problem is similar to that faced by researchers working in the hermeneutic position.
3 The emphasis on emancipation has similar problems as those noted for the critical theory position.
4 The role of males in adopting a feminist position has not been adequately addressed. In the South African context this issue is especially problematic owing to the low representation of qualified and experienced female researchers.

5.5 Relevant position/s for South Africa

The positions that we would like to promote in South Africa are those that emphasize social change. This is especially relevant in the current post-apartheid dispensation where a great deal of emphasis is being placed on the transformation of social, economic, and political institutions, organizations, and practices. To this end, both the critical theory and feminist positions are applicable. Both these positions provide relevant frameworks for community psychology researchers to address the rigorous demands of conducting research and generating knowledge, as well as meeting the needs of communities. In addition, both positions advocate an eclectic approach to the use of research methods.

5.5.1 Methodological eclecticism

The position taken in this chapter is that any research method most suitable for a specific purpose and context (whatever the paradigmatic origin), and which has a relevant practical application, should be used. Hammersley (1996) refers to this approach as methodological eclecticism. When used together, qualitative and quantitative data provide enriching information, and serve as verification for information that is obtained through one paradigm on its own (Leedy, 1993). Typically in practice, the purpose of the study, the nature of the data, and the problem for research dictate the research method applied. A simple rule is that if data is verbal, the method is qualitative, whereas if data is numeric, the method is quantitative. The question, however, about who decides on the nature of the data to be collected or the focus of the problem remains unresolved. For example, in planning an intervention programme for addressing the AIDS epidemic in a community, a quantitative approach would involve identifying the number of people with AIDS and where they are located. A qualitative approach, however, would examine the conditions under which people who have AIDS are living, while an eclectic approach would address both aspects noted.

Hammersley (1996) notes that methodological eclecticism takes three forms: triangulation, facilitation, and complementarity. The concept of triangulation provides one way to combine the qualitative and quantitative paradigms. Triangulation is defined as a:

> procedure designed to reconcile the two major methodologies by eclectically using elements from each of the major methodologies as they contribute to the solution of the problem (Leedy, 1993, p.145).

Triangulation is noted as a process that:

1 involves the use of several frames of reference or perspectives in the analysis of data;
2 attempts to obtain data through a variety of sampling strategies;
3 makes use of multiple observers, coders, interviewers; and
4 uses two or more methods of data collection procedures within a single study.

With the technique of facilitation, one method is used as an initial basis for the development of the research methodology.

For example, qualitative interviews can be used to generate hypotheses, or to ascertain what types of questions should be included in the survey. Later, additional information or greater meaning regarding some responses from a survey can be obtained from in-depth interviews with respondents.

In the technique of complementarity, two different methods are used to provide different types of data that complement each other. Hammersley (1996) notes that qualitative research is sometimes regarded as being better able to produce information about interactional processes and about participants' perspectives, whereas quantitative research is presumed to be better at documenting frequencies and causal patterns.

6 Epistemology, methodology, and community psychology research

In this section, the relationship between epistemology, methodology, and the selection of specific methods for conducting community psychology research is discussed. Included in this discussion is a brief comment on the research relationship itself. However, first the role of the community psychology researcher in the context of the relationship between the researcher and individuals, groups, or communities he or she studies, needs to be clarified.

6.1 Role of community psychology researchers

Community psychology has retained many of the characteristics of the traditional scientific model (Loo, Fong, and Iwamasa, 1988). However, as community research developed, various questions arose about the applicability of the philosophy, principles, and practices of traditional research to the problems and questions of interest to community psychology (Kingry-Westergaard and Kelly, 1990; Seidman, 1983). Shin (1990) observes that community psychology is an oxymoronic title because it deals both with community, vis-à-vis ecological contexts, and with psychology, a discipline that traditionally has concentrated on the individual. She writes:

> Although community psychologists may be concerned with relationships between settings or with effective functioning of groups or organisations as targets of research or intervention, we study these higher levels of analysis not just for their own sake but for their impact on individual well-being. Were we to lose this ultimate connection to the individual, we would cease to be psychologists; but when we confine ourselves to the individual level, we lose our community identity (Shin, 1990, p. 113).

There are no ready answers to this dilemma. For example, what epistemology will adequately account for the complexities and dynamisms of community phenomena? If a particular framework is used, how does it stand against competing frameworks or how will it take account of the individual-setting interaction? If collaborative research is meant to be a *sine qua non* of community research, then how should these relations be understood as part of what is being studied? If knowledge is socially constructed, that is, individuals understand their world through an interactive and reflexive process of interpretation, then how is the social context of knowledge to be understood? Indeed, if community psychology research is concerned with action in the world, then what is the relationship between action and knowledge? Given the traditional model's limited applicability, it follows, then, that the 'normal science' activity of incremental building of knowledge by a group of researchers, all working on a few big questions within a single, shared theoretical orientation, is an inauthentic description of community psychology, both now and in the future.

Community psychology itself has to grapple with developing creative ways for understanding the complexity of communities, as this is not easily addressed by a traditional model of scientific knowledge. Heller (1988) made the observation that despite the avowed claim of researching communities, community psychologists frequently remain primarily concerned with the study of individuals. He pointed out that for most community psychologists, community represents the location of their research rather than its focus. Hughes, Seidman, and Williams (1993) similarly argue that despite criticisms by community psychologists of social programmes and policies that do not take account of the social context of the populations, they appear to be unaware of the contradictions of using traditional research methodologies in their work. These observations reflect the tension between studying individuals in isolation from their context and researching the multiple layers and complexities of individuals enmeshed in particular social contexts.

The contextualist approach to community research is perhaps best captured by Shadish's (1986) concept of *critical multiplism,* which argues that every research method has its unique set of biases and that no single approach can provide an adequate understanding of human events. In short, each method is only partially valid in providing methodological answers to community psychology research. This includes the significant contributions made by feminist writers about the importance of including a distinctly female point of view (Harding, 1987; Hare-Mustin and Marecek, 1988; Jackson and Van Vlaenderen, 1994).

A key assumption underlying the research process in community psychology is that one is concerned with systemic variables. Systemic variables are variables that affect the community as a whole. Systemic variables tend to have large-scale effects, that is, they generate and influence opportunities for resources or constraints. Racism is one such systemic variable. Poverty is another. Kelly (1988) argues for the use of a systems perspective in research as it encompasses multiple levels of a phenomenon, emphasizing the interrelationships between the components involved.

> The use of the concept of system in understanding behaviour makes it possible for research topics to be investigated as multivariate phenomena. A systems perspective promotes awareness of the interrelationships between the components of a system

and thereby lessens the chance of the research investigator focusing upon any individual component or unit (Kelly, 1988, p.107).

Kelly (1988) points out that using the concept of a system not only increases the number of different variables relevant for analysis but also moves the research away from primarily psychological variables. Consideration can then also be given to those aspects that influence people's lives, such as economic, social structural, and physical environment variables. Importantly, by concentrating on systems, it is possible to examine available resources in other domains of a person's or community's life. How the parts of the system interact determines the processes by which an intervention will be absorbed or deflected. Richter and Griesel (1994), for example, noted in their study of South African children that infections adversely affect nutritional status while nutritional status affects vulnerability to and the severity of infections. Inevitably, a child's nutritional status is related to conditions of poverty. This double hazard is suffered by almost one-third of all African, coloured, and Indian children below the age of fourteen years in South Africa (Hansen, 1984). One response of the new South African government has been to address children's nutritional status through its school-feeding schemes. Nevertheless, at some stage it must inevitably take into account poverty as the underlying issue contributing to the nutritional status of children.

According to Heller et al. (1984), the role of community psychology researchers should be to research the issues and problems that are stimulated by the community, to use research as a tool for social action, to yield products that are useful to the community, and to evaluate the effects of change on the individual or group. Thus the primary purpose of community psychology research should be to meet community needs. However, Heller et al. (1984) argue that researchers have contributed little to communities in return for the studies they conduct with and in communities. These authors acknowledge that the role ascribed to researchers may cause conflict, especially among academics, where researchers value very highly the traditional role of detached scientist and the opportunity to test hypotheses and build theory. Community organizations and neighbourhoods, however, are relatively unconcerned with the world of theory; they value action taken to improve conditions that affect their daily lives (Heller et al., 1984).

From the above discussion it would seem that the implication for researchers working in the context of community psychology is very clear: select the methodology that meets the needs of the communities. Even within this context, however, a great deal of flexibility is available to researchers. Whether the decision is to use a positivist, hermeneutic, critical theory, or feminist perspective, the epistemological position of the researcher inevitably affects not only the research process but the consequences of that process as well.

6.2   The research relationship

Since community psychology emphasizes non-hierarchical partnerships, it is inevitable that questions of resources and power differences will emerge. Researchers inevitably have power and better access to resources, which bring about inequalities between them and the population concerned. However, community psychologists have tended to pay lip service to the notion that research relationships must be horizontal. Some community psychologists believe that there should be no differences between researcher and participants (Brown and Tandon, 1983; Gruber and Trickett, 1987). Bond (1990) argues that this is a dishonest portrayal of real differences in power and resources between researcher and participant. She argues that research relationships are not horizontal, that is, based on equity, but are characterized by power differences. Seedat, Cloete, and Shochet (1988) point out similarly that the differences in skills between researcher and participant will not disappear by simply declaring that one is one of the people, since the skills differentials will still be in place.

Given these real differences, the researcher has a great responsibility. Bond (1990) argues that the researcher must work toward a 'respectful, mutually beneficial relationship' (p. 185) by actively questioning what participation means, developing mutual respect, recognizing and acknowledging power differences, and maintaining the focus of research on the social problem rather than on the individual *per se*. One distinct way that researchers in community psychology have articulated the research relationship is in terms of an empowerment agenda. This means that the researcher should be guided by a commitment to:

identifying, facilitating, or creating contexts in which heretofore silent and isolated people, those who are 'outsiders' in various settings, organisations, and communities, gain understanding, voice, and influence over decisions that affect their lives (Rappaport, 1990, p.52).

(This subject matter is more fully discussed in Chapter 9 by Kelly and Van der Riet.)

6.3 Selecting appropriate research methods

Only once the above issues have been adequately addressed can the researcher select the appropriate research method. In terms of the eclectic approach, any method/s appropriate to addressing the objectives of the research study can be used for obtaining information.

Other factors (Duffy and Wong, 1996; Heller et al., 1984) that may influence the selection of methods when conducting community psychology research include:

1 How much is already known of the phenomenon in question, that is, is the study an exploratory study to gain greater insight into a new phenomenon?

2 What are the practical and ethical constraints confronting the researcher? Can the study be conducted without informing participants of the purpose of the study but without contaminating the outcome, and thereby violating the rights of communities?

3 What are the researcher's objectives in conducting the study? Is it to obtain information to facilitate transformation, or is it meant to test a specific hypothesis?

4 What level of analysis is appropriate for the phenomenon under study, that is, at the individual, group, or organizational level?

5 What is the level of co-operation from the communities involved in the study?

6 What is the time frame within which the study has to be completed?

Research methods

The various methods commonly used in community psychology research include the following:

1 Correlational research, which provides information on the association or relationship between two or more variables (Leedy, 1993).

2 Quasi-experimental research, which allows the researcher to conduct studies in real life situations where the researcher is able to manipulate some independent variable but cannot randomly assign subjects to experimental or control groups (Orford, 1992).

3 True-field experimental research, in which the researcher conducts the study in a natural setting and is able to manipulate some independent variable and randomly assign participants to different groups, for example in a school setting (Rosnow and Rosenthal, 1996).

4 Ethnographic research, which includes any method that describes social or cultural phenomena based on direct systematic observation, for example, becoming a participant in

the group under investigation (Vogt, 1993).

5 Epidemiology studies, which includes research that deals with the occurrence and distribution of disease and other health-related conditions in human populations (Duffy and Wong, 1996).

6 Action research is regarded as a methodology where the researcher moves from the role of a chronicler of social activity to that of an agent of social change. Key features of an action research approach is that it is participatory, practical, emancipatory, interpretative, and critical in its approach. (See Chapter 9 by Kelly and Van der Riet.)

7 Needs assessment is a systematic process of obtaining specific information necessary for making decisions for bringing about positive change as desired by the majority.

8 Case study method involves gathering and analysing data about an individual example. This is a way of studying a broader phenomenon, on the assumption that the 'case' is in some way typical of the broader phenomenon. The case may be an individual, an event, a community, or any other possible object of analysis.

9 Programme evaluation entails research using any of several methods designed to test the effectiveness or impact of a social programme or intervention.

7 Research and community psychology in South Africa

This section deals with a few issues specific to community psychology research in South Africa. Research practices in general, and social science research in particular, especially for the generation and use of knowledge, are intricately linked to dominant ideologies (Neuman, 1997; Scot and Usher, 1996). In South Africa, this has meant that research practices were primarily used for the promotion and the maintenance of the status quo, especially under the apartheid regime (Appel, 1989; Bulhan, 1993, 1981; Muller and Cloete, 1986; Savage, 1981; Webster, 1982). Thus researchers have had an extremely negative impact on the development of communities, primarily because community psychology research studies have failed to promote or advance a social action agenda. Community psychology has also been criticized for failing to adequately theorize the relationship between the individual and society (Seedat, Cloete, and Shochet, 1988). Arguably, Seedat, Cloete, and Shochet (1988) contend that community psychology does not go far enough in challenging socio-political and economic realities that disempower individuals, groups, and societies. They claim that community psychology has instead lowered its sights to helping groups and communities to have greater control over their lives.

Despite general acknowledgement that the social and political milieu has markedly influenced developmental outcomes for millions of South African children, the bulk of psychological research in this country is skewed away from this issue. It is claimed that apartheid policy has in fact normalized the racist and exploitative structure of South African society (Dawes and Donald, 1994). The task of community psychology is to refocus and re-energize our research agenda around systemic influences, including poverty, racism, and sexism, that shape much of our lives. Included in this call is a need to develop theory and practice relevant to the context and circumstances of South Africans (Berger and Lazarus, 1987; Seedat, Cloete, and Shochet, 1988). This is perhaps the biggest challenge that face researchers in South Africa today.

South Africa is a complex society, and research practices that fail to acknowledge these complexities are bound to provide solutions that are short-term or temporary. For example, the complexity of a community is hinted at in the work of Dawes and Donald (1994), who ask the simple question: 'Why do so many African children drop out of school in South Africa?' The research response first has to understand historical and structural inequalities introduced into the education system by apartheid policies. Poverty is a key factor in the type and level of education African school children received during the apartheid years. The ability of families to feed, clothe, and educate their children has been compromized by the low education and skill levels of parents and further eroded by their inability to secure long-term employment that ensures a steady income. In such an instance, the methodology employed would most likely use both quantitative (surveying the extent of the problem) and qualitative approaches (how they understand their own problems and how they could possibly change them).

8 Conclusion

Community psychology research is difficult to do, probably for the reason that it requires more than being an expert researcher. Likewise social change is a difficult endeavour, especially when scarce resources require a greater willingness from community psychologists to engage in research practices that are empowering.

In seeking empowering partnerships with participants, the skill, ingenuity, and integrity of the researcher will no doubt be tested. A crucial aspect for any researchers doing research in a community psychology setting is therefore to ensure that they are aware of some of the fundamental assumptions made in the research process and the likely impact that these assumptions may have on the communities in question. While the critical theory and feminist positions appear to be relevant in addressing the needs of disadvantaged South African communities and for working towards social change, even these approaches need to be examined for their appropriateness within and across specific community contexts.

Given South Africa's past, there is a desperate need for researchers to turn their attention to issues such as poverty, violence, and racism. This is likely to be an appropriate beginning for developing theoretical frameworks and intervention approaches that explain the relationship between the individual and society in all its complexity. While the critical and feminist positions may be offered as powerful models for social change, it is within the context of working with South Africa's diverse communities that new epistemologies should be developed. A model that empowers and contributes to new understandings of old problems may be a strong incentive for collaborative research. Local knowledge and local practice are critical to improving the fit between theory and practice.

Exercises

1 A major problem currently affecting your community is the poor matriculation results. As someone with some research expertise, you are approached by the school governing board for assistance to address this problem.
2 Organize yourselves into groups of at least four to discuss how you would approach this request. Each person should specifically select one of the epistemological positions noted in this chapter. Each member should present to the rest of the group how he or she would approach this problem from a specific epistemological position. Identify the various methods that you would use, and list the various issues that could influence you/your team as community psychology researchers.
3 After the various positions have been presented, identify, if possible, the 'best' position to adopt in addressing the issue at hand.

References

ALCOFF, L. and POTTER, E. (1993). *Feminist epistemologies.* New York: Routledge.
APPEL, S. W. (1989). Outstanding individuals do not arise from ancestrally poor stock: Radical science and the education of black South Africans. *Journal of Negro Education, 58,* 544–557.
ARY, D., JACOBS, C. L., and RAZAVIEH, A. (1990). *Introduction to research in education.* Florida: Holt, Rinehart and Winston.
BARKER, R. G. (1968). *Ecological psychology: Concepts and methods for studying the environment of human behaviour.* Stanford, CA: Stanford University Press.
BERGER, S. and LAZARUS, S. (1987). The views of community organisers on the relevance of psychological practice in South Africa. *Psychology in Society, 7,* 6–23.
BOND, M. A. (1990). Defining research relationship: Maximizing participation in an unequal world. In P. Tolan, C. Keys, F. Chertok, and L. Jason (Eds.), *Researching community psychology: Issues of theory and methods.* Washington, DC: American Psychological Association.
BOZALEK, V. and SUNDE, J. (1994). Shaking off the textbook paradigm: The value of feminist approaches in the research curriculum. *Perspective in Education, 15,* 69–82.
BRANNEN, J. (1992). Combining qualitative and quantitative approaches: An overview. In J. Brannen (Ed.), *Mixing methods: Qualitative and quantitative research* (pp. 3–38). England: Ashgate Publishing.
BREAKWELL, G. M. (1995). Research: Theory and methods. In G. M. Breakwell, S. Hammond, and C. Fife-Schaw (Eds.), *Research methods in psychology* (pp. 5–15). Newbury Park, CA: Sage.
BROWN, D. L. and TANDON, R. (1983). Ideology and political economy in inquiry: Action research and participatory research. *Journal of Applied Behavioural Science, 19,* 277–294.
BRYMAN, A. (1984). The debate about quantitative and qualitative research: A question of methods or epistemology. *The British Journal of Sociology, 35,* 75–93.
BULHAN, H. A. (1981). Psychological research in Africa: Genesis and function. *Race and Class,* xxiii(i), 25–41.
BULHAN, H. A. (1993). Imperialism in studies of the psyche: A critique of African psychological research. In L. J. Nicholas (Ed.), *Psychology and*

oppression: Critiques and proposals (pp. 1–34). Johannesburg: Skotaville.

CASTELLS, M. and DE IPOLA, E. (1976). Epistemological practice and social sciences. *Economy and Society,* 5, 111–143.

COOK, T. D. and SHADISH, W. R., JR. (1986). Program evaluation: The worldly science. *Annual Review of Psychology,* 37, 193–232.

CRABTREE, B. F. and MILLER, W. L. (1992). *Doing qualitative research.* Newbury Park, CA: Sage.

CRESSWELL, J. W. (1994). *Research designs: Qualitative and quantitative approaches.* Thousand Oaks, CA: Sage.

DANE, F. C. (1990). *Research methods.* Pacific Grove, CA: Brooks/Cole.

DAWES, A. and DONALD, D. (Eds.). (1994). *Childhood and adversity: Psychological perspectives from South African research.* Cape Town: David Philip.

DUFFY, K. G. and WONG, F. Y. (1996). *Community psychology.* Boston: Allyn and Bacon.

GRUBER, J. and TRICKETT, E. J. (1987). Can we empower others? The paradox of empowerment in the governing of an alternative public school. *American Journal of Community Psychology,* 15, 353–371.

GUBA, E. and LINCOLN, Y. (1991). What is the constructivist paradigm? In D. Anderson and B. Biddle (Eds.), *Knowledge for policy: Improving education through research* (pp. 158–170). New York: The Falmer Press.

HAMMERSLEY, M. (1992). Deconstructing the qualitative-quantitative divide. In Brannen (Ed.), *Mixing methods: Qualitative and quantitative research* (pp. 39–56). England: Ashgate Publishing.

HAMMERSLEY, M. (1996). The relationship between qualitative and quantitative research: Paradigm loyalty versus methodological eclecticism. In J. T. E. Richardson (Ed.), *Handbook of qualitative research methods* (pp. 159–174). Leicester: The British Psychological Society.

HANSEN, J. (1984). *Food and nutrition policy with relation to poverty: The child malnutrition problem in South Africa.* Second Carnegie Inquiry into Poverty and Development in Southern Africa, Paper No. 205. Cape Town.

HARDING, S. (1987). Introduction: Is there a feminist method? In S. Harding (Ed.), *Feminism and methodology* (pp. 1–14). Bloomington: University of Indiana Press.

HARE-MUSTIN, R. T. and MARECEK, J. (1988). The meaning of difference: Gender, theory, postmodernism and psychology. *American Psychologist,* 43, 455–464.

HELLER, K. (1988). *The return to community.* Invited address presented to the division of community psychology at the 96th annual meeting of the American Psychological Association, Atlanta, GA, August 1988.

HELLER, K., PRICE, R. H., REINHARZ, S., RIGER, S., and WANDERSMAN, A. (1984). *Psychology and community change: Challenges of the future.* Chicago, IL: The Dorsey Press.

HENWOOD, K. L. and PIDGEON, N. F. (1993). Qualitative research and psychological theorizing. In M. Hammersley (Ed.), *Social Research: Philosophy, politics and practice* (pp. 14–32). Newbury Park, CA: Sage.

HOLTZMAN, W. H. (1997). Community psychology and full-service schools in different cultures. *American Psychologist,* 52(4), 353–371.

HUGHES, E., SEIDMAN, E., and WILLIAMS, N. (1993). Cultural phenomena and the research enterprise: Toward a culturally anchored methodology. *American Journal of Community Psychology,* 21, 687–704.

JACKSON, C. A. and VAN VLAENDEREN, H. (1994). Participatory research: A feminist critique. *Psychology in Society,* 18, 3–20.

JAYARATNE, T. E. (1993). The value of quantitative methodology for feminist research. In M. Hammersley (Ed.), *Social research: Philosopy, politics and practice* (pp. 109–123). Newbury Park, CA: Sage.

KELLY, J. G. (1988). *A guide to conducting prevention research in the community: First steps.* New York: The Haworth Press.

KINGRY-WESTERGAARD, C. and KELLY, J. G. (1990). A contextualist epistemology for ecological research. In P. Tolan, C. Keys, F. Chertok, and L. Jason (Eds.), *Researching community psychology: Issues of theory and methods* (pp. 23–31). Washington, DC: American Psychological Association.

LEEDY, P. D. (1993). *Practical research: Planning and design* (5th ed.). New York: Macmillan.

LEWIN, K. (1948). *Resolving social conflicts.* New York: Harper & Row.

LOO, C.; FONG, K., and IWAMASA, G. (1988). Ethnicity and cultural diversity: An analysis of work published in community psychology journals, 1965–1985. *Journal of Community Psychology, 16*, 332–349.

MIES, M. (1993). Towards a methodology for feminist research. In M. Hammersley (Ed.), *Social research: Philosophy, politics and practice* (pp. 64–82). Newbury Park, CA: Sage.

MITROFF, I. (1983). Beyond experimentation: New methods for a new age. In E. Seidman (Ed.), *Handbook of social intervention* (pp. 163–177). Beverly Hills, CA: Sage.

MORROW, R. A. (1994). *Critical theory and methodology.* London: Sage.

MULLER, J. and CLOETE, N. (1986). *The white hands: Academic social scientists, engagement and struggle in South Africa.* Paper presented at the XIth World Congress of Sociology, New Delhi, India.

NEUMAN, W. L. (1997). *Social research methods: Qualitative and quantitative approaches* (3rd ed.). Boston: Allyn and Bacon.

ORFORD, J. (1992). *Community psychology: Theory and practice.* Chicester: Wiley.

POPPER, K. R. (1968). *The logic of scientific discovery.* New York: Harper.

PRILLELTENSKY, I. (1997). Values, assumptions, and practices: Assessing the moral implications of psychological discourse and action. *American Psychologist, 52*, 517–535.

RAPPAPORT, J. (1990). Research methods and the empowerment social agenda. In P. Tolan, C. Keys, F. Chertok, and L. Jason (Eds.), *Researching community psychology: Issues of theory and methods* (pp. 51–63). Washington, DC: American Psychological Association.

RICHTER, L. and GRIESEL, R. (1994). Malnutrition, low birth weight and related influences on psychological development. In A. Dawes and D. Donald (Eds.), *Childhood and adversity: Psychological perspectives from South African research* (pp. 66–91). Cape Town: David Philip.

ROBINSON, V. (1993). *Problem-based methodology: Research for the improvement of practice.* Oxford: Pergamon.

ROSNOW, R. L. and ROSENTHAL, R. (1996). *Beginning behavioural research: A conceptual primer.* Englewood Cliffs, NJ: Prentice Hall.

SAVAGE, M. (1981). Constraints on, and functions of, research in sociology and psychology in contemporary South Africa. In J. Rex (Ed.), *Apartheid and social research* (pp. 45–65). Paris: UNESCO Press.

SCOT, D. and USHER, R. (1996). *Understanding educational research.* New York: Routledge.

SEEDAT, M., CLOETE, M., and SHOCHET, I. (1988). Community psychology: Panic or panacea. *Psychology in Society, 11*, 39–54.

SEIDMAN, E. (Ed.). (1983). *Handbook of social intervention.* Beverly Hills, CA: Sage.

SHADISH, W. R. (1986). Planned critical multiplism: Some elaborations. *Behavioural Assessment, 8*, 75–103.

SHADISH, W. R. (1990). Defining excellence criteria in community research. In P. Tolan, C. Keys, F. Chertok, and L. Jason (Eds.), *Researching community psychology: Issues of theory and methods* (pp. 9–20). Washington, DC: American Psychological Association.

SHIN, M. (1990). Mixing and matching: Levels of conceptualization, measurement, and statistical analysis in community research. In P. Tolan, C. Keys, F. Chertok, and L. Jason (Eds.), *Researching community psychology: Issues of theory and methods* (pp. 111–126). Washington, DC: American Psychological Association.

TOLAN, P., KEYS, C., CHERTOK, F., and JASON, L. (Eds.). *Researching community psychology: Issues of theory and methods.* Washington, DC: American Psychological Association.

USHER, R. (1996a). Feminist approaches to research. In D. Scot and R. Usher (Eds.), *Understanding educational research* (pp. 120–142). New York: Routledge.

USHER, R. (1996b). A critique of the neglected epistemological assumptions of educational research. In D. Scot and R. Usher. (Eds.), *Understanding educational research* (pp. 9–32). New York: Routledge.

VOGT, W. P. (1993). *Dictionary of statistics and methodology*. Newbury Park, CA: Sage.

WEBSTER, E. (1982). The state, crises and the university: The social scientist's dilemma. *Perspectives in Education*, 6, 1–13.

WILLIAMS, M. and MAY, T. (1996). *Introduction to the philosophy of social research*. London: UCL Press.

9

Participatory research in community settings: processes, methods, and challenges

Kevin Kelly

Mary van der Riet

Study objectives

By the end of this chapter you should have:

- examined the unique characteristics, processes, methods, challenges, and problems associated with the conduct of social research in community settings;
- read about the emergence of the Participatory Research (PR) approach;
- found out what is distinctive about this approach;
- examined the core processes and methods of PR;
- explored some of the difficulties involved in conducting PR; and
- developed a critical understanding of the approach.

1 Emergence of the participatory research approach

Central to the participatory research (PR) approach is the careful maintenance of an ongoing relationship between social researchers and community representatives, in the interests of assisting the planning and implementation of transformation processes aimed at meeting community needs, alleviating problems, and facilitating community development. In this chapter, after describing the emergence of participatory research as a distinctive paradigm and outlining the foundational characteristics of the paradigm, we explore the challenges of doing participatory research in societies in democratic transition. We then go on to describe three broad processes in the interaction between researchers and communities. Some unique methods are described that have been developed specifically for facilitating these processes in community research settings. The chapter includes reference to some of the challenges and problems involved in doing research in and with communities. Some of these problems are understood to present unsolved and ongoing challenges to the development of the participatory research paradigm.

1.1 The participatory research movement

A scientific paradigm may be understood as a comprehensive system for gaining knowledge of the world, whereby is prescribed the way in which information of the world is gathered, organized, and interpreted. In 1981, Peter Reason and John Rowan published a collection of essays that brought together ideas from a number of different, emerging fields under a common banner, which became known as new paradigm research. They defined it as follows:

> New paradigm research involves a much closer relationship than that which is usual between the researcher and the researched: significant knowledge of persons is generated primarily through reciprocal encounters between subject and researcher, for whom research is a mutual activity involving co-ownership and shared power with respect both to the process and to the product of the research (Reason and Rowan, p. 489).

In the community development field the term participatory research at about the same time became the rallying point of the new paradigm, and was used to refer to an emerging approach to research that involves a close, collaborative working together of researchers and those who are the subjects of study. In the field of community development the term PR has been defined thus:

> We have used the term (participatory research) to emphasize the necessity to involve those persons who are the supposed beneficiaries of research in the entire research process. We are specifically talking about the participation of the working classes, the peasants, the exploited and the poor in an analysis of their own reality (Hall, Gilette, and Tandon, 1982, pp. 7-8).

The methods used in participatory research are designed to bring the researcher to understand the specific qualities of a given context or person and the experiences, issues, and problems that are unique to that context or person. The emphasis is on the term 'understand', and participatory researchers in community settings interact, listen, observe, reflect, and question with a view to gaining an insight into what it is like to be a member of a particular community or to be in a particular kind of situation. Understanding in this sense means to gain knowledge of a person's life or a community's situation as if you are the other person or community you are trying to understand; that is, from their point of view. Understanding from the point of view of being in that situation, as one of them, or being the other person, is sometimes termed empathy.

PR involves a fundamental accountability of the researcher to the way in which a community understands itself and its problems, but the participatory researcher is also committed to developing the self-understanding of the community in ways that did not exist prior to the PR intervention. So the goal is not simply to show people what they already understand or to lead them to an expression of needs that they are already aware of. The goal of the research goes

160

beyond this. It is to extend self-understanding in ways that did not previously exist. It will be shown how participatory researchers do this by using their position as skilled outsiders to develop the capacity of communities to think about their problems in new ways, which allow for new kinds of social action on the part of communities.

In PR the method of enquiry is usually conceived of as being a dialogue between researcher and community. The researcher as an outsider enters into a process of dialogue with the community and this dialogue is a research process; that is, it is a form of research that occurs in the context of a relationship between different parties, and is characterized by the exchange of views and reciprocal interaction.

The approach of PR is a challenge to the idea of the researcher being neutral and uninvolved. PR is explicitly engaged in bringing about change; it is done for a social purpose, rather than only to find out about something. Thus PR on women's issues may be done specifically in order to empower women or solve their problems. Thus the research is seen as part of a social process or project.

Before going further in describing what PR entails, it is necessary to pause and examine the term participation and its centrality in the community development and health fields.

1.2 Participation in the community development and health fields

Theories and strategies of development have historically promoted the expansion of physical and economic resources in the context of increasingly centralized planning and control over the distribution of resources (Coetzee, 1987). This so-called modernization approach emphasized the stimulation of economic growth and production, and it was supposed that the development of resources in the economic system as a whole would result in the eventual spread of benefits to the nooks and crannies of the system. This approach has gradually been superseded and it is now fairly widely recognized that modernization has not been successful as a strategy of development in the countries with developing economies. Recently theorists have challenged the idea that the injection of resources into an otherwise unchanged system would necessarily lead to development and there appears to be much evidence to support the refutation of this approach (Korten, 1990; Rahnema, 1990).

Proponents of the more recently emerging 'people-centred development' paradigm have adopted an alternative strategy for development. This approach sees development as a process whereby members of a society increase their personal and institutional capacities to mobilize and manage resources. This is intended to lead to sustainable improvements in the quality of life that are consistent with the peoples' own aspirations (Korten, 1990). People-centred development calls for people to be involved in decisions about development interventions and the implementation thereof (Brown, 1985). Community participation in the determination of priorities, identification and allocation of resources, and the selection of problem-solving strategies lies at the heart of this approach to development (Brown, 1985; Erasmus, 1992).

There are numerous definitions of 'participation' to be found in the literature on development. Cohen and Uphoff (1977) describe participation as people's involvement in decision making about what should be done and how, in implementation of the project, in sharing in the benefits of a project, and in evaluation of the project. In reality one would not usually expect to find all members of a community involved in all aspects of the project, and it is more usual to find that the majority of a community only enjoy the benefits of the project. Cohen and Uphoff (1977) maintain that in examining how participation occurs in a particular project, consideration should be given to (a) where the initiative starts (from above or below), (b) what inducements for participation are involved (how voluntary or coerced it is), (c) the structure, and (d) the channels of participation. Furthermore, they suggest that consideration should be given to (e) duration and (f) scope of participation.

The issue of participation has also become a central concept in the context of community health projects. Through the development of the 'primary health care' (PHC) movement, a need to understand what the notion of participation means has emerged. Participation has been described as the cornerstone of PHC (Kasege, 1991) and is referred to in the founding document of PHC, the Alma Ata Declaration, which was adopted by the World Health Organization in 1978. A clause in the declaration reads: 'The people have the right to participate individually and collectively in the planning and implementing of their health care.' In this respect the PHC approach

to development is an elaboration of the 'people-centred development' approach and is set against the 'modernization' equivalent in the health terrain, an historically profession-led, top-down approach to health planning and service delivery. Rifkin (1986) reviews over 200 case studies of PHC projects and suggests a classification of health projects according to different forms of participation involved. She suggests that there are three broad approaches to community participation in health projects: (1) the formal health system reorients itself towards providing more accessible professional services to a community, which involves little direct community participation; (2) projects adopt a specific health services orientation that involves direct community consultation about their health services; (3) an approach that sees health as inseparable from living conditions and control over resources. This approach involves a comprehensive strategy of community development in which community self-reliance is a key element.

The various attempts to involve communities in expressing their needs and finding their own solutions inevitably require the meeting of funders, developers, and governments with the people. Standing in between these stakeholders are the researchers and facilitators who practice PR.

2 Cornerstones of participatory research in community settings

Apart from PR involving an ongoing relationship between researcher and community, which has the qualities of a dialogue, there are two other fundamental ideas in PR that set it apart from other research models, and give it the status of a distinctive paradigm. All three of these characteristics may be present in research that does not deliberately support the participatory ethos, but in PR they are the very foundation of the research process. We will now go on to discuss the second and third of these under the headings 'Praxis: research as action' and 'Research as empowerment'.

2.1   Praxis: research as action

In the paradigm of the scientific experiment the effects of the experimenter's presence would typically be controlled so that the object of research could be seen as it would be were the researcher not present. Under ideal conditions the researcher would have little or no effect on what is observed. To a certain extent researchers are able to overcome the effects of their own presence, that is, to overcome a phenomenon that is known in the context of experimental work as experimenter effects. However, those promoting PR have argued that it is ultimately not possible to overcome such effects and that we should acknowledge the effects and see them as inevitable, so that they can at least be taken into account. They have shown that even the asking of questions of a person can make the person think differently about a situation and thus have a reflexive effect. The term 'reflexive' is used here to refer to the way in which the process of conducting the research can have an impact upon the context of that research. The understanding and theories that we develop through

research also have a reflexive effect in that they influence how we see the options for action that are available.

Participatory researchers eagerly accept that research is reflexive. They recognize that the theories that are developed in research and the self-understanding that communities and individuals develop through processes of self-enquiry have an effect on the actions they are likely to take. Participatory researchers then harness reflexivity and use it as an instrument of change. The word praxis is often used to describe the circular relation between understanding and practice. Praxis may be defined as a form of social intervention that is at one and the same time an idea and an action. Because ideas about social life offer certain kinds of possible solutions and exclude others, they are also invitations to act in certain ways and not to act in others. When an individual or community is involved in trying to analyse its own problems, the participatory researcher sees the work of understanding and analysing as the beginning of a path of action. The importance of this to the PR process will become more evident later in the chapter when we discuss the development of critical perspectives in PR, and particularly in the discussion of the work of Paulo Freire.

2.2   Research as empowerment

In the development field it is generally understood that the need for development in a community follows from a situation where that community lacks access to the ability to mobilize resources to develop in a desired direction. The community may have become alienated from the resources that are needed in order for it to develop. The nature of such alienation invariably involves marginalization of the community from the means of exercising power in the political, economic, technical, and intellectual arenas. In general the need for PR is thus motivated by the need to bring about some form of co-operative action between a community and an outside resource or agent, in the hope of improving the conditions of existence of the community. It is not surprising, therefore, that the term 'empowerment' and the term 'participation' are so closely interwoven (Kieffer, 1984; Swift and Levin, 1987; Werner, 1988). Indeed, participatory processes are usually conceived of as a means to developing a community in such a way that the community begins to participate more actively, in one way or another, in tasks and benefits associated with access to resources and increased decision-making power. This implies, according to Freire (1972), a changing relationship between those who have been historically dominant and those who have been marginalized from the exercise of power. It is surprising, therefore, that more has not been written about the relational dynamics between participants in development projects. There is a lack of literature dealing with how participatory relationships are formed and sustained between parties who are grossly different in terms of access to skills, resources, education, political power, and the sense that their own individual efforts can make a difference. The participatory researcher stands between funders, developers, and governments on the one hand and communities on the other; and attempts through research pro-cesses to assist the community to mobilize itself to a point of being able to overcome its own marginalization and to assume positions of greater power. Participatory researchers see one of their primary tasks as identifying the inherent capacity of people in terms of what resources and skills they have and what capacities they lack in the process of bringing about their own development. Following this, participatory researchers envisage the development process as necessitating engagement in a community building process, which involves the acquisition of new capacities for action, a process known as capacity building. Capacity building, which can take many forms (Van Vlaenderen and Gilbert, 1992), 'enables' people to participate actively in development processes and usually entails some form of skills enhancement. This can mean many different things, ranging from training in skills for proposal writing, workshop facilitation, and literacy, through management and administration skills. It would also typically involve developing the capacity to be aware of problems. The last of these is a central focus in the Freirian method, which will be discussed below. Under optimal conditions of community building one would expect to find an increased involvement of those who previously did not have the capacity to participate actively in all phases of participatory project development.

It is common to hear community researchers express frustration at the lack of engagement on the part of the community. Paulo Freire (1972) speaks of apathy as a characteristic of communities who have come to accept that their situation is unlikely to change in any meaningful way. The challenges to communities in South Africa in the post-apartheid era have called on different skills and capacities than were needed in the fight against apartheid. Building of capacity to contribute meaningfully to the process of reconstruction and development has become of foremost importance in PR in South Africa. However, community researchers face a dilemma between doing the work of capacity building and demonstrating concrete progress to funders. It is helpful for participatory researchers in such circumstances to realize that capacity-building is progress and that real progress is in any case determined at the community end of the PR relationship, and not at the researcher's end.

It is in this sense that the building of capacity is both a means and an end in community development. It is a means insofar as it is necessary in order to assist a community in engaging with existing resources and mobilizing development resources and activities. It is an end insofar as the enhancement of the capacity to develop is actually the desired outcome. In the people-centred approach, development is seen as being achieved by the community itself, rather than delivered to the community by an outside agency. Thus speaking, development can be seen as a process, and not a product that can be passed from one group of people to another. To the extent that a community develops the capacity to develop itself, the function of those agencies that attempt to seed or initiate development is gradually diminished. Chesler (1991) describes the need to mobilize consumer activism in health care through the medium of self-help groups. The effectiveness of self-help groups, or any other community-based health interest groups, in bringing about meaningful change in the health system is dependent upon their organizational and communicative capacity (the ability to communicate their needs effectively in the hallways of power) to engage in dialogue at a level where structural changes in the health system can be brought about. In development projects this is often a problem. It often happens that, as projects move beyond the initial needs assessment phase, the community whose needs have been assessed becomes increasingly disengaged from project activities, because they often do not have the capacity to engage in project planning beyond expression of their needs.

It is arguable that not all development projects require the same degree of capacity building. In the health field, for example, it is necessary to distinguish between projects that involve a comprehensive process of community health development, and those that are more task specific or 'selective' in orientation (Rifkin and Walt, 1986; Foster, 1982). In the latter case the specific objectives of the development process are pre-determined. In the former case the initial objectives are very general and oriented towards facilitation of a comprehensive process of community development. Following Kieffer (1984) and Korten (1980), such comprehensive processes of community development always require capacity building, and this takes time, perhaps years. For participatory researchers this may also mean doing research that is not in their field of research. Participatory researchers need to balance their own needs for order, structure, and planning with the realities of how needs are shaped and developed during the PR intervention.

As much as participatory researchers might want to have egalitarian relationships with communities where there are no power differences between themselves and the communities they work with, in reality they do have a greater capacity and hence more power at many different levels. In the following section we discuss these power differentials and in so doing we will introduce a problem inherent to the PR model, which needs to be carefully thought about.

3 Dialogue and participation in the transition context

In the process of rapid democratic transition, as in South Africa, there may occur a pressure for equally rapid transformation of existing public services through 'community participation' in the planning and implementation of new services. The recent history of South Africa is such that within a matter of a few years only, the idea of community participation in political and social processes has replaced a system of unilateral, government-dominated public service policy formulation and implementation. Having evolved over such a short period of time, attempts at increasing community participation have accentuated the difficulties involved in the co-operative working together of parties who are grossly different in terms of their relative capacities to engage in planning and implementing new service programmes. The 'transition' situa-

tion also typically involves the working together of people who were, until fairly recently, deeply committed to political struggle rather than co-operation. The history of this struggle and the legacy of the past inevitably continue to cause a degree of suspicion and mistrust and will arguably do so for some time to come. These factors militate against the development of shared understanding and co-operative action, and there is a need for greater understanding of how these problems undermine community development initiatives, and how they can be overcome.

In PR there is a strong need to take into account the context out of which a project emerges. The 'context' may involve the history of previous encounters with participatory researchers or other experts, as well as the broad socio-political history of the society. For example, in South Africa certain kinds of institutions, such as hospitals, continue to be seen as places of power and élitism, and initiatives arising out of these institutions are likely to be regarded with suspicion in some communities. A research process should always be understood as being situated or embedded in a larger process, which will have an effect on factors such as motivation and trust.

Frequent reference to the 'dialogical model' of communication can be found in the participatory development literature, which suggests a similarity between the concepts of 'participation' and 'dialogue'. 'Dialogue' is seen as a kind of communication context that enables participation. The problem with this model is that it sees dialogue as a 'means' through which participation should proceed, but in reality the community development situation almost implies that at the outset there will be different capacities for engaging in dialogue amongst participants. This is obviously more apparent in situations of sudden transition, such as may be found in recently democratized countries.

Habermas (1984) suggests that dialogue requires an equality of participatory capacity and in our opinion this makes problematic the use of the term 'dialogue' to refer to the 'means' of community development, where the capacity for engaging in the participatory process is inevitably less for some of the participants; that is, where 'partners' differ greatly in terms of access to legitimate and dominant modes of participation. Habermas's (1984) 'theory of communicative action' outlines the 'speech conditions' that are likely to lead to dialogue. These conditions refer to communication contexts where there is no domination of the dialogue by one of the participants to the dialogue, or by one of the perspectives represented, and there is an equality of discursive opportunity between participants. By 'discursive opportunity' is meant the opportunity and capacity of participants to express themselves effectively in the context of the communicative exchange.

Often it seems that people have equal opportunities, but there are deep structural reasons why they are not in fact equal. Such reasons may include certain ways of speaking enjoying more legitimacy in the context. So language that seems more educated, or more ordered, or more in keeping with professional, academic, and scientific standards may overshadow other ways of speaking, which then do not enjoy the same kind

of influence. This means that certain voices remain marginalized, unless these people get someone to speak for them. The capacity for communicative engagement is one that is not easily learned because it is largely a product of education and experience, and this means that capacity building for effective communication is not easily achieved.

Schrijvers (1991), in an article entitled *Dialectics of a dialogical ideal*, is somewhat pessimistic about the possibility of dialogue in development contexts. She outlines the difficulties involved in bringing about dialogue in the context of two participants wielding different degrees of power in a research situation. She suggests that dialogical forms of communication can be established most easily if there are only small power differentials in the research situation, a condition she describes as 'studying sideways' as opposed to 'studying down' or 'studying up'.

There are many other reasons why imbalances of power may be present and that would make 'studying sideways' difficult. Environmental and societal conditions under which PR takes place can have a significant negative impact on the relevance and effectiveness of a participatory initiative (see box on p. 168).

Freire (1972) provides a conceptual way of overcoming the problem of using dialogue as a method in a context where dialogue is not easy to establish. He suggests that dialogue is both a 'means' of communication and a 'goal' towards which communication strives; that is, it is both a method and a goal. To the extent that the context is 'anti-dialogical', or not conducive to dialogue (Freire, 1972), we might say that dia-

Factors influencing effectiveness and relevance of PR

- Lack of skills, available communication channels, and transportation infrastructures.
- Prevailing ideologies, which may be supportive or not of democratic procedures.
- Social stratifications that exclude certain people from taking leading roles (e.g., women in some communities).
- Deferential attitudes toward authority and beliefs opposing social equality.
- Historical factors where the people involved have had a previous experience of participation that was perceived to have had a negative outcome.

(Cohen and Uphoff, 1977)

logue is not a means so much as an ideal towards which participatory projects should strive.

It is exactly in those situations where dialogue is not easily attained that participatory methodology is usually proposed by funders as the most appropriate approach. Almost by definition development work requires joint action and decision making between partners who differ in their degree of familiarity with and access to dominant modes of participation, and hence in their 'capacity' to take an active role in participatory research and development initiatives.

This returns us to the earlier discussion of capacity building. If we are not to be naive in hoping to bring about dialogue between researchers and communities we should not assume that the community is empowered to participate in a dialogue about the development goal at the outset of the process. Many of the methods that follow are explicitly designed to build the capacity for dialogue; they are dialogue enabling. Furthermore PR processes should ideally be accompanied by education and training efforts that gradually improve the resources of the community so that they are more likely to be able to participate in an effective way in all aspects of the research process, including proposal writing, meeting facilitation, decision making, conflict resolution, administration, co-ordination, and management. But it should be remembered that lack of empowerment in these areas is often the reason for the community needing outside assistance in the first place, and properly designed PR processes will attempt to develop participatory or dialogical capacity as one of the fundamental objectives of a project.

The reader might consider whether participatory approaches are ways of coaxing oppressed communities into a world of technology, science, and 'Western democracy' that negates communities' 'indigenous' modes of decision making, advocacy, and action. This is a question well worth debating and one that is debated in the literature of PR. One response to this criticism might be to say that the ability to make one's needs known and have them responded to does require development of the capacities mentioned, but this does not necessarily negate the legitimacy of a community's own modes of doing things. Indeed, in good PR these action resources would be harnessed and would be fundamental to the action initiative. The South African struggle against apartheid attests to this. Oppressed South Africans achieved their ends using their own means. It is, however, worth considering whether a marginalized and isolated community in the rural Eastern Cape of South Africa would be as effective as a national movement with international support.

4 Processes and methods

4.1 Getting involved as a researcher

How does a participatory researcher generally engage with a community, in order to facilitate dialogue, empowerment, and reflexivity? One issue to consider in addressing this question is the gap that exists between academic and community settings. Most research projects use terms and follow conventions that are familiar to researchers but very foreign to the everyday life context of a community. The way in which a researcher bridges this gap is a key element in effective participatory engagement. The researcher needs to be attuned to a number of key communicative processes that, in more conventional research, are not considered at all. To make the shift to a participatory model, it is crucial for PR practitioners to engage in a process of self-reflection about their own role and behaviour in the research setting. In this section we will make explicit some issues that, when taken note of by the researcher, will significantly alter the researcher's behaviour in the research setting. It is these issues that affect the power relations in the research setting and will shift the power balances

towards a more dialogical ideal. It should, however, be remembered that the ideal in such situations is rarely attainable. It is rather an objective that is constantly striven for.

In examining how we set about establishing a satisfactory relationship between the researcher and the research context, it is useful to outline a framework for thinking about the ways in which researchers get involved in community contexts. As mentioned previously, Cohen and Uphoff (1977) argue that consideration should be given to where the initiative starts, from above or below, or from within or outside of the community.

It is useful to think in terms of three broad modes of initiation: (1) the researcher contacts members of a community; (2) the researcher is asked by an outside party (e.g., the government, a non-governmental organization, or a donor agency) to engage with the community; and (3)the community calls on a researcher to undertake research in the community. In addition, these modes of initiation are broadly linked to the researcher's motive for involvement. These might be mainly academic purposes (the first mode of initiation); to influence policy (mostly the second mode of initiation); or to engage in a learning, empowering, and conscientizing process (the second and third modes of initiation). By conscientizing we mean a process that allows the participants to see their situation and its problems, challenges, and potentials in a different way.

The PR approach is aligned with this last motive, in which the primary aim of the research is the development of individual capacity within the community to understand their life situation, and development of their own potential to take action to improve the quality of their lives. In the PR approach, participation implies that outside researchers and local participants are involved in a joint enquiry, an educational process, and a programme of action related to problems of mutual interest (Van Vlaenderen, 1993). Ideally all parties become learners, they share control over the research process, they commit themselves to constructive action as opposed to detachment, and their participation promotes empowerment as well as understanding (Brown, 1985). This may seem to imply that the researcher is the 'expert' conscientizer who has something to give the 'unschooled' community. This is not intended and we will presently describe how central the community's own knowledge and understanding of problems are to the entire process of PR.

Engagement of a researcher in a research project following the participatory model is a collaborative effort that would lead under optimal circumstances to increased participation by the community at all levels. Throughout the process the researcher endeavours to create a context for eventual withdrawal. The researcher's engagement in this is concerned with producing circumstances that prepare the community for independence. This is not an easy process to successfully achieve and there is always the difficulty that outside consultants, such as researchers, will result in a form of dependency. The degree of engagement and distance is an issue that should be held in consciousness by the PR practitioner at all times. Both of these qualities serve positive functions and both have negative consequences. Balancing distance and engage-

ment and keeping a dynamic tension between them is probably the greatest art involved in PR. Let us look at this in the process of gaining and maintaining access to the community; negotiating an understanding of and agreement to the objectives of the research; and negotiating the nature and results of the engagement with the community through the research process.

4.1.1 Gaining and maintaining access to the community

Thornton and Ramphele (1988) argue that communities are not homogenous entities. Communities have multiple subgroups, each with differing access to power and resources within the larger community. A common mistake is for the researcher to make contact with the most visible and articulate member or group of the community, but, they argue, 'visibility may serve as a strategic substitute for representation' (Thornton and Ramphele, 1988, p. 32). Chambers (1985) comments that it is easier for researchers to talk to people who are most like them: who are well educated, who speak their language, and who are confident and articulate. However, these individuals might not be truly representative of the community's interests. They might represent particular political interests, or they might represent only the youth, or the male members of a community. Contact with these individuals might create suspicion and mistrust of the researcher by excluded groups. Van Vlaenderen and Nkwinti (1993) comment that it is difficult to make an *a priori* assessment of local dynamics. An understanding of local dynamics will only come in time, through close co-operation with the community. Once the initial contact has been made, the researcher should encourage and ensure the participation of representatives of all groupings in the community, for example, women and the elderly.

This process, which can be called building and maintaining rapport with the community, must be seen as an ongoing process, and not only a preliminary stage of the research. In essence, this process entails a sensitive 'listening' to all views expressed by individuals in the community, whether these be verbal or shown in behaviour. It is time-consuming and requires patience and insight. For example, should numerous meetings with representatives from the community fail to take place, the researcher should attempt to understand why this is happening. Perhaps the community has not yet reached a consensus decision on an issue, and does not want to present an image of disunity to the researcher. Perhaps there are underlying tensions about the issue that is being researched, and no individual in the community is prepared to confront the researcher with these.

PR relies upon and builds on the capacity and legitimacy of local community organizations. Usually PR leads to the development of a project team consisting of representatives of the community, the researcher, and the developers. A difficulty may arise in such contexts where decisions are made that, although they might express the views of the project organization, do not necessarily represent the community and certainly not the range of views existent within the community. This problem of representation is very central to PR. In any situation where

people claim to be representing others, there is the possibility of misinterpreting the real needs of others or speaking on their behalf in ways that are less than accurate.

The PR practitioner can deal with these issues by continuously questioning the understanding that emerges as to its accountability to community opinion and particularly new and emerging bodies of opinion. This has to be balanced against a tendency of PR practitioners to want to get on with the business of implementation of a project and perhaps completion of their involvement. The dialogical process should never be laid to rest and should always be open to finding new directions and to being corrected. Kelly and Van Vlaenderen (1996) stress the need to encourage a culture of reflection upon dialogical processes in the context of developmental projects.

Researchers often believe that their research is of the same importance in the lives of the community members as it is in their own. It may happen that in a PR process, more pressing issues overshadow the community's interest in the PR process. There needs to be a sensitivity to the ongoing life process in the community. For example, members of a rural community might have to travel long distances to towns for pensions and salaries and therefore might be absent from the village during parts of the research process. In fact, paying attention to these local fluctuations in mood and availability often generates important, although informal, research data. It is this process that enables the researcher to 'get a feel' of the local dynamics of the situation, as well as the issues, tensions, and disagreements, which are important in the lives of

171

people in this community, but which might not otherwise be expressed to the researcher. The process of rapport building is often constrained by lack of time and financial resources. In conventional research it is usually considered as a peripheral activity, but in PR it is central and it is necessary that this process be budgeted for in the initial research proposal. Donors, unfortunately, are often reluctant to fund this stage of the research. Researchers in this paradigm need to motivate strongly to donors for support during this phase, representing this phase as a critical and integral part of the research.

4.1.2 Negotiating research objectives

A second crucial issue in laying the foundation for the development of trust and co-operative action, and one that is part of the rapport-building process, is *negotiating an understanding of, and agreement to, the objectives of the research for the community*. In a development research project reported by Van Vlaenderen and Nkwinti (1993), the researchers explained in a community meeting that they did not provide funds, but were tasked to assist the community to identify its needs and the priorities among them. The community debated this and was divided about the usefulness of co-operating with the researchers and unclear about what it expected from the researchers. The community requested time to discuss these issues amongst themselves. At a second meeting, the researchers facilitated a brainstorming session about the needs, problems, expectations, and questions of all participants and tried to clarify common themes extracted from the multitude of problems

and issues raised. Van Vlaenderen and Nkwinti (1993) reported that, although the process was very slow and difficult, it had the effect of making the community members feel 'listened' to and thus become more open to the process of engagement. It also helped the researchers to develop a more realistic picture of the development challenges in this context. Through engagement in this process the researcher develops a relationship with the community through which good participation is facilitated. This lays a solid foundation to the rapport between community and researcher and an opportunity to begin the process of capacity building.

4.1.3 Negotiating outcomes of the research

In addition to negotiating the objectives of the research, the researcher needs to *negotiate the nature and projected outcome of the community's engagement in the research process*. Researchers are frequently seen as better resourced than community members and the researcher needs to be careful not to raise expectations that cannot be met. This can be done by being explicit about what can be provided, and what the community members will have to provide for themselves. Being clear about the limitations of the outcomes of the research is also important.

4.1.4 Local knowledge

We now move on to examining what it is that the researcher should aim at in research in community settings. PR assumes that communities have well established *systems of knowledge and information, and carefully developed techniques of management and problem solving,* which have been their survival resource in harsh conditions (Van Vlaenderen, 1993). This local knowledge resource is the basis from which participants engage in the research process. This concept of local knowledge has its roots in new developments in cognitive psychological theory, which suggest that there are differences in the way people think as a result of their different socio-cultural contexts. This idea has historical roots in the theory of Russian psychologist Lev Vygotsky, who in the 1920s argued that all our higher mental functions, including our knowledge, skills, and strategies of survival, have social origins. This implies that expertise in managing the challenges and conditions of life in a particular context are rooted in that context. Gilbert (1995) argues that local knowledge is the *everyday knowledge of a community of practice; the collection of ideas and assumptions that are used in a community of practice to guide, control, and explain actions within the specific setting.* Eminent anthropologist Clifford Geertz (1983) argues that local knowledge can be understood as *common sense operating as a cultural system;* it is a body of colloquial wisdom.

In order for any research intervention to be well grounded, thorough, and within the grasp of a community's potential, there is a need to acknowledge and tap into the community's local knowledge resources. The researcher should initiate and play an active role in the process of accessing local knowledge, indigenous technologies, survival strategies, and resources, which will serve as a foundation for the development of an appropriate action plan. Exposing and building on indigenous knowledge and resources have two effects: it reduces the likelihood that a programme intervention will de-skill and undermine the local people and increase their dependency on external suppliers and experts; and secondly, it serves to highlight areas of values and beliefs that might be obstructing critical reflection on the part of the community about a particular problem. However, there is a corollary to this argument. The researcher, too, has a 'local' knowledge, one that makes researchers competent in their own setting. Researcher's engaging in processes requiring community participation should understand that their own ways of doing things and understanding things are no more intrinsically valuable or correct than the community's and should not be imposed by way of 'expert' advice or guidance. Marsden (1990), O'Dea (1985), Puckett and Reese (1993), Rogoff and Lave (1984), and Scribner (1986) are useful references on everyday cognition, local knowledge, and practical thinking.

4.1.5 Modes of engagement

The mode of engagement of the researcher is the third main component of laying the ground for the development of trust and co-operative action. We mention the modes of the researcher as activist and consultant, and explore more in depth the researcher as ethnographer.

A researcher may engage as an activist in a particular field, in which case the researcher will be quite forthright about the intention to change social conditions in a particular direction. Much feminist research has been conducted along these lines, where feminist researchers have engaged in research on women's issues, not as impartial researchers, but in order to facilitate change in a way that is most likely to be effective and to be in the interests of women. A consultant, on the other hand, would tend to be less driven by particular social causes and would become involved in order to impart skills or render services as a detached professional. There are wide ranges of ways in which researchers can get involved, and the way in which the researcher enters the context and engages with the different stakeholders cannot be strictly prescribed in ideal terms that cut across all situations. However, amongst the approaches to social science research that provide insight into the different possibilities of engagement, the one that is most noteworthy is the anthropological method of ethnography.

4.1.5.1 Research as ethnography

Spradley (1979) argues that ethnography is the 'work of describing a culture. The essential core of this activity aims to understand another way of life from the native point of view. . . . Rather than studying people, ethnography means learning from people' (p. 3). Within the ethnographic approach, there are a variety of techniques that allow the researcher to become the 'learner'; amongst these are 'going native' (directly experiencing what it is like to live as a native to that context), and cultivating the ability to ask naive questions, such as an apprentice would. However, a core principle in ethnography centres on the way in which the researcher is involved in the everyday activi-

ties of the community. This is not necessarily structured involvement. It could involve a 'listening survey'. This is not the traditional survey in which the researchers decide beforehand which facts they are going to find out about, and use very precise questionnaires. Rather, in this approach, the researcher listens primarily to unstructured conversations in which the community members feel relaxed and talk about things that they are most concerned about. This occurs in places such as markets, buses, homes, school playgrounds, shopping centres, and taverns. The researcher as ethnographer listens especially for feelings about meeting basic needs, relationships between people, community decision-making processes, education and socialization, recreation, and beliefs and values (Hope and Timmel, 1984). This means that research methods are adapted to the context of work and the researcher simply gets involved in such a way as to be maximally exposed to how the community functions at all levels.

In the tradition of ethnography, anthropologists conducting research go and live in the 'field', or the community setting. They immerse themselves in a setting, trying to remain as unobtrusive as possible, whilst observing how people perform their everyday activities. In this sense, whilst they participate in the activities of the community, they are also observers. For example, if the researcher wished to understand the role of women in a community, he or she would live in a home in the community for perhaps a few months, and make daily records of his or her observations of the activities and functions of women in a particular community of practice. In some PR approaches, participant observation involves becoming a participant. The researcher might ask to be taught the tasks that a woman does, in order to more fully understand them. More directed forms of enquiry are also part of the ethnographic approach.

Spradley (1979) refers to the use of the 'grand tour' type question – a questioning technique in which you ask the research subject to guide you through a familiar everyday activity. In the 'researching women' example, the researcher would meet with individual women in their work contexts and ask them to describe very generally what their jobs entail. A woman might identify particular tasks that she does each day, for example, collecting water or firewood, making meals, and looking after children. A 'mini-tour' question would be a more focussed question on something that arises from the 'grand-tour' response. For example, the researcher in an urban context might discover that some tasks a woman does are done collectively, like caring for children in informal playgroups. The researcher would then ask the woman to describe a typical day on which this is done: who is responsible for the children and why, where are they looked after, what do they do with the children? The researcher would pay particular attention to words and phrases that she uses, because it is these contextual terms, the 'slang' or colloquial terms of the woman, that will provide opportunities for insight into the meaning of the experience of being a woman in that context.

Spradley (1979) argues that 'the essential core of ethnography is (the) concern with the meaning of actions and events to the people we seek to understand' (p. 5). In the

process of being an ethnographer, the researcher becomes a learner, a student of the 'culture' of the research community. Ellen (1984) and Spradley (1979; 1980) are two excellent sources on the ethnographic approach.

So far we have highlighted the issues and methods in the process of getting involved with the community. A second aspect of processes and methods is that of fostering community involvement.

4.2 Fostering community involvement

There are two central tensions that need to be addressed in fostering community involvement. The one involves identification of a coherent, distinctive community; and the other concerns awareness of the inherent heterogeneity of communities. The challenge to PR is to involve all parts of the community in the research process, whilst acknowledging the stratifications within communities, and the different affiliations of sectors within the community.

Any community, in order to be a distinctive community, necessarily has some form of homogenous identity that makes it distinctive and sets it apart from other communities. Thornton and Ramphele (1988) argue that the term 'community' is used 'to denote aggregations of people who have something in common, such as a common residence, geographic region, and shared beliefs, or who claim membership in a common lineage structure, or who are distinguished by similarities of economic activity or class position' (p. 30). In a very well-defined community (e.g., the mentally ill or aged who live alone far from clinics in a particular community) it is relatively easy to outline the target community and its needs. Some communities are more homogenous than others and in doing research in such communities we would expect to be able to define what the community's needs are without having to encounter very many tensions or differences of opinion. Research in very specific communities is often like this.

However, coherent communities may also have considerable heterogeneity within their ranks. It is all too easy to overlook the complexities and tensions within a community in attempting to develop general statements that may be applied to the community as a whole. For example, in developing an understanding of the needs of the aged in a particular community, it would be easy to make general statements about this group and overlook, for example, the specific needs of the aged who are disabled or mentally ill, or to overlook the different needs of the married and the single.

We suggest that there are different steps in the process of managing these tensions. Firstly, it is necessary to be wary of individuals or small groups of people who claim to represent the interests of the community. At the outset of a research process the volunteers who become involved, or the community leaders, or the representatives appointed by the committee tend not to be representative of the community in general. In fact, it often makes little sense to speak of the needs of the community in general. A community represents a conglomeration of a range of different needs: those of the young, the old, women, men, employed, and unemployed are some of the categories that may be represented within a community.

Even if those who step forward to participate are legitimate representatives, what they stand for needs to be evaluated in respect of the extent to which there is an ongoing dialogical process between themselves and the broader community that they represent.

Secondly, within the process of community consultation, the researcher should attempt to evaluate the different interest groups within a community with respect to the issue at stake. It is always necessary to identify distinctive differences or stratifications within the community. For example, in the case of assessing the health service needs it may be necessary to distinguish between two groups on the basis of a criterion that superficially seems to have little to do with health, but that makes a great difference when one goes into questions about the accessibility of health services. For example, there might need to be taken into account the stratification between those who have access to transport or resources to pay for transport, and those who do not. If we neglect to do this, the way in which we go about conducting research may lead us to a biased evaluation of the characteristics of the community.

Thornton and Ramphele (1988) argue that development projects world-wide have been known to reinforce inequalities in the countries where they have been initiated, by not paying sufficient attention to the patterns and problems of existing social relations. For example, those who actually carry the burden of child care and who make decisions on health care issues are often ignored in favour of 'leaders', usually males, with special interests of their own (Chambers, 1985). Women are particularly vulnerable to being further disadvantaged by 'community' development projects. 'Whenever there is a need for voluntary community action it is the women, who are already over-burdened, that have to give their often non-existent leisure time for communal efforts like village health work, building toilets, promoting literacy, etc.' (Thornton and Ramphele, 1988, pp. 34–35).

Thirdly, having evaluated the groupings involved, it becomes important to ensure participation of the different groupings. Here we come to a practical challenge that is critical to the success or failure of PR. How can the researcher foster the involvement of the uninvolved? It is clear that appropriate dialogue is very difficult in a context of unequal capacity. We stated that dialogue is not a means so much as an ideal towards which participatory projects should strive. Below we outline three techniques that attempt to address this issue by establishing environments that are 'dialogue enabling'.

There are a wide range of facilitation methods for fostering community involvement. These methods range from general techniques for facilitating communication and interaction within groups, to more comprehensive methods. Many examples of the former methods can be found in the *Community workers' handbook* (Hope and Timmel, 1984), based on the work of Paulo Freire. These include 'ice-breaking exercises', listening skills, and group games for exploration of relational dynamics.

A number of comprehensive PR systems have been developed, which provide some solutions to the problem of initiating dialogue in community settings. For example,

the 'planning for real' approach caters specifically for non-verbal interaction; it deliberately employs methods that do not rely on verbal articulation. The 'participatory rural appraisal' approach draws on the idea that dialogue can be developed through participation with others in activities that show what the community knows. It also facilitates the researcher gaining access to the marginalized sections of a community. These two methods for fostering community involvement are outlined below.

4.2.1 Planning for real

The 'planning for real' approach developed under the auspices of the Neighbourhood Initiatives Foundation in Britain as a community planning process. It is based on the concept of making three-dimensional models of geographic areas, and providing opportunities for members of a community to participate in the reconceptualization of these areas through an 'alternative currency to words' (Gibson, 1980, p. 204). By this is meant that in the process of interaction with the community development task, the other community members, and the researcher, an individual community member does not have to be articulate,' well-educated, or confident in speaking in front of other people. An alternative way of expressing one's views is facilitated. In this way it helps residents of communities and professionals to work out and then share in implementing joint plans of action for neighbourhood regeneration.

A typical 'planning for real' exercise consists of the following steps. A model of the town is constructed and set out in a public

177

place, such as a local hall. Each building or space, for example a park, is drawn on movable cards. Through public advertising of the event, members of the community are invited to stroll into the hall and contribute their views on the siting of, for example, the library, or a sports field, or a new community centre. This they do non-verbally, through moving the cards marked with diagrams of these structures. This technique puts everybody on an equal footing as they move around the model shifting cards as they see fit. Instead of the 'eyeball-to-eyeball confrontations' (Gibson, 1993, p. 5) of traditional community meetings, which benefit those who are fluent and confident in speaking publicly, everyone's views converge on the subject matter – the model and its possibilities. Once an individual has placed a card with a suggestion on a particular spot, the suggestion is depersonalized. The suggestion does not 'belong' to anyone anymore but is in the public space of the model and has a legitimacy and status that is unconnected to the person's social status. With a physical model of their neighbourhood to play with, timid people can physically put down their ideas. The contribution of the 'experts' such as engineers, town planners, lawyers, and city treasurers in the community is limited in this part of the process. This professional advice serves as a back-up where experts are 'on tap', not 'on top'. Community initiative is encouraged and facilitated. The foundation of the approach is the acknowledgement of local knowledge and commitment.

Once contribution to the model is complete, follow-up groups are formed to work out the main recommendations in more

detail, to negotiate between conflicting interests and priorities, and to put them across with the weight of the whole community behind them.

Gibson (1993) argues that seeing what could be done, and what should be done, is the key that unlocks commitment. Experts and ordinary people working together using this method generate a sense of mutual confidence and staying power, which provides the motive force. In addition, no one has to make any concessions, or run the risk of appearing to condescend (Gibson, 1980, p.204). In fact, Gibson reports that a group of architects were surprised at the latent capacities the model suddenly revealed in their clients when they used it with a housing co-operative in Liverpool.

Planning for real can help the community to see things and plan in relation to a comprehensive and integrated vision, to co-ordinate its actions with the backing of 'on tap' professionals, and to concentrate its resources on a realistic development programme that has roots in the community. The programme therefore has a better chance of surviving and being safeguarded by the community, than would a programme planned by and delivered to the community by outside agencies.

4.2.2 Participatory rural appraisal (PRA)

Participatory rural appraisal (PRA), sometimes referred to as participatory learning and action (PLA), is a research methodology involving various activities that emerged out of a need to do research more rapidly with results being more immediately available to be used by communities and development workers to make decisions.

The emphasis on participation developed as a result of disenchantment with the way that development initiatives would often lead to information being taken out of the community and being collated and interpreted in the researchers' offices. Key responsibilities for information collection and interpretation often rest with outsiders. When the techniques used are compatible with the local dynamics of the moment, and when the methods complement rather than replace indigenous forms of expression and problem solving, participation is maximised.

PRA is a methodology with a specific philosophy about the role of people in their own development. The focus is not just on gathering information, but the recognition of how empowering the process of gathering this information can be. PRA uses a variety of tools that have an emphasis on activities. One of the underlying assumptions in PRA is that activity encourages people's commitment to the process, it accesses those who are not literate and who are often marginalized in the community, and it emphasizes collective work, which provides a more secure environment for participation than, for example, interviewing an individual. Some of these techniques are mapping, drawing Venn diagrams, walking across a piece of land and drawing up a 'transect', doing livelihood analyses and semi-structured interviews (see Theis and Grady, 1991). These tools are outlined in the box on page 180. These methods aim at equipping communities with the necessary tools for identifying, analysing, and solving their own issues. Although used predomi-

Participatory rural appraisal

Participatory rural appraisal can be used to:
- assess the development needs of a community;
- identify priorities for further research/development action;
- assess the feasibility (social and technical) of planned interventions;
- implement development action; and
- monitor development action.

It is based on the following principles:
- It optimises trade-offs: what needs to be known against measuring only as accurately as necessary.
- It offsets the bias of urban outsiders with that of the local rural reality.
- Where necessary the processes and goals of the study are modified en route.
- It emphasises learning from and with the rural people, gaining from indigenous physical, technical, and social knowledge.
- Local people perform the activities: choose the methods, draw the diagrams and maps, run the workshops, and adapt the methods to the local conditions.

nantly in rural settings, the methods could be used in many different contexts, for example, urban communities, the business sector, and in non-governmental organizations. Engaging with a community in these activities develops an awareness within people of their own life situation and of their own potential to take action to improve the quality of their lives.

Visual representation of problems, situations, and histories is a major part of the PRA approach. It is significant in two senses. Firstly, visual material helps to demystify the research process by making the collection of information and its analysis visible, obvious, and available to the group of people engaged in the exercise. Secondly, visual representations of information, or pictures of one's surroundings, enable one to take a new perspective on the situation. Readers might think of times when they have seen their town on a map, and been made aware of the type of land that surrounds it, and the distances between their own town and surrounding towns. In addition to providing this chance to see the 'overall picture' instead of just one's own perspective, collective production of visual material facilitates communication and dialogue between members of communities; makes knowledge and ideas public; provides a holistic picture of events; and allows for information to be owned, verified, and added to by participants. Because the visual representation is drawn up by a group, an individual becomes aware of how his or her own knowledge overlaps, or is different to that of other people in the community. Visual representations facilitate the involvement of the more marginalized members of a community, the non-literate, and very shy members, because it relies less on formal education than, for example, a written survey questionnaire would.

Tools of participatory rural appraisal

- Direct observation of events, processes, relationships, or people.
- Semi-structured interviews are informal, guided discussions with key informants, or groups of community members.
- Ranking and scoring are analytic tools that order information according to importance or preference.
- Participatory planning, budgeting, and monitoring of the research process.
- Group discussions and analysis of information.
- Diagramming is probably the most significant of the PRA techniques because it facilitates communication and stimulates discussion. Some of the diagramming techniques are:
  - mapping, which accesses information on resources, infrastructure, and demography. Maps are drawn on all surfaces, from paper to using sticks and stones on the ground;
  - transects, which are diagrams of land use obtained by systematically walking with an informant through an area whilst asking questions and observing;
  - seasonal calendars and daily routine charts are diagrams that articulate the main activities, problems, and opportunities in a community through the daily or annual cycle;
  - time trends and historical profiles encapsulate people's accounts of the past and may include major epidemics, droughts, or changes in customs and land use;

– flow diagrams and Venn diagrams highlight the institutional relationships in a community or group of people, and assist in identifying and solving problems by analysing how they are interconnected;
– livelihood analysis diagrams are used to interpret the behaviours, decisions, and coping strategies of households. For example, a pie chart might be used to analyse the income and expenditure of a group in the community.

PRA is a very powerful process, but depends greatly on the quality of facilitation. Chambers (1992) argues that it can, unfortunately, be seen as a quick fix for complex and deeply entrenched problems, or used too routinely and rigidly with not enough attention to development process dynamics. Skilled and sensitive facilitation is necessary, as purely technical use of methods does not constitute a development research process.

4.3 Developing a critical perspective

In this section we will discuss an often overlooked but crucial aspect of PR. This involves the introduction of critical perspectives into contextual research. We hope to bring readers to the point of seeing that the act of understanding a context involves both standing in that context, and taking the perspective of standing outside of the context. Standing outside, and the benefits of this perspective, sometimes referred to as a 'distanciated' perspective, are very important in PR, as is the perspective of 'standing in' or 'the insider's perspective'.

The role of critique in social research is well explained by the critical theorist Jurgen Habermas (1972) who, in his book *Knowledge and human interests*, describes psychoanalysis as the paradigm for the critical social sciences. While he has been criticized for using this analogy, and we should be careful of applying the analogy in a general way, it nevertheless is useful for making a particular point. He understands psychoanalysis as being a method for bringing about self-reflection, where what is taken for granted, or given at face value, is reflected on with a view to exposing the limits and false conceptions we have about ourselves. In psychoanalysis the patient comes to see the limitations of his or her self-understanding and develops new forms of self-understanding, which can be the basis for new kinds of action. This can be conceived of as a process of critical enquiry, which leads to the sweeping away of misconceptions and the letting go of old beliefs, assumptions, and taken-for-granted meanings, to be replaced by alternative conceptions.

When we ask people what they feel, or what they desire; and ask them to account for their opinions or attitudes, and the motives for their actions; what can we expect in terms of them being able to respond to our enquiry? The answer to this question from a critical perspective is that we cannot expect them to be able to completely account for themselves. This is not as patronizing as it may seem and there are good reasons to believe that the psychological life of an individual or group cannot be completely understood if one only has access to the empathic perspective (see section 1.1). The outsider's perspective helps us to understand ourselves better and this idea lies at the heart of the PR endeavour. In a satisfactory PR process the researcher or facilitator and the community continually have their understanding of events and processes challenged and enlarged, as they begin to understand an event through the insider's and outsider's perspectives, respectively.

Let us consider a few examples of how understanding of a situation may be improved if we for a moment stand outside of the situation and view it from a distance. We are concerned here with what can be said, for example, of a moment in time by virtue of the perspective of hindsight. A different kind of example is the way in which someone may know a person so well that we might say that he or she knows the other person better than that person knows him- or herself. It might be said that in some respects a parent is better positioned to know who a child is, and what the child is becoming, by virtue of seeing the child in his or her complete life history context, which is something that the child is unable to do. The child knows him- or herself only in the context of the present and its immediate surrounds. By virtue of being in a situation, of living in a moment, we are often prevented from seeing the broader contexts in that our experience is mounted, and prevented from understanding the meanings that we live in a 'received' or taken-for-granted way.

The above gives reason to believe that sometimes we can better understand experiences by getting a distance from them. The PR practitioner attempts to move back and forth between understanding something from the empathic perspective and seeing the situation from a distance. By bringing distanciated perspectives to communities, the practitioner attempts to bring the community to a fuller and better understanding of its predicament and then to assist the community to translate this understanding into programmes of action.

The critical theory model sees its theories as transforming social life when these theories are introduced into people's self-understanding. Thus critical theory relies on reflexivity (see section 2.1) to bring about social change. More particularly, the critical model aims to change social life by overcoming the state of alienation that distances human beings from an understanding of the 'true' state of their being and that prevents them from understanding their condition. By showing people the shortcomings of their self-understanding, it is intended that they will begin to understand in ways that are less compliant with the forces of social domination, and this will make them more inclined to resist and know how to change these conditions. Thus theoretical perspectives may sometimes enhance our self-understanding. The models for understanding social life developed by theoreticians can help to illuminate for us the reasons why we do things, beyond the way in which we spontaneously and naturally understand ourselves.

Freire (1972) suggests that the historical understanding that a community has of its own conditions of life may be the very reason why the community is unable to find creative solutions that are likely to change these conditions. Freirian method is radically committed to praxis, and the method is based on the need to bring a community to think differently and particularly critically about the causes of the negative conditions that prevail in the community.

'True reflection leads to action but that action will only be a genuine praxis if there is critical reflection on its consequences' (Paulo Freire, 1972, p. 41). This quotation sets the stage for understanding Freire's action-reflection cycle, which consists of a model for ensuring that critical consciousness becomes part of the PR effort. Reflection on action involves an appraisal of both successes and failures. The successes are celebrated and enhance motivation, whilst the failures and mistakes make for the need to more deeply understand the causes of a problem and the necessary solutions that will lead to the desired transformation of daily life. The continual reflection upon the consequences of actions and the evaluation thereof is envisaged as an ongoing process that should accompany all actions at all times. However, it is an ideal process and its implementation is sometimes far from the ideal. It is sometimes much easier to blindly proceed with a programme of action than to be self-critical and go back to planning and redesigning the intervention.

As a participatory researcher one feels the pull of both sides of the continuum, from being an involved participant to being a distanciated observer. Funders will often demand an objective, 'standing outside' perspective, whereas community members will demand empathy, engagement, and concern. One prescription that seems to provide

some guidance in mediating these competing pulls is that the researcher should maintain a moving, flexible relation to both sides and be critically aware of the need to be influenced by both sets of demands. Furthermore, researchers should be self-reflective and transparent concerning their own 'needs' and academic demands.

As has already been said, the process of critical reflection is a strongly developed feature in the work of Paulo Freire, the philosophical foundations of which are laid out in Freire's (1972) *Pedagogy of the oppressed*. This short but challenging book has laid the foundation for a great deal of practical work in the community development field. An interesting and valuable Freirian method is discussed below, and you will be able to see how the method involves a practical implementation of many of the points made above.

4.3.1 The dialogical method of Paulo Freire

Paulo Freire popularized the word conscientization to represent the awakening of critical awareness or consciousness. Critical consciousness is characterized by the development of a critical understanding of culture that goes beyond everyday understanding of problems.

The first stage of a typical Freirian intervention begins with researching the peoples' thematic universe. The themes are the ideas, values, hopes, and concepts by which people live. Freire intends by his methods to take these themes and show the contradictions and tensions within them. In particular it is intended that the method lead to an understanding of how a people's understanding can limit their experience and make them 'fatalistic' in the sense of not expecting anything different.

These themes are then coded into a representation that depicts some of the central constituent elements of a community's thematic universe. This may be in the form of a painting, a photograph, a poem, a poster, or any other method of representation.

This representation is presented back to a community in a group discussion context conducted by a facilitator, PR practitioner, or, as Freire calls it, an animator. People are required to describe what is happening in the code and to 'unpack' the story of the code. Codes are typically structured so as to present ambiguous images to people, which will lead to much discussion and differing interpretations.

Having begun to divulge their ways of understanding what is happening in the code, and having begun to develop a grasp of the themes through which they think about the code, the facilitator then turns to ask them if the kind of situation depicted in the code occurs in their own community. Having already entered into talking about the code from the perspective of their own thematic universe, they easily begin to talk about their everyday reality in terms of the themes that matter to them. Thus the method begins with understanding an external situation and then examines how these ways of understanding work to structure everyday reality. Once this reflection is under way it is the facilitator's task to challenge the understanding that underlies everyday action. Through this the participants in such exercises are brought to realize that their understanding constitutes a problem and they are challenged to deepen and broaden this understanding. The process of beginning to see their understanding of situations as limited is termed 'problematizing their understanding'. Once they have understood that their own understanding of the situation is what limits effective action, alternative ways of understanding are explored and then developed for their practical import. Practical courses of action are developed on this basis.

It is not always easy for a group to discuss freely those issues that are most deeply important to them. Real life is often 'too close' to understand, and it helps to project one's understanding onto an external image, before turning to understand one's own situation. The code enables us to step back a couple of paces, look at the problem from a distance, and to think about it in new, problem-solving ways.

5 Conclusion

In this chapter we have examined the unique characteristics, processes, methods, and problems associated with the conduct of social research in community settings. The emergence of the 'participatory research' paradigm has challenged researchers to rethink their motives for doing research and to adopt a more needs-driven and problem-oriented approach to conducting research. The need to involve communities in the research process places on researchers a set of demands generated within the community or context of the research, which reshapes the way that the research process is designed and how it is managed.

In this chapter we discussed the importance of research as action, or praxis. We also discussed the empowering qualities of the PR process in which the community increases its control over access to resources and decision making. We mentioned that this might involve the participatory researcher engaging in a process of capacity building, which we view as both a means and an end in community development. Establishing environments that enable dialogue is an extremely important part of participatory research. In discussing the facts that threaten its establishment we argued that dialogue is not a means so much as an ideal towards which participatory projects should strive.

We then discussed three broad processes in the interaction between researchers and communities. This included the mechanisms of facilitating dialogue, empowerment, and reflexivity when getting involved as a researcher. We discussed the process of building rapport and of negotiating the terms of engagement with the community. We commented on the importance of valuing the local knowledge of the community and of acknowledging the local knowledge of the researchers. In discussing modes in which the researcher could engage with the community, we commented on the researcher as activist, consultant, and ethnographer. We argued that in the process of being an ethnographer the researcher becomes a learner, a student of the 'culture' of the research community. The point was also made that it is important to understand the complexity of the term 'community' and to be aware of the heterogeneity of communi-

ties. We identified two methods of fostering community involvement: planning for real and participatory rural appraisal. The importance of a critical perspective in contextual research was highlighted in our discussion of Freire's action-reflection cycle and dialogical method.

Contemporary social theory shows us that human beings have available to them multiple ways of understanding their own needs and realities. When we begin processes of social or psychological research we necessarily begin the enquiry by trying to understand how people currently understand themselves and their past, present, and future. The greater part of what we seek in such enquiry is yet to be formulated, and will often only be discovered with imaginative reflection, by adopting new ways of thinking and different perspectives. In this sense the outcome of such enquiry is formed in a dialogue between the enquirer and the context of enquiry. Viewed in this way, participatory social research is a forward-looking, productive, and creative endeavour. It involves developing new hybrids between local knowledge and other, perhaps new, possibilities of understanding.

Thus the answer to a participatory research question is not something waiting there to be seized upon like an essential truth, and upheld as a discovery about what a community feels or thinks. It is to be established and not simply found. It is arrived at by mixing what a community already thinks and feels with the possibilities of experience and action that arise through the research process itself. In this sense it is a constructive and creative process. It has been shown in this chapter that the 'distance' of the researcher and the researcher's ability to ask positively motivated but critical questions is a vital part of the research process and particularly so in relation to the establishment of new forms of action.

Exercises

1 In small groups think of a situation in the past about which you now, after time has passed, have come to feel very differently about.

  1.1 Can you relate your example to the difference between insider and outsider perspectives?

  1.2 Does knowing a situation like it **really is** mean knowing it only from the perspective of the person experiencing the situation?

  1.3 Does the outsider's perspective also have something to offer?

2 Can you identify other factors that would militate against dialogue? What about psychological factors that make it difficult to express yourself in certain kinds of situations? Try to imagine and analyse situations where you experience insecurity or lack of confidence, or perhaps the feeling that you will be treated negatively if you express your feelings.

3 It could be argued that giving value to local knowledge is merely romanticizing what is old and conservative. It could also be argued that romanticizing such knowledge serves to keep, for example, the rural poor in their place, and deny them access to technology and progress. What do you think is the value of listening to, recording, and working with local knowledge? What are the problems and constraints of local knowledge?

4 In the environment around you, at your university, college, or town, identify a job that you do not know much about (for example, how a hawker makes a successful sale, or how a waitress manages many different orders). Ask a person in that job to describe a part of the job they find most difficult. Listen carefully to how they describe the job. What words do they use that are unfamiliar to you? This is their 'slang' or colloquial expressions. What techniques do they use to manage the difficult situation? Ask questions that help the person to tell you more, for example, 'Can you give an example of how that happens?'

References

BROWN, L. D. (1985). People centred development and participatory research. *Harvard Educational Review,* 55, 69–75.

CHAMBERS, R. (1985). *Rural poverty: Putting the last first.* London: Longman.

CHAMBERS, R. (1992). *Rapid appraisal: Rapid, relaxed and participatory.* Discussion Paper 311. Brighton: Institute of Development Studies, University of Sussex.

CHESLER, M. A. (1991). Mobilizing consumer activism in health care: The role of self help groups. *Research in Social Movements, Conflicts and Change,* 13, 275–305.

COETZEE, J. K. (1987). *Development is for people.* Johannesburg: Southern.

COHEN, J. M. and UPHOFF, N. T. (1977). *Rural*

development. *Participation: Concepts and measures for project design, implementation and evaluation.* New York: Rural Development Committee.

ELLEN, R. F. (Ed.). (1984). *Ethnographic research: A guide to general conduct.* London: Academic Press.

ERASMUS, K. (1992). *Saints or sinners: NGO's in development.* Paper presented at the biennial conference of the Development Society of Southern Africa, Grahamstown.

FOSTER, G. (1982). Community development and primary health care: Their conceptual similarities. *Medical Anthropology Cross Cultural Studies in Health and Illness,* 6, 183–195.

FREIRE, P. (1972). *Pedagogy of the oppressed.* Harmondsworth: Penguin.

GEERTZ, C. (1983). *Local knowledge: Further essays in interpretive anthropology.* New York: Basic Books.

GIBSON, T. (1980). Sooner done than said. *The Architect's Journal,* July, 204–205.

GIBSON, T. (no date). *Planning for real: User's guide.* Telford, UK: Neighbourhood Initiatives Foundation.

GIBSON, T. (1993). *Meadowell community development.* UK: Social Welfare Research Unit, University of Northumbria.

GILBERT, A. (1995). *Small voices against the wind: Local knowledge and social transformation.* Unpublished paper presented at the Fourth International Symposium on the Contributions of Psychology to Peace, University of Cape Town, 25–30 June 1995.

HABERMAS, J. (1972). *Knowledge and human interests.* London: Heinemann.

HABERMAS, J. (1984). *Theory of communicative action, Vol. 1.* Boston: Beacon.

HALL, B., GILETTE, A., and TANDON, R. (Eds.). (1982). *Creating knowledge: A monopoly? Participatory Research in development.* Toronto: Participatory Research Network Publication.

HOPE, A. and TIMMEL, S. (1984). *Community workers' handbook (1,2,3).* Zimbabwe: Mambo Press.

KASEGE, D. C. O. (1991). *Community empowerment: The key to health for all.* Keynote address at Namibian National Primary Health Care Workshop, 16–28 February 1991.

KELLY, K. J. and VAN VLAENDEREN, H. (1996). Dynamics of participation in a community health project. *Social Science and Medicine,* 42, 1235–1246.

KIEFFER, C. H. (1984). Citizen empowerment: A developmental perspective. *Prevention in Human Sciences,* 3, 9–36.

KORTEN, D. (1980). Community organisation and rural development: A learning process approach. *Public Administration Review,* Sept/Oct, 480–503.

KORTEN, D. (1990). *Getting to the 21st century: Voluntary action and the global agenda.* Connecticut: Kumarian Press.

MARSDEN, D. (1990). Using local knowledge. *Community Development Journal,* 25 (3), 266–271.

O'DEA, P. (1985). Immunizing with knowledge: The epistemology of traditional health theories, a neglected dimension in development. *Assignment Children,* 69–72, 417–428.

PUCKETT, J. M. and REESE, H. W. (Eds.). (1993). *Mechanisms of everyday cognition.* Hillsdale: Lawrence Erlbaum.

RAHNEMA, M. (1990). Participatory action research: The 'last temptation of saint' development. *Alternatives,* 15, 199–226.

REASON, P. and ROWAN, J. (Eds.). (1981). *Human Inquiry.* London: John Wiley & Sons.

RIFKIN, S. B. (1986). Lessons from community participation in health programmes. *Health Policy and Planning,* 1, 240–249.

RIFKIN, S. and WALT, G. (1986). Why health improves: Defining the issues concerning 'comprehensive primary health care' and 'selective health care'. *Social Science and Medicine,* 23, 559–566.

ROGOFF, B. and LAVE, J. (Eds.). (1984). *Everyday cognition: Its development in social contexts.* Cambridge, MA: Harvard University Press.

SCHRIJVERS, J. (1991). Dialectics of a dialogical ideal: Studying down, studying sideways and studying up. In *Constructing knowledge: Authority and critique in social science* (pp.162–179). London: Sage.

SCRIBNER, S. (1986). Thinking in action: Some characteristics of thought. In R. J. Sternberg and

187

R. K. Wagner (Eds.), *Practical intelligence: Nature and origins of competence in the everyday world* (p.13–30). Cambridge: Cambridge University Press.

SPRADLEY, J. (1979). *The ethnographic interview.* New York: Holt, Rinehart and Winston.

SPRADLEY, J. (1980). *Participant observation.* New York: Holt, Rinehart and Winston.

SWIFT, C. and LEVIN, G. (1987). Empowerment: An emerging mental health technology. *Journal of Primary Prevention,* 8, 71–94.

THEIS, J. and GRADY, H. M. (1991). *Participatory rapid appraisal for community development: A training manual based on experiences in the Middle East and North Africa.* London: International Institute for Environment and Development.

THORNTON, R. and RAMPHELE, M. (1988). The quest for community. In E. Boonzaier and J. Sharp (Eds.), *South African keywords: The uses and abuses of political concepts.* Cape Town: David Philip.

VAN VLAENDEREN, H. (1993). Psychological research in the process of social change: A contribution to community development. In *Psychology in developing societies,* 5 (1). New Delhi: Sage.

VAN VLAENDEREN, H. and GILBERT, A. (1992). Participatory research for capacity building in rural development: A case study. In P. Styger and M. Cameron (Eds.), *Development in transition: Opportunities and challenges.* Pretoria: Development Society of Southern Africa.

VAN VLAENDEREN, H. and NKWINTI, G. (1993). Participatory research as a tool for community development. *Development Southern Africa,* 10, 211–228.

VYGOTSKY, L. S. (1978). *Mind in society: The development of higher psychological processes.* Cambridge, MA: Harvard University Press.

WERNER, D. (1988). Empowerment and health. *Contact,* 102, 1–9.

10 Social programme evaluation

Charles Potter
Johan Kruger

Study objectives

After studying this chapter you should have an understanding of:

- the definition, scope, and nature of programme evaluation;
- the development of the field of programme evaluation, and its current status in Western countries, Africa, and particularly South Africa;
- particular research methodologies used in programme evaluation;
- applications to community psychology; and
- practical considerations when implementing programme evaluation.

1 Introduction

1.1 Aims and scope

There has been increasing interest in *programme evaluation* as a fertile area of research in the social sciences. One of the major reasons for the interest in this area among community psychologists is the potential impact of evaluations on the socio-political contexts of programmes, as well as their potential as a means of developing a social psychology that is relevant to community needs. Programme evaluation offers various ways of bringing the psychologist out of the laboratory, the lecture theatre, or the consulting room. More importantly, it provides a means of influencing the work of different stakeholders involved in social programmes, improving the quality of human services, and improving the welfare of communities.

Evaluations can be conducted for different purposes and can be formative when undertaken for the sake of developing and fine-tuning a programme, or summative when undertaken in order to make a judgement regarding outcomes and effectiveness, or both. Due to the different vested interests involved, evaluations are often ideologically and politically charged, requiring both tact and negotiation on the part of the evaluator. As Cronbach and associates (Cronbach et al., 1980), House (1973), and Patton (1990) have argued, evaluations have a political dimension, which is present whether or not the evaluator wishes to have political influence. As social programmes are closely linked to social priorities and political decisions (Greene, 1994; Weiss, 1973), programme evaluation involves a form of research that is closely linked to the realities of social and community development and the politics of resource allocation and power.

This chapter is intended as an introduction to students of community psychology and the other social sciences. The authors begin by defining programme evaluation and its relevance to community psychology, and then provide an overview of the development of the field in Western countries and its current status in Africa, and particularly in South Africa. Various definitions and conceptions of programme evaluation are then presented. Thereafter different approaches and methodologies employed by programme evaluators are detailed. In the final sections of the chapter, applications to community psychology and various practical considerations when implementing evaluation programmes are highlighted.

1.2 What is programme evaluation, and what is its relevance to community psychology?

Programme evaluation is research conducted with two major purposes. The first purpose is to consider issues and questions concerning the development of social programmes. Many issues and theories are normally involved in social development, and one purpose of evaluation research is to establish and describe the ways in which those involved in a particular social programme go about their work, the issues with which they deal, and how they confront these issues. This evidence is often highly relevant to developing or substantiating social theory.

A second purpose of programme evaluation is to analyse evidence about the impact of social programmes in order to answer specific questions about its development. These questions are normally concerned with programme implementation and outcomes, as well as with the quality of service provided. They usually have an accountability dimension, relating both to use of resources as well as whether the programme is providing an effective service in relation to social needs.

For the community psychologist, involvement in programme evaluation provides a number of ways in which theories concerning social developments can be linked to practice. As Shadish (1990a, 1990b) has pointed out, there are many similarities in community research and programme evaluation, and both have common origins in the experimental tradition in the social sciences. Both fields have grown in breadth and stature over the past thirty years, and both fields can benefit from mutual exchange of ideas, as well as mutual critique of practice. For the community psychologist, involvement in programme evaluation thus provides a number of relevant ways of engaging in the development and improvement of social programmes, of developing theory, and of testing theories of

Systematically evaluating a fire-safety education programme

McConnell, Leeming, and Dwyer (1996) evaluated a fire-safety programme for 443 pre-school children from ten child-care facilities. Children in six centres received the eighteen-week training programme called Kid Safe. Children in four other centres were assigned to the delayed-treatment condition and constituted the comparison group. All the children were pre-tested on a comprehensive fire-knowledge test. The same test was readministered after the programme. All the children in the treatment group showed significantly greater knowledge gains from pre-test to post-test than the children in the comparison group. The findings supported the value of training pre-school children in fire safety as an important strategy for injury prevention.

community development and research in practice.

Programme evaluation typically assists in the identification and solving of social problems. One recent example is the AIDS/HIV crisis, which began in the 1980s and has now become a pandemic, turning southern Africa into one of the leading AIDS/HIV infected areas in the world.

2 Origins and current status of programme evaluation as a form of social science research

2.1 Programme evaluation in Western countries

The origins of evaluation as a field distinct from the testing movement can be traced to the 1930s, when Ralph Tyler and his colleagues (1942) suggested that programmes could be evaluated in their own terms, through examination of the attainment of their objectives. Following Tyler, objectives-based evaluation became the norm, with the majority of subsequent evaluation approaches being developed in reaction to the Tylerian form of evaluation (Madaus, Scriven, and Stufflebeam, 1983; Madaus and Stufflebeam, 1989).

Programme evaluation as a field achieved its greatest impetus to growth in the 1960s and early 1970s, when demands for educational and social reform led to a search for new forms of education in Britain and the United States, and to the so-called war on poverty in the United States (Madaus et al., 1983; Shadish, 1990b). This was accompanied by a widespread increase in government and private sector spending on education, mental health, and other social programmes, and calls for their evaluation.

2.2 Programme evaluation in Africa

A 1998 search on the PsycLIT database (Silverplatter International N.V.) reveals that

191

from 1974 to 1997 only fifteen articles and one book chapter were indexed under 'programme evaluation' and 'Africa', out of a total of 4 721 articles and books that were indexed under 'programme evaluation'. Only one of the articles came from Nigeria, three from the United States, and the remaining eleven, as well as the book chapter, from South Africa. Overall, this represents less than half a per cent of the international literature on programme evaluation on the PsycLIT database. The same trends are evident on other psychology-related databases such as Medline and the Social Sciences Index.

The lack of a systematic data base in the international psychological literature is one indicator of the underdevelopment of programme evaluation in Africa. Others are the lack of government and public interest in the field, accompanied by lack of stress on accountability in governance, a lack of universities and other training institutions teaching courses in programme evaluation, and the lack of professional associations, networks, and academic journals supporting the development of the field. Asamoah (1988) comments that the under-utilization of programme evaluation research in Africa deprives policy makers of empirical data on which to base decisions. She also discusses the socio-economic conditions in Africa that pose many methodological and cultural challenges to researchers who wish to undertake evaluation research.

While African and North American contexts vary considerably, it can be inferred that growth of programme evaluation in Africa is most likely to occur in those contexts in which there is demand for evalua-tions for accountability purposes, supported by government, private sector, or international donor agency funding. Increased demand is likely to lead to increased public, academic, and professional interest in the area, which, in turn, will enable the field to develop and become self-sustaining. There are indications that this is the case in South Africa today.

2.3 Programme evaluation in South Africa

Louw (1998) suggests that programme evaluation in southern Africa can be characterized as diffuse and fragmented, with the lack of university and non-formal training courses, the lack of researchers working full-time in the area, and the lack of a broad-based professional association contributing to the underdevelopment of the field.

Many programme evaluations conducted in South Africa have thus been conducted by persons without specific training in the area. While an evaluation association, The Association for the Study of Educational Evaluation in Southern Africa, has existed since the early 1970s, it has been mainly dedicated to educational assessment rather than programme evaluation. Courses in programme evaluation have also been organized nationally by agencies such as Wits Centre for Continuing Education and the South African Association for Academic Development (SAAAD), as well as locally by non-governmental organizations such as the Forum for Adult Educators.

Increased interest can also be inferred from the number of evaluations that have been conducted in recent years. These include measurement-based and systematic approaches; interpretive and naturalistic approaches to educational programmes, community development programmes, and evaluations of social responsibility programmes mounted by industry; and participatory, critical emancipatory, and empowerment evaluations.

What are the factors on which this recent interest and growth in the field of programme evaluation in South Africa are based, and what factors are likely to ensure its continuance? In the context of social change, which has characterized the move from apartheid government to a democracy, the state is placing increasing emphasis on transformation through social development (Corder, 1997). In addition, despite a number of recent setbacks in this area, the private sector and international donors are continuing to support NGOs and CBOs, creating the socio-economic conditions in which an increased number of programme evaluations are likely to be commissioned (Potter, 1996). There is also evidence of an increased number of courses in which educational and programme evaluation are taught by South African universities and NGOs, as well as increased activity in the South African evaluation association. It can thus be argued that a number of contextual, political, socio-economic, and cultural factors are currently combining to encourage a climate in which growth of programme evaluation as a field is likely.

The conceptual foundations of these different approaches to programme evaluation are detailed in the next section.

3 Methodological approaches

There are a number of ways in which evaluation issues and questions can be addressed, and a number of ways in which researchers work with those involved in social programmes. These reflect different ways in which evaluation research can be defined, as well as different ways in which programme evaluations can be conducted. There are a number of different types of programme evaluation, which differ both in their methodological as well as their epistemological assumptions (House, 1983). The community psychologist needs to know the different forms of evaluation models available, so that an appropriate approach can be chosen to suit the purposes for which the evaluation is being conducted, and the nature of the programme being evaluated.

3.1 Systematic and measurement-based approaches

Systematic and measurement-based approaches are frequently used in evaluation. They offer logical frameworks that can be translated easily into evaluation designs, and research models that are clear and understandable to the different stakeholders in a programme. There are firm conceptual links between systematic and measurement-based approaches to evaluation. Both are based on positivist assumptions, in which programmes are conceptualized as entities producing effects that can be observed or measured, using the methodologies of social science research (Neuman, 1997).

Systematic evaluation offers a conceptualization of a programme as an integrated system that can be observed or measured. Aspects of the system could form the focus of evaluation, as well as different stages in its development. This type of conception of evaluation was particularly strong in the 1960s and early 1970s, and underpins many of the definitions of evaluation commonly used today (e.g., Heiman, 1995; Posavac and Carey, 1989; Rossi and Freeman, 1985; Shaugnessy and Zechmeister, 1997). The link between programme evaluation and accountability has been a strong one, not only in influencing increased demand for evaluations, but also in the conceptualization of evaluation as an activity linked to programme development. This is one of the reasons why the majority of published evaluations are based on systematic and measurement-based approaches based on quasi-experimental assumptions (Lipsey et al., 1985).

A number of models of evaluation are systematic in character, social programmes being conceptualized as entities reflecting a number of different stages or phases 'in planning and implementation'. The most influential of these has been the objectives-based approach suggested by Tyler et al. (1942), who suggested that a programme's aims form a rationale for the programme's subsequent development, and thus could also form a set of criteria against which the programme's outcomes could be evaluated.

There are other systematic models directed at the developmental aspects of a social programme. Stufflebeam (1968, 1972) proposed a comprehensive evaluation model involving four types of evaluation, namely, context, input, process, and product evaluation.

More recently, two writers have offered a comprehensive approach, which they define as: 'The systematic application of social science procedures in assessing the conceptualisation and design, implementation and utility of social intervention programmes' (Rossi and Freeman, 1985, p. 20). Rossi and Freeman's framework involves needs assessment, programme planning, progress evaluation, and outcomes evaluation, with the programme's aims being used as evaluative criteria, and measurement and cost-benefit analyses being used to establish its effects and value.

Systematic assumptions also underpin the theory-driven approach to evaluation proposed by Chen (1990), and Chen and Rossi (1983), for example. Chen defines programme theory as: 'A specification of what must be done to achieve desired goals, what other important impacts may also be anticipated, and how these goals and impacts may be generated' (Chen, 1990). Similar assumptions underpin the systematic evaluation framework suggested by Shaugnessy and Zechmeister (1997), in which different forms of evaluation are conducted, relating to different phases in the development of a programme, namely:

1   Needs assessment (descriptive evaluation), which is usually conducted by means of surveys or situational analyses undertaken by means of questionnaires, interviews, and/or observation, to determine a particular area of need requiring intervention. It often also incorporates analyses of documents or archival data, as well as analyses of previous research or evaluations of the work of other programmes working in the area in

which intervention is likely to take place.

2 Programme planning (formative evaluation), which is directed at the process of programme conceptualization and the feasibility of programme plans. It usually examines programme aims and purposes, and whether these relate to needs, as well as programme policy and whether the intervention as planned is feasible.

3 Formative evaluation, which is directed at the process of programme implementation. It usually incorporates a process of programme monitoring, to establish whether the intervention is being implemented as planned. In formative evaluation, the evaluator attempts to identify aspects of the programme that are working well, aspects of the programme that are problematic, and aspects of the programme requiring modification or improvement.

4 Summative evaluation, which has a retrospective focus, and usually incorporates an attempt to establish the outcomes, effects, or impact of the programme by observation or measurement. Summative evaluations examine evidence relating to indicators of programme effectiveness, and for this reason often incorporate quasi-experimental or *ex post facto* research, as well as some form of cost-effectiveness or cost-benefit analysis.

In practice, as with other systematic evaluation models, these different forms of evaluation research are often combined in a single evaluation design. Despite having different emphases, they share a common conceptual basis, reflecting the view that evaluation is a systematic activity, that programme development and programme evaluation are closely linked, and that impacts and effects can be observed or measured. For the purposes of measuring effects, the quasi-experimental approaches suggested by Campbell and Stanley (1963) and Cook and Campbell (1979) are often used in practice.

While there has been widespread interest in other more contextual and person-oriented evaluation approaches, there are many researchers whose work is still influenced by the Tylerian rationale for programme evaluation (Madaus and Stufflebeam, 1989). The evidence from the literature would suggest (Lipsey et al., 1985) that the majority of published evaluations have been conducted on measurement-based assumptions. In the literature, systematic assumptions concerning the nature of programme development are also widely held, and underpin a number of the definitions of programme evaluation found in psychology textbooks (Heiman, 1995; Shaugnessy and Zechmeister, 1997).

Systematic and measurement-based approaches to evaluation are thus useful for the community psychologist, as these have formed the basis of community research as it has traditionally been taught and practised (Tolan et al., 1990), and are readily understood both by programme sponsors as well as those involved in social programmes. The community psychologist may find that systematic and measurement-based conceptions of programme evaluation correspond with his or her her own view of programme development, and of evaluation. However, it may be necessary to distinguish the 'perceived need' of the community from 'actual need', or the need as perceived by the evaluator or health professional. This difference can have a major impact on service delivery and utilization.

One difficulty with a systematic and measurement-based conception of programme evaluation is that it is aimed at the programme as an entity, rather than on the different conceptions, aspirations, and values of those involved in the programme. As House (1973, 1977) and Hamilton and his colleagues (Hamilton, 1976; Hamilton et al., 1977; Parlett and Dearden, 1977) have pointed out, this carries with it the danger of assuming that there is value-consensus among the different stakeholders involved in a social programme.

This is stressed by Posavac and Carey (1989), who define programme evaluation as a collection of methods, skills, and sensitivities necessary to determine whether a human service is needed and likely to be used, whether it is sufficiently intense to meet the identified need, whether the service is being offered as planned, and whether the human service actually does help people in need without undesirable side effects. This assumes focus on the perceptions of a programme's clients, as well as the perceptions of other programme stakeholders.

3.2 Interpretive and naturalistic approaches

The point should be made that community development, community research, and programme evaluation are not easy. Differing values and ideologies are often involved in social programme development. Different stakeholders in a programme also have varying degrees of power and influence in society. Issues in community development do not resolve easily, and have high potential for value conflicts (Tolan et al., 1990).

A number of approaches to evaluation have thus been developed that do not assume value consensus in programmes, and that assume that social programmes are interventions that are both ideological as well as political in nature (House, 1973; 1977).

In reaction to what was perceived as increased central control by the bureaucracy and government in Britain, a number of critiques of systematic and measurement-based approaches to evaluation were advanced in the early 1970s by a group of evaluation theorists who came to be known as the 'new wave' evaluators (e.g., Hamilton et al., 1977; Parlett, 1974; Parlett and Hamilton, 1972; Stenhouse, 1975). The objections of this loose alliance of social scientists to the dominant positivist tradition in evaluation were based on epistemological concerns as well as issues of ideology, suggesting the need for evaluators to be sensitive to the political and power relationships in social programmes.

Many evaluation approaches of the period involved a rejection of what the 'new wave' evaluators termed 'the numbers game' (Hamilton et al., 1977), in favour of approaches that dealt with interpersonal and transactional issues. The alternative methodologies suggested were broad-based and holistic in character, involving use of qualitative methods, based on the interpretive and reflexive paradigms adopted within social anthropology and sociology. There was a growth of interest in holistic and

An interpretive evaluation of a peer-based mentoring programme for students

Mahatey, Kagee, and Naidoo (1994) implemented a pilot peer-based student mentoring programme at an historically black university, aimed at addressing some of the negative effects of apartheid. Firstly they developed a comprehensive understanding of the problem and its solutions. They assumed that students needed: to develop 'deep-level' cognitive skills; to undergo a conceptual change in their understanding of learning; to learn adequate study skills; positive role models; and an environment that provides support and promotes personal well-being. Fifty-five mentors were trained. A comprehensive evaluation strategy included weekly management and supervision meetings, evaluations after each workshop for mentors and students, and an extensive formal evaluation including both qualitative (focus groups) and quantitative (questionnaires) data-gathering methods from both students and mentors. Both students and mentors had indicated that they benefited socially and academically from the programme, and thought that it had contributed to their personal development and growth.

interpretive evaluation methodologies (Guba and Lincoln, 1989; Patton, 1982; Stake, 1980; Weiss, 1983a, 1983b).

Interpretive and naturalistic approaches stress the complexity of the transactional issues involved in social programmes, as well as the different realities and vested interests of different stakeholders. Many of these issues could not be established through observation or measurement, suggesting the need for a different paradigm based within an interpretive and naturalistic research tradition (Denzin and Lincoln, 1994; Guba and Lincoln, 1981; Hamilton et al., 1977), which could be sensitive to the different values, needs, and requirements of programme stakeholders.

One of the most influential evaluation models in the interpretive and naturalistic tradition has been the illuminative evaluation approach suggested by Parlett and Hamilton (1972). Illuminative evaluation is based on the assumption that a social programme represents a complex culture. Dimensions, layers, and specific transactions within the programme can best be understood and interpreted through repeated engagement, using the strategies and observational methodologies of the social anthropologist. Another influential model was the responsive evaluation model proposed by Stake (1983), who suggested procedures for taking the vested interests of different stakeholders in a programme into account in the process of evaluation design, implementation, and reporting. This approach formed the conceptual underpinning of the responsive constructivist or fourth generation evaluation approach suggested by Guba and Lincoln (1989).

Interpretive and naturalistic evaluation models are based on the assumption that social programmes need to be understood before they can be evaluated. There is thus a hermeneutic as well as a political process involved, the political dimension being there whether the evaluator wishes it or not (Shadish 1990a; 1990b; Weiss, 1973, 1982). For this reason there is value in evaluation approaches that are able to take different frames of reference, vested interests, as well as knowledge needs into account.

There has thus been a growth of interest in multi-method and eclectic approaches that combine qualitative and quantitative data (Williams, 1986), as well as approaches based on the logic of critical multiplism (Cook, 1985; Houts, Cook and Shadish, 1986; Shadish, 1986; Shadish, Cook, and Houts, 1986), which assumes that all methodological approaches are limited and need to be supplemented by others. In addition, there has been interest in the value of case studies (Burgess, 1984; Stake, 1978; Walker, 1980), process studies (Cronbach, 1963), and the ethnography in evaluation research (Fetterman, 1989).

Of interest to the community psychologist are the similar debates, manifesting an interest in holistic, interpretive, and naturalistic approaches, found in the literature on community research (Tolan et al., 1990).

In this regard a recent special issue of the *American Journal of Community Psychology* (Vol 26(4), Aug 1998) was dedicated to the issue of qualitative research in community psychology. This publication covered the usefulness of interpretive and naturalistic approaches as discussed in this section, as well as the critical and empowerment approaches discussed in the section following.

3.3 Critical and empowerment approaches

Critical and empowerment evaluation approaches are often associated with conflict theory, feminist analysis, and radical psychotherapy (Neuman, 1997), and are based on critiques that have characterized positivist thinking as being narrow, anti-democratic, and non-humanist. These approaches also view interpretive thinking as being too subjective and relativist in treating people's ideas as more important than the actual conditions that they are dealing with, and the imbalances of power and influence in society that combine to bring about these conditions. Both traditional and interpretive traditions in research have been criticized for the researcher's lack of involvement in social issues.

Critical social science is based on more activist assumptions relating to knowledge and human interests (Habermas, 1971), and views researchers as being either conscious or unconscious agents of the operation of wider social forces, which act to reinforce or reproduce the existing social order. Critical evaluation is based on the notion that critical awareness gained through reflection informs practical action, which is then critically evaluated (Carr and Kemmis, 1986; Grundy, 1984; Lakomski, 1988). Critical theory is formed through what is termed praxis, which involves an on-going reflective process undertaken both individually and collectively in groups (Freire, 1972). This process is normally facilitated through the researcher's active participation in the process.

There are a number of approaches to programme evaluation based on the re-

A participatory and action research approach to literacy in rural communities.

Kriegler, Ramarumo, Van der Ryst, and Van Niekerk (1994) describe a multi-site, multi-method project consisting of a situation analysis and culminating in a kind of systems intervention programme to break the illiteracy cycle in the context of a rural print-bereft community. Action research was conducted within a participatory empowering framework, using qualitative methods underpinned by the epistemological bases of ethnography. The results proved that even a short-term literacy programme based on appropriate principles can be effective in establishing and enhancing the emerging literacy behaviour of black nursery-school children. The latter compared favourably with older Grade 1 children after a twenty-three-week exposure to the programme, implemented by care-givers who, although not fully literate themselves, were empowered by way of in-service training to support emergent literacy.

searcher's involvement in facilitating a process of reflection by participants in a social programme. The notions of research-based teaching and self-evaluation suggested by Stenhouse (1975, 1983) are based on processes of participative action research aimed at improving practice. The responsive evaluation approach developed by Stake (1980, 1983) is based on establishing stakeholder concerns and issues through a participative process that involves programme stakeholders in evaluation design, implementation, and reporting. The democratic approach to evaluation suggested by the work of Mac-Donald (1978) and Simons (1987) is based on the active participation of the researcher in facilitating a process of self-discovery through action research, which enables greater knowledge, power, and self-determination among programme participants to emerge.

Other approaches address the development of critical awareness in programme participants. The critical action research framework suggested by the work of Carr and Kemmis (1986) is concerned with developing the ability of participants to critically analyse the power relationships implicit in the transactions in which they are involved. The empowerment evaluation approach developed by Fetterman, Kaftarian, and Wandersman (1996) is based on the direct involvement of the researcher in developing the capacity of those involved in social programmes to solve problems, access resources, and gain increased power and influence in society.

In both critical and empowerment approaches to evaluation the researcher becomes an active participant in the programme, with the programme evaluator acting as a catalyst to empowering persons involved in social programmes to be active in solving their own problems. This is done by a process of analysis of the underlying sources of social relations, with the aim that this process becomes empowering for others (Freire, 1972). The critical social researcher is thus action oriented, working to change the world and transform the social order. Research becomes a transformative endeavour, with both political as well as emancipatory dimensions (Kincheloe and McLaren, 1994).

For this reason, these types of participatory evaluation are often associated with work in low-income countries (Choudhary and Tandon, 1988; Hall, 1978;), and in those contexts undergoing rapid transformation or social change. A common theme in these approaches concerns the developmental and educative value of evaluation, as a means to enabling persons involved in social programmes to further their work, enhance their power through gaining access to skills and knowledge, and to overcome their problems.

Critical and empowerment approaches to programme evaluation have implications for the community psychologist, both due to the centrality of the concepts of empowerment to community psychology (Rappaport, 1987; Zimmerman, 1995), and the fact that in community research, neither the research process nor the subject of a research investigation occurs in a vacuum. Glenwick et al. (1990) have pointed out that there is a reciprocal relationship between the individual and the social system or environment. As Rappaport (1987, 1990) suggests, empowerment is a process that is multi-directional, being embedded in people, organizations, and communities.

4 Issues and applications

4.1 The politics and ethics of evaluation

Programmes and programme evaluators are imbued with political significance and power (Shadish 1990a). Politics in this sense does not necessarily refer to 'political party politics', but rather to the tensions inherent in personal interaction. Social programmes are themselves the creatures of political decisions. They are proposed, defined, debated, enacted, and funded through political processes, and in implementation they remain subject to political pressures – both supportive and hostile (Weiss, 1973).

The community psychologist needs to continually keep the political dimension in mind. Following case studies of research and development programme evaluations in the United States and Canada, Melkers and Roessner (1997) conclude that the political systems and the organizational politics of evaluation in the two countries significantly impact on the reasons for financing evaluations of science and technology programmes, the methods employed by evaluators, and the manner in which evaluations are eventually used. The associated political as well as ethical issues that programme evaluators face (Becher, 1974; Becher and MacLure, 1978a, 1978b; House, 1973; 1977; 1983; Weiss, 1973) reflect different accountability pressures (Lacey and Lawton, 1981). This includes the need for the evaluator to answer to different clients and stakeholders in the programme and the evaluation (moral accountability); responsibility on a scientific and ethical level to him- or herself, peers, and colleagues (professional account-ability); and accountability to those who have commissioned the evaluation, who are usually those with political and economic power (contractual accountability).

A useful way of establishing the political dimension of an evaluation is to conduct a stakeholder analysis (Potter, 1991, 1996, 1999). This implies attempting to establish whose interests are served by the evaluation, and what the informational needs of each set of stakeholders are relative to the focuses of the evaluation, and the evaluation issues and questions. On the basis of the analysis, it should then be possible to map out the vested interests in the evaluation, and the purposes for which it has been commis-sioned. In this respect, the classification of programme evaluations proposed by Mac-Donald (1978, 1993) is also helpful, with evaluations being characterized as either bureaucratic, autocratic, or democratic. Whereas bureaucratic evaluations are con-ducted in terms of the needs of those in positions of managerial power and influence, autocratic evaluations are con-ducted for the evaluator's own needs, pur-poses, or ends. Democratic evaluations are conducted in terms of the needs and pur-poses of all stakeholders in a programme.

In using such a classification or stake-holder analysis, Elliot's (1980) caution should be noted. Elliot comments that the asso-ciation of answerability, responsibility, and accountability with particular audiences, in-cluding clients, professionals, and employ-ers, is not a simple one. Such classifications may thus obscure the complexity of the political and ethical issues confronting the programme evaluator.

On an ethical level, Gredler (1996) sug-gests that programme evaluations should attempt to maximize good outcomes, avoid harmful procedures, assure participant anony-mity, and maintain confidentiality and privi-leged communication. In addition, the researcher faces social equity issues in the sense of ensuring for all stakeholders in a programme equitable assignment to treat-ments, equitable access to the evaluator's time and attention, and equitable design

Monitoring and accountability

An adult literacy campaign in the Western Cape received R50 million in donor funding. One year later only R10 million is left and no-one can show where the rest of the money went or how effectively it was used. This caused a big outcry and public outrage. Supposing you received this funding, what systems and processes would you put into place to establish whether the money was well-spent, whether the programme achieved its goals and was beneficial to the recipients, whether there were no unanticipated negative outcomes, and to keep all stakeholders relatively happy? Remember that adult literacy adds significant value to recipients' lives, including enhanced self-esteem, improved control over their environ-ment, and enhanced ability to adapt to an industrialized and information society. What are the ethical con-siderations for the evaluator in this instance?

and measurement. The pluralistic nature of stakeholder approaches requires careful consideration of the associated issue of conflicting perspectives and the multiple social meaning attributed to evaluations.

From this perspective, evaluation embraces issues of social justice, in the sense of the public's right to know, and the imperative that evaluation should be useful not only to those with informational needs, but also the public (Patton, 1982). Evaluators should understand their craft as a new form of cultural authority that requires studying the profound implications of values as a prerequisite for sound professional practice.

4.2 Methodology

For the community psychologist, it is important to know that programme evaluation is an applied science in which there are many unresolved issues. Cook and Shadish (1986) have called programme evaluation 'the worldly science', implying that evaluation requirements are stated first, and methodologies follow. However, as Shadish (1990a) comments, methodology is important. The tensions concerning what constitutes appropriate evaluation methodology remain largely unresolved, there being many different approaches associated with the work of different evaluation theorists (Shadish et al., 1986).

The context of the majority of evaluations is one in which notions of control in the experimental sense are normally absent. For these reasons, evaluations, which by definition normally have a formative emphasis, require different and more flexible methodologies than those offered by traditional science. At the same time, the criticisms of the rigour of evaluations based on qualitative methods is a recurring theme (Joint Committee on Standards for Educational Evaluation, 1981). The role of the evaluator relative to the programme being evaluated is also a major issue. Lipsey (1993, p. 7) suggests that programme theory is 'a set of propositions regarding what goes on in the black box during the transformation of input to output, that is how, via treatment inputs, a bad situation is transformed into a better one.' The black box approach to change means that we know what inputs we give as an intervention, and we then look to see whether the outputs change as expected, but it is not necessary to know what processes and events happen inside the box (which could be, for argument's sake, a person, a group of people, or a community). The black box model is seductive, as the problems, subjects, programme components, and implementation of the programme are usually very complex and show great variation.

In the black box model only the inputs and outputs need be defined; no thought is given to the actual process of change. However, in this model the selection of variables is informed by the researcher's implicit understanding of the problem. He or she may well select the wrong input and output variables, for reasons such as ease of measurement, availability of data, or habit. This gives an artificial and very constricted view of what is going on. An example of this would be the selection of age, ethnicity, sex, and test scores in the prediction of drop-outs at school, at the cost of major factors that are more difficult to define and measure, such as motivational and personal conflicts involving work, family, and non-academic career opportunities (Lipsey, 1993).

4.3 Getting started

The novice programme evaluator may find the various aspects of programme evaluation confusing and difficult to reconcile. The following systematic model (Figure 1) provides a useful conceptual framework for developing, managing, and evaluating a programme.

The developmental approach for the evaluation of health education models (Nutbeam, 1996, p. 317-319; Nutbeam, Smith, and Catford, 1990) can be usefully applied within a systematic approach to programme evaluation in community psychology and public health. During phase 1 epidemiological and demographic research are used to determine the causal basis of health problems and the scope of intervention, as well as to do a community needs assessment to clarify priorities and opportunities for intervention.

In phase 2 solutions are generated through social, behavioural, and organizational research to improve understanding of the target populations, and of the modifiable personal, social, and environmental characteristics, which would form the content of the intervention. The intervention theory development also identifies possible methods for achieving change, and the potential for different applications in different settings and with different groups.

Phase 3 refers to solution testing, where a systematic approach to the development and testing of an intervention can lead to a successful and sustainable solution to a defined health problem. According to Nutbeam et al. (1990), outcome evaluation is more prominent at the initial stages of phase 3, mainly in order to firstly establish

Figure 1 Stages of research and evaluation. Adapted from Nutbeam, Smith, and Catford (1990), and Nutbeam (1996)

1 Problem definition	2 Solution generation	3 Solution testing		4 Solution maintenance	
		Innovation testing	Intervention demonstration	Intervention dissemination	Programme management
Epidemiology and demography & Community needs assessment	Social, behavioural, and organizational research & Intervention theory development	Assessment of outcome Understanding of process			Cost-benefits assessment (financial, psycho-social, political) & Performance monitoring and quality control
What is the problem?	How might the problem be solved?	Does the solution work?	Can the programme be repeated and refined?	Can the programme be widely reproduced?	Can the programme be sustained?

whether desired end points are achieved. This is often achieved by means of experimental or quasi-experimental methods. However, process evaluation is, at the same time, also important and becomes increasingly important in order to understand which variables influence the change process and to broaden the findings and relevance of findings to practitioners and policy makers. This also refers to the black box problem, and having to explain why a programme was successful or unsuccessful as opposed to only establishing that a programme was successful or unsuccessful. In turn, this enables the exporting of the programme by different managers to other people in other times and places. Demonstration research represents a shift to more real-life environments, identifying the contextual variables, conditions for success, and analysis of costs relative to benefits. Such studies are of greater relevance and interest to practitioners and policy makers.

Phase 4 relates to solution maintenance, which includes dissemination research and quality control. Attention is given to ways of implementing the successful programme extensively, promoting its use among practitioners, and establishing the optimal conditions for success in different settings. This kind of information is of greatest interest to managers and practitioners because it helps define 'what needs to be done, by whom, to what standard and at what cost' (Nutbeam, 1996, p. 319).

Paradoxically, the volume of reported research decreases from phase 1 to phase 4, as the usefulness and relevance of the findings to practitioners increase. Nutbeam, (1996, p. 319) emphasizes that there is a need for researchers to follow through the developmental sequence as indicated in Figure 1, in order to:

> promote the transfer of new knowledge from basic research into intervention program development, and to ensure that evidence of success from experimental research is systematically tested in real life conditions and disseminated in ways which are sensitive to the needs of practitioners who need to know how to create the conditions for success … (the practitioners in this case being the community psychologists).

Although the developmental model of evaluation is systematic in orientation, it can be used as a planning tool that is operationalized using any of the systematic and measurement-based, interpretive, or participatory-activist approaches, or a combination of approaches.

5 Summary and conclusions

In this chapter we have discussed programme evaluation as an emerging area of social science research, which is of great relevance to the community psychologist. A number of types of evaluation research have been outlined, as well as specific models and approaches used in conducting evaluations of social programmes. Similarities between the focuses of community research and programme evaluation have been pointed out.

In South Africa, as in many other countries, the field of programme evaluation in the 1990s reflects increasing diversity as well as increasing sophistication. As an alternative to systematic and measurement-based evaluation designs based on positivist assumptions, there has been a growth in interest in qualitative methods (Miles and Huberman, 1994) and in multi-method and eclectic approaches (Williams, 1986), as well as post-experimental multiplist perspectives (Cook, 1985; Cook and Shadish, 1986; Shadish et al., 1986), which attempt to integrate the use of quantitative and qualitative data in evaluation research.

However, critics of evaluation cite the large number of evaluation studies that have been conducted without any theoretical basis, as well as the minimal contribution made by programme evaluation to theory. Advocates of evaluation suggest that there is a theory implicit in every programme, and that those conducting evaluations should be encouraged to treat their work as both an applied and theoretical endeavour. This issue is of particular relevance to community psychology, in the sense that theories of community psychology could contribute to the development of evaluation as a field, and conversely, that programme evaluations could contribute to the development of community psychology. In this respect, community psychology has much to gain from, as well as to contribute to the field of programme evaluation.

Another issue relates to the standards, quality, and rigour of programme evaluations (Joint Committee on Standards for Educational Evaluation, 1981). Many evaluations are commissioned for accountability purposes, implying an examination of programme impact and effects. Given the expectation that social programmes will lead

Why do evaluators fail?

- Volatility: evaluation occurs in a continually changing decision-making milieu. The resources, priorities, and influence of stakeholders change.
- Failure to deal with unanticipated problems.
- Scientific vs. pragmatic postures: inability to adapt from an academic social research perspective to an applied social pragmatist approach, in order to obtain information that is 'good enough under the circumstances' to answer programme questions.
- Funders seem to view programmes as one-shot enterprises.
- Evaluators are called in too late.
- Because of ethical and/or political concerns it is often difficult to develop the most rigorous designs.
- Social science research is still in its youth.
- Educational researchers and evaluators themselves cannot agree about the appropriateness of research designs for evaluation.

(Adapted from Fitz-Gibbon and Morris, 1987; Rossi and Freeman, 1985.)

to social benefits, it is necessary to establish that specific interventions are indeed related to or a cause of change in the beneficiaries. This is especially difficult in community settings, as many effects of programmes cannot be directly observed or measured.

Given the context of social development, and the social disparities and poverty that characterize societies in many areas of the African continent, it is likely that the community psychologist will opt for some form of participatory evaluation, based within a critical/emancipatory paradigm, as most likely to lead to the empowerment of those involved in social programmes. In terms of this paradigm, the evaluator takes an activist role, acting to directly improve the programme through assuming various roles, including advocacy for the programme's work, as well as developmental work undertaken with the aim of empowering those involved in the programme to cope with the problems they encounter. This approach is of relevance to evaluation in low- to middle-income countries, and has particular relevance to the community psychologist working in community settings in Africa.

Exercises

1 A group of concerned volunteer teachers from a far-away rural town approach you, and ask your assistance in setting up a therapeutic centre for their school children. The nearest psychologists and remedial teachers are 200 km away. You have a free hand to help them but can only go there once a month. How will you help set up this community centre? What will the driving assumptions of this project be? How would you structure the summative, formative, process, outcome, and impact evaluations of this programme? Use a time-line to indicate at which time evaluation processes start and stop.

2 How does the black box theory relate to the objectives-based approach to evaluation? Which approaches address the inside of the black box?

3 A social worker was interested in reducing the amount of prejudice expressed by the members of the community with which she worked. She designed what she thought would be an effective programme for changing prejudicial attitudes, which initially would be implemented at a pilot level in a community centre. A corporate sponsor agreed to support the development and implementation costs over a two-year period, provided that the programme was properly evaluated. The sponsor stipulated that they needed hard quantitative evidence, as well as evidence of support from the programme's various stakeholders. The programme plan provided for each implementation to take place over six weekends, in which a number of sessions would be conducted dealing with issues relating to analysing the nature of prejudice, as well as ways of dealing with prejudice. This would be followed by an applied project in which each participant would work with three families over a further six-week period in the area in which they lived. Progress made in the programme would be monitored by means of an evaluation conducted by a team of evaluators consisting of a community psychologist, an adult educator, and a community worker.

3.1 What would an appropriate evaluation design be to meet the needs and vested interests of the programme planners, the users of the programme, as well as the corporate sponsors?

3.2 Do an analysis of all the stakeholders and their evaluation and informational needs.

3.3 What type of evaluation/research questions would you have about the programme?

3.4 What process would you follow so that you could also solicit and include in your evaluation design the evaluation/research questions of the programme's stakeholders?

3.5 Propose a time frame and budget for the evaluation. Assume that you are doing the evaluation yourself.

4 Apply the three major evaluation streams discussed in the chapter (e.g., systematic and measurement-based; interpretive and naturalistic; and critical and empowerment) to the six phases of research in Nutbeam's adapted model (refer to the section 'Getting started').

Note

1 The authors would like to thank Johann Louw for his comments on the first draft of this chapter, and for his contributions during a workshop on programme evaluation at the Centre for Peace Action; Willy de Haes from the Rotterdam Health Services for drawing our attention to Nutbeam's model of research and evaluation; Jennifer Greene from Cornell University for her kind support; and most importantly, the staff of the Centre for Peace Action for their commitment to promoting peace through intervention and evaluation, and whose work gave the impetus and practical input for materials in this chapter.

References

AMERICAN JOURNAL OF COMMUNITY PSYCHOLOGY (1998). Special Issue. *Qualitative research in community psychology.* 26(4).

ASAMOAH, Y. (1988). Program evaluation in Africa. *Evaluation and Program Planning,* 11(2), 169–177.

BECHER, R. A. (1974). *Styles of curriculum development and curriculum evaluation.* Edinburgh: Scottish Council for Research in Education.

BECHER, A. and MACLURE, S. (Eds.). (1978a). *The politics of curriculum change.* London: Hutchinson.

BECHER, A. and MACLURE, S. (Eds.). (1978b). *Accountability in educating.* Windsor: NFER.

BURGESS, R. (Ed.). (1984). *The research process in educational settings: Ten case studies.* Lewes: Falmer.

CAMPBELL, D. T. and STANLEY, J. C. (1963). *Experimental and quasi-experimental designs for research.* Boston: Houghton Mifflin.

CARR, W. and KEMMIS, S. (1986). *Becoming critical: Knowing through action research* (2nd ed.). London: Falmer.

CHEN, H. T. (1990). *Theory-driven evaluations.* London: Sage.

CHEN, H. T. and ROSSI, P. H. (1983). Evaluating with sense: The theory-driven approach. *Evaluation Review,* 7, 283–302.

CHOUDHARY, A. and TANDON, R. (1988). *Participatory evaluation.* New Delhi: Society for Participatory Research in Asia.

COOK, T. D. (1985). Postpositivist critical multiplism. In L. Shotland and M. M. Mark (Eds.), *Social science and social policy* (pp. 458–499). Beverly Hills, CA: Sage.

COOK, T. D. and CAMPBELL, S. T. (1979). *Quasi-experimentation: Design and analysis issues for field settings.* Chicago: Rand McNally.

COOK, T. D. and SHADISH, W. R. (1986). Program evaluation: The worldly science. *Annual Review of Psychology*, 37, 193–232.

CORDER, C. K. (1997). The reconstruction and development programme: Success or failure? *Social Indicators Research*, 41(1–3), 183–203.

CRONBACH, L. J. (1963). Course improvement through evaluation. *Teachers College Record*, 64, 672–683.

CRONBACH, L. J., AMBRON, S. R., DORNBUSCH, S. M., HESS, R. D., PHILIPS, D. C., WALKER, D. F., and WEINER, S. S. (1980). *Toward reform of program evaluation*. San Francisco, CA: Jossey-Bass.

DENZIN, N. K. and LINCOLN, Y. S. (Eds.). (1994). *Handbook of qualitative research*. Thousand Oaks, CA: Sage.

ELLIOT, J. (1980). *SSRC Cambridge Accountability Project: A summary report*. Cambridge: Cambridge Institute of Education (mimeo).

FETTERMAN, D. M. (1989). *Ethnography: Step by step*. Beverly Hills, CA: Sage.

FETTERMAN, D. M., KAFTARIAN, S. J., and WANDERSMAN, A. (Eds.). (1996). *Empowerment evaluation: Knowledge and tools for self-assessment and accountability*. Thousand Hills, CA: Sage.

FITZ-GIBBON, C. T. and MORRIS, L. L. (1987). *How to design a program evaluation* (2nd ed.). Newbury Park, CA: Sage.

FREIRE, P. (1972). *Pedagogy of the oppressed*. Harmondsworth: Penguin.

GLENWICK, D. S., HELLER, K., LINNEY, J. A., and PARGAMENT, K. I. (1990). Criteria of excellence. I. Models for adventuresome research in community psychology: Commonalities, dilemmas and future directions. In P. Tolan, C. Keys, F. Chertok, and L. Jason (Eds.), *Researching community psychology* (pp. 76–87). Washington, DC: American Psychological Association.

GREDLER, M. E. (1996). *Program evaluation*. Englewood Cliffs, NJ: Prentice Hall.

GREENE, S. (1994). Qualitative program evaluation: Practice and promise. In N. K. Denzin and Y. S. Lincoln (Eds.), *Handbook of qualitative research* (pp. 530–544). Thousand Oaks, CA: Sage.

GRUNDY, S. (1984). *Beyond professionalism: Action research as critical pedagogy*. Unpublished Ph.D. thesis, Murdoch University.

GUBA, E. G. and LINCOLN, Y. S. (1981). *Effective evaluation: Improving the usefulness of evaluation results through responsive and naturalistic approaches*. San Francisco, CA: Jossey-Bass.

GUBA, E. G. and LINCOLN, Y. S. (1989). *Fourth generation evaluation*. Newbury Park, CA: Sage.

HABERMAS, J. (1971). *Knowledge and human interests*. Boston: Beacon.

HALL, B. L. (1978). Breaking the monopoly of knowledge: Research methods, participation and development. In B. L. Hall and J. Roby Kidd (Eds.), *Adult learning: A design for action* (pp. 155–168). Oxford: Pergamon.

HAMILTON, D. (1976). *Curriculum evaluation*. London: Open Books.

HAMILTON, D., JENKINS, D., KING, C., MACDONALD, B., and PARLETT, M. (Eds.). (1977). *Beyond the numbers game*. London: MacMillan Education.

HEIMAN, G. A. (1995). *Research methods in psychology*. Boston: Houghton Mifflin.

HERRICK, V. E and TYLER, R. W. (Eds.). (1950). *Toward improved curriculum theory*. Chicago: The University of Chicago Press.

HOUTS, A. C., COOK, T. D., and SHADISH, W. R. (1986). The person-situation debate: A critical multiplist perspective. *Journal of Personality*, 54, 52–105.

HOUSE, E. R. (1973). *School evaluation: The politics and process*. Berkeley, CA: McCutchan.

HOUSE, E. R. (1977). The politics of evaluation in higher education. In F.G. Caro (Ed.), *Readings in evaluation research* (pp. 94–101). New York: Russell Sage Foundation.

HOUSE, E. R. (1983). Assumptions underlying evaluation models. In G. F. Madaus, M. Scriven, and D. L. Stufflebeam (Eds.), *Evaluation models: Viewpoints on educational and human sciences evaluation* (pp.45–64). Boston: Kluwer-Nijhoff.

JOINT COMMITTEE ON STANDARDS FOR EDUCATIONAL EVALUATION. (1981). *Principles and by-laws*. Michigan: Western Michigan University Evaluation Center.

KINCHELOE, J. L. and MCLAREN, P. L. (1994). Designing social inquiry: Scientific inference in qualitative research. In N. K. Denzin and Y. S. Lincoln (Eds.), *Handbook of qualitative research* (pp. 138–157). Thousand Oaks, CA: Sage.

KRIEGLER, S., RAMARUMO, M., VAN DER RYST, M., and VAN NIEKERK, K. (1994). Supporting emergent literacy in print bereft rural communities. *School Psychology International*, 15(1), 23–37.

LACEY, C. and LAWTON, D. (1981). *Issues in evaluation and accountability*. London: Methuen.

LAKOMSKI, G. (1988). Critical Theory. In J. P. Keeves (Ed.), *Educational research, methodology and measurement: An international handbook* (pp. 54–58). London: Pergamon.

LIPSEY, M. W. (1993). Theory as method: Small theories of treatments. In L. B. Sechrest and A. G. Scott, *Understanding causes and generalising about them* (pp. 5–38). San Francisco: Jossey-Bass.

LIPSEY, M. W., CROSSE, S., DUNKLE, J., POLLARD, J., and STOBART, G. (1985). Evaluation: The state of the art and the sorry state of the science. In D. S. Cordray (Ed.), *Utilising prior research in evaluation planning: New directions for program evaluation* (No 27, pp. 7–28). San Francisco: Jossey-Bass.

LOUW, J. (1998). Programme evaluation: A structured assessment. In J. Mouton and J. Muller (Eds.), *Theory and method in South African human sciences research: Advances and innovations* (pp. 255–268). Pretoria: Human Sciences Research Council.

MACDONALD, B. (1978). Accountability, standards and the process of schooling. In A. Becher and S. MacLure (Eds.), *Accountability in education* (pp. 127–151). Windsor: NFER.

MACDONALD, B. (1993). A political classification of evaluation studies in education. In M. Hammersley et al., *Social research: Philosophy, politics and practice* (pp. 105–108). London: Sage.

MADAUS, G. F., SCRIVEN, M., AND STUFFLEBEAM, D. L. (Eds.). (1983). *Evaluation models: Viewpoints on educational and human services evaluation*. Boston: Kluwer-Nijhoff.

MADAUS, G. F., STUFFLEBEAM, D. L., and SCRIVEN, M. (1983). Programme evaluation: A historical overview. In G. F. Madaus, M.

Scriven, and D. L. Stufflebeam (Eds.), *Evaluation models: Viewpoints on educational and human services evaluation* (pp. 3–22). Boston: Kluwer-Nijhoff.

MADAUS, G. F. and STUFFLEBEAM, D. L. (1989). *Educational evaluation: Classic works of Ralph W. Tyler*. Boston: Kluwer Academic Publishers.

MAHATEY, N., KAGEE, A., and NAIDOO, T. (1994). Mentoring for learning: The student development programme at UWC. In B. Leibowitz and M. Walker, *Voices, development and learning*. Ad Dialogues, 3. Cape Town: University of the Western Cape.

MCCONNELL, C. F., LEEMING, F. C., and DWYER, W. O. (1996). Evaluation of a fire-safety training program for preschool children. *Journal of Community Psychology*, 24(3), 213–227.

MELKERS, J. and ROESSNER, D. (1997). Politics and the political setting as an influence on evaluation activities: National research and technology policy programs in the United States and Canada. *Evaluation and Program Planning*, 20(1), 57–76.

MILES, M. B. and HUBERMAN, A. M. (1994). *Qualitative data analysis: An expanded sourcebook*. Beverly Hills, CA: Sage.

NEUMAN, W. L. (1997). *Social research methods: Qualitative and quantitative approaches* (3rd ed.). Boston: Allyn and Bacon .

NUTBEAM, D. (1996). Achieving 'best practice' in health promotion: Improving the fit between research and practice. *Health Education Research*, 11(3), 317–326.

NUTBEAM, D., SMITH, C., and CATFORD, J. (1990). Evaluation in health education: A review of progress, possibilities, and problems. *Journal of Epidemiology and Community Health*, 44, 83–89.

PARLETT, M. and HAMILTON, D. (1972). *Evaluation as illumination: A new approach to the study of innovatory programmes*. Occasional Paper of the Centre for Research in the Educational Sciences. Edinburgh: University of Edinburgh.

PARLETT, M. and DEARDEN, G. (Eds.). (1977). *Introduction to illuminative evaluation: Studies in higher education*. Cardiff-by-the-Sea, CA: Pacific Soundings Press.

PATTON, M. Q. (1982). *Practical evaluation.* Beverly Hills, CA: Sage.

PATTON, M. Q. (1990). *Qualitative evaluation and research methods* (2nd ed.) Newbury Park, CA: Sage.

POSAVAC, E. J. and CAREY, R. G. (1989). *Program evaluation* (3rd ed.). Englewood Cliffs, NJ: Prentice-Hall.

POTTER, C. S. (1991). What is evaluation? An operational framework. In P. Irwin and E. Janse van Rensburg (Eds.), *Evaluation in environmental education* (pp. 30–37). Grahamstown: Rhodes University and South African Environmental Education Association.

POTTER, C. S. (1996). Four white men and a dog: The implications of the ANC's draft policy framework for education and training for the training of evaluators in South Africa. *Journal of Educational Evaluation,* 4, 23–38.

POTTER, C. S. (1999). Programme evaluation. In M. T. Terre Blanche and K. D. Durheim (Eds.), *Research in practice* (pp. 209–226). Cape Town: UCT Press.

RAPPAPORT, J. (1987). Terms of empowerment/ exemplars of prevention: Toward a theory for community psychology. *American Journal of Community Psychology,* 13(2), 121–148.

RAPPAPORT, J. (1990). Research methods and the empowerment social agenda. In P. Tolan, C. Keys, F. Chertok, and L. Jason (Eds.), *Researching community psychology* (pp. 51–63). Washington, DC: American Psychological Association.

ROSSI, P. H. and FREEMAN, H. E. (1985). *Evaluation: A systematic approach* (3rd ed.). Beverly Hills, CA: Sage.

SHADISH, W. R. (1986). Planned critical multiplism: Some elaborations. *Behavioural Assessment,* 8, 75–103.

SHADISH, W. R. (1990a). Defining excellence criteria in community research. In P. Tolan, C. Keys, F. Chertok, and L. Jason (Eds.), *Researching community psychology* (pp. 9–20). Washington, DC: American Psychological Association.

SHADISH, W. R. (1990b). What can we learn about problems in community research by comparing it with program evaluation? In P. Tolan, C. Keys, F. Chertok, and L. Jason (Eds.), *Researching community psychology* (pp. 201–223). Washington, DC: American Psychological Association.

SHADISH, W. L., COOK, T. D., and HOUTS, A. C. (1986). Quasi-experimentation in a critical multiplist mode. *New Directions for Program Evaluation,* 31, 29–46.

SHAUGNESSY, J. J. and ZECHMEISTER, E. B. (1997). *Research methods in psychology* (3rd ed.). New York: McGraw-Hill.

SILVERPLATTER INTERNATIONAL N.V. PsychLIT on CD-Rom.

SIMONS, H. (1987). *Getting to know schools in a democracy: The politics and process of education.* London: Falmer.

STAKE, R. E. (1978). The case study method in social inquiry. *Educational Researcher,* 2(2), 148–152.

STAKE, R. E. (1980). Program evaluation, particularly responsive evaluation. In W. B. Dockrell and D. Hamilton (Eds.), *Rethinking educational research* (pp. 72–87). London: Hodder and Stoughton.

STAKE, R. E. (1983). Responsive evaluation. In *International Encyclopaedia of Education,* Vol. 7, 4349–4351.

STENHOUSE, L. (1975). *An introduction to curriculum research and development.* London: Heinemann.

STENHOUSE, L. (1983). The curriculum as hypothetical. In J. Ruddick and D. Hopkins (Eds.), *Research as a basis for teaching: Readings for the work of Lawrence Stenhouse* (pp. 70–71). London: Heinemann Educational Books.

STUFFLEBEAM, D. L. (1968). *Evaluation as enlightenment for decision-making.* Columbus, OH: Ohio State University, Evaluation Center.

STUFFLEBEAM, D. L. (1972). The relevance of the CIPP evaluation model for educational accountability. *SRIS Quarterly,* 5, 3–6.

TOLAN, P., KEYS, C., CHERTOK, F., and JASON, L. (Eds.). (1990). *Researching community psychology: Issues of theory and methods.* Washington, DC: American Psychological Association.

TYLER, R. W., SMITH, E. R., and THE EVALUATION
STAFF. (1942). *Purposes and procedures of the evaluation staff. Appraising and recording student progress. Vol III, Adventure in American education.*
New York: Harper.

WALKER, R. (1980). The conduct of educational case studies: Ethics, theory and procedures.
In W. B. Dockrell and D. Hamilton (Eds.),
Rethinking educational research (pp. 30–63).
London: Hodder and Stoughton.

WEISS, C. H. (1973). Where politics and evaluation meet. *Evaluation*, I, 37–45.

WEISS, C. H. (1982). Policy research in the context of diffuse decision making. *Journal of Higher Education*, 53, 619–639.

WEISS, C. H.(1983a). Toward the future of stakeholder approaches in evaluation. *New Directions for Program Evaluation*, 17, 83–96.

WEISS, C. H.(1983b). The stakeholder approach to evaluation: Origins and promise. *New Directions for Program Evaluation*, 17, 3–14.

WILLIAMS, D. D. (1986). Naturalistic evaluation.
New Directions for Program Evaluation, 30.

ZIMMERMAN, M. A. (1995). Psychological empowerment: Issues and illustrations. *American Journal of Community Psychology*, 21(2), 581–598.

211

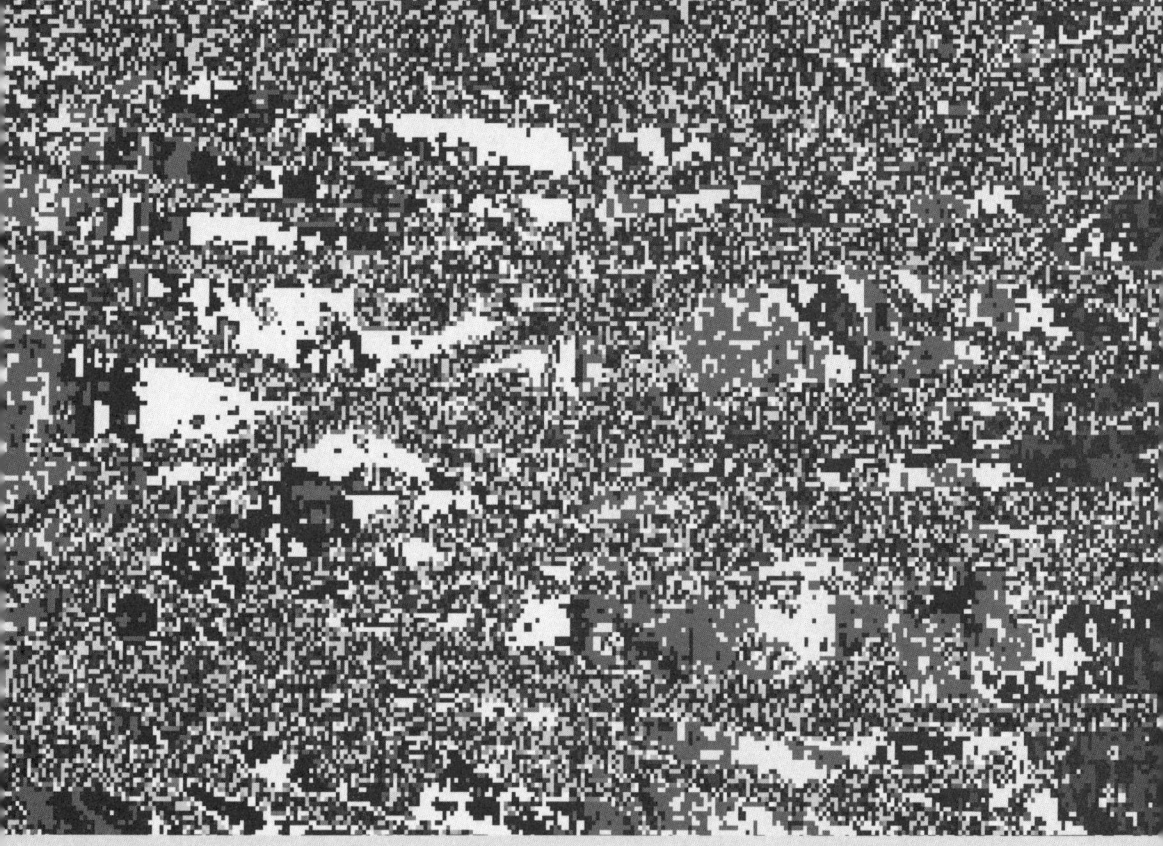

SECTION III

Practice in
community
psychology

Community
Psychology

Public health and community psychology: a case study in community-based injury prevention

Alexander Butchart

Johan Kruger

Study objectives

After studying this chapter you should have:

- an understanding of what public health is and how it works in an applied setting;
- an understanding of the terms epidemiology and demography, and the related concepts incidence, prevalence, morbidity, and mortality;
- an understanding of how the evidence produced by epidemiology is converted into concrete action for community development;
- an awareness of the limitations and potential sources of error that can bias the design and effects of public health interventions; and
- the background to begin further reading and study in public health.

1 Introduction

Among the least developed connections between community psychology and related disciplines is the link to public health. As a scientific approach to disease prevention and the promotion of individual and social well-being, public health operates beyond the clinics, nurses, and doctors usually associated with the idea of health. Instead, public health targets all points where matter, energy, and information are exchanged between people and their human, social, and physical environments, for it is through this exchange that individual and group health status is determined.

To manage this exchange for the improvement of well-being, public health employs a range of strategies aimed at altering individual behaviour and community lifestyle, the social and political context of harmful beliefs and practices, and dangers in the physical environment. It is therefore a profoundly social activity with powerful implications for individuals and communities, as conveyed by Last's definition of public health as:

> the combination of science, skills and beliefs that are directed to the maintenance and improvement of the health of all the people through collective or social action. The programmes, services, and institutions involved emphasise the prevention of disease and the health needs of the population as a whole. Public health activities change with changing technology and social values, but the goals remain the same: to reduce the amount of disease, premature death and disease-produced discomfort and disability in the population (Last, 1988, p.107).

Implicit in this definition are the three main elements of public health. First, it addresses health not at the level of the individual, but at the level of the entire population. Where clinical medicine treats disease within a person, public health aims to prevent problems before they occur by working at the aggregate level with issues such as the social norms shaping the acceptability of smoking, community access to adequate sanitation, or the protection of people from such harmful by-products of economic activity as pollution, firearms, and alcohol. Second, because they frequently target major social processes (like poverty, violence, and substance abuse), beyond the ability of a single community or discipline to alter, public health interventions draw upon the resources of multiple disciplines (e.g., psychology, building science, and medicine), and many different social sectors (e.g., professionals, church groups, community residents). Third, to collect the information for aggregate-level change, public health requires methods that can define

---

Figure 1 Public health model of a scientific approach to prevention

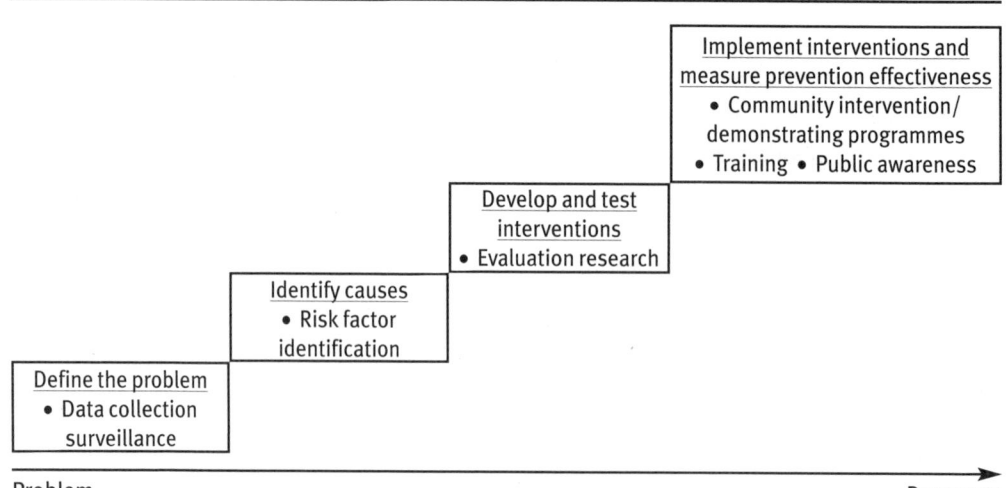

Problem   Response

problems at the population level in ways that open them up to interventions involving multiple disciplines and sectors.

Public health integrates these components into a four-stage model of a scientific approach to prevention (see Figure 1). The first stage involves problem definition. It includes obtaining information about the demographic characteristics of persons who manifest the problem, details about the geographical location and time at which they were injured or infected, and details about the severity of their problem and its financial costs. Stage two identifies the causes of the problem and what its risk factors may be. In other words, where stage one asks 'who, where, when, what, and how', stage two tries to answer the question 'why?' In stage three the information from steps one and two is used to develop interventions, which are then tested to see if they are effective in reducing the size of the target problem. The final stage is to implement interventions shown to be effective, and to continue measuring the impact of the programme on the target problem. To do this, steps four and three use information produced in steps one and two, which by monitoring changes in the size and nature of the target problem, serve as important evaluation mechanisms.

Built around a South African case study of public health as applied to community-oriented injury prevention, this chapter explores the basic concepts, models, and tools that underlie such interventions. First, it explores the concepts of injury, injury prevention, and the safe community approach to delivering safety promotion. Second, it examines the methods of epidemiology and

demography, and concepts such as incidence, prevalence, morbidity, and mortality, which are the core tools used by public health to define its problems, design its interventions, and measure intervention effectiveness. The practical meaning of these ideas in the context of a community intervention aimed at reducing injuries due to violence and other causes is then demonstrated in the case study. Throughout, this chapter critically reflects on the weaknesses and strengths of the method, and concludes by suggesting how the fusion of public health and community psychology could be extended fruitfully beyond injury to many other problems.

2 Injury prevention and Safe Communities

2.1 Injuries: an emerging threat to health

Following the World Health Organization (WHO), the estimated contribution of injuries to the global burden of disease will increase from 14,3 per cent in 1990 to 20,9 per cent by the year 2020, unless action is taken to prevent this emerging threat to health (see Table 1). While the proportional burden of disease due to injuries is likely to increase in all countries as a result of success in preventing communicable diseases, it is projected that in sub-Saharan Africa the injury-related disease burden will more than double, due not only to reductions in communicable conditions, but also because of increased violence and transport-related injuries.

Table 1 Disability adjusted lost years of life by main categories of cause in 1990, with alternative projections for 2020

	GLOBAL		SUB-SAHARAN AFRICA	
	1990	2020	1990	2020
Communicable, maternal, and peri-natal	42,7	17,4	64,5	33,0
Non-communicable	43,1	61,8	20,8	35,8
Injuries	14,3	20,9	14,7	31,2

SOURCE: Ad Hoc Committee (1996)

Over the past few decades, public health has expanded from an emphasis on infectious and non-communicable diseases, such as tuberculosis, cardiovascular problems, and nutritional disorders, to embrace the emerging problem of deaths and disabilities due to injuries (Rosenberg and Fenley, 1991). Following WHO's working group on the classification of external causes of injury:

> Injury is a bodily lesion at an organic level resulting from acute exposure to energy (this energy can be mechanical, thermal, electrical, chemical or radiant) interacting with the body in amounts that exceed the threshold of physiological tolerance. In some cases an injury results from an insufficiency of any of the vital elements (in drowning, strangulation, or freezing) (WHO, 1989, pp. 110-111).

Two broad classes of injury are distinguished by the presumed intentionality of cause, namely, unintentional injuries and intentional injuries. To eliminate the idea that injuries are due to fate or other unpredictable events, the term unintentional injury is preferred over the term 'accident' (Langley, 1988), and to distinguish this work from the areas of psychological counselling and emergency medicine, the term injury is used in preference to 'trauma'.

As the burden of disease due to infectious conditions declines in high-income and some low-income countries, there has been increasing recognition of injury as a major source of death and disability (Ad Hoc Committee, 1996). Particularly in Scandinavia and Europe, but also in the United States and Australia, this has led to sustained prevention programmes that are returning clear evidence of success in preventing injuries due to unintentional causes, such as burns (Ytterstad, 1995), transport collisions (Engel and Thomsen, 1992; Ytterstad and Wasmuth, 1995), and events occurring in the home and at schools (Victorian

Health Promotion Foundation, 1996). Although less convincing, there is also tentative evidence that such programmes may be effective in reducing levels of interpersonal violence, using a mix of educational, enforcement, and engineering strategies (Farrington, 1993; Gainer, Webster, and Champion, 1993; Laird, Syropolous, and Black, 1996; Mcdowell, Loftin, and Wiersma, 1992).

Central to the success of these initiatives is their sensitivity to local variations in the injury profile and conditions in which injuries occur (Svanström and Svanström, 1989; Lindqvist, 1993). Injuries result from events that damage the body through sudden energy transfers into or out of it, and repeated scientific investigations of when, where, and how they occur have shown that injuries are not randomly distributed, but follow clear patterns that allow their occurrence to be predicted at the population level.

Perhaps more so than many other diseases, the distribution of injuries and injury causes varies widely between different communities, neighbourhoods, and social sectors, as defined in terms such as gender, age, income, and occupation. While injuries must therefore be understood as a global problem, their prevention requires responses that are sensitive to these local-level variations.

It is this recognition that underlies the aims of WHO's 'Safe Communities' movement (see box on this page), and its emphasis upon enhancing the ability of people around the world to develop effective injury prevention programmes based upon recent and reliable local level information. Safe Communities programmes combine the bottom-up input of individuals and groups most affected

Safe Communities

An international movement affiliated to WHO's Global Programme on the Prevention of Violence and Injury, the Safe Communities movement grew out of the innovations of Scandinavian injury prevention workers. In the late 1960s, injury research and prevention programmes were developed at Lund University in Sweden, engaging sociologists, anatomists, psychologists, epidemiologists, architects, and specialists in systems analysis and social medicine. By the early 1970s, the interdisciplinary approach modelled by the group found application in field research investigations, one of which was the Falköping study in Sweden's Skaraborg county. After two years of intervention, this programme was shown to have reduced injuries by almost 30 per cent overall, and in some groups by as much as 45 per cent (Karolinska Institute, 1992). Since then, further pilot interventions were developed throughout Sweden and similar programmes initiated in Norway and Denmark to establish a Scandinavian network of community-oriented injury prevention programmes.

In 1989 the First World Conference on Accident and Injury Prevention was held in Stockholm, Sweden. This had as an important outcome the 'Manifesto for Safe Communities' (WHO, 1989), which marked expansion of the Safe Communities movement into the global safety arena. After noting that all human beings have an equal right to health and safety, and that to be effective in promoting safety, all demonstration projects for injury prevention must include community-level programmes, the manifesto identified four Safe Community action areas: (1) the formulation of public policy for safety whereby governments are committed to investing greater human and financial resources in safety promotion; (2) the creation of environments that support injury prevention activities through local and international networks for sharing knowledge and experience; (3) strengthening community action against injuries through training, technical advice, financial assistance, and help in programme evaluation; and (4) broadening the range of public services involved in safety promotion to ensure that all relevant sectors coordinate their efforts to achieve optimum results.

After reviewing community safety programmes in various high- and low-income countries, twelve criteria were developed that stipulated the requirements that a community or organization should meet in order to be declared a 'safe community'. These emphasize the need for combining epidemiological information, community involvement, and cross-sectoral participation, and provide a framework in which the diverse activities of programmes in different countries can find a common language. As of 1997 the Safe Communities network consisted of twenty-one programmes in nine

countries, and had held six international conferences.

The Safe Communities website is at: http://www.ki.se/phs/wcccsp/safecom/main.html.

by the injury problem with top-down interventions involving safety legislation, the elimination or modification of high-risk products, and the rehabilitation of dangerous environments. As for all public health problems, a prerequisite for the local-level targeting of injury prevention activities is the availability of information that describes the causes, nature, and extent of the problem, and risk factor information for the identification of intervention targets (Annest and Mallonnee, 1995). The technique by which problem definition and causal identification proceed is known as epidemiology.

2.2 Epidemiology and demography

Derived from the Greek words for 'upon' and 'people', epidemiology means the 'study of people'. It developed in the mid-1800s during attempts to control outbreaks of infectious diseases such as cholera and bubonic plague. John Snow's revolutionary approach to the 1853–1854 outbreak of cholera in London was widely regarded as the scientific beginning of epidemiology (Lilienfeld and Lilienfeld, 1980; Yach and Botha, 1986). Against the conventional reason of the time that viewed cholera as an air-borne disease, Snow postulated that it was carried by the water consumed by people. To test this, he observed the geographical distribution of cases and questioned sufferers as to where they got their drinking water. These observations all pointed to the 'Broad Street pump' as the single source of infection, and in what was probably the first attempt at preventive medicine, Snow removed the pump handle to stop further contamination.

Contemporaneous with epidemiology's emergence were wide-ranging developments in the science of demography. Demography is the science of population statistics, and the method by which the characteristics of a population are defined, such as its size, its gender and age distributions, and the average life expectancy. Initiated in the late 1700s, it was with the mid-1800s expansion of urban populations within the industrializing cities of western Europe that the value of demography for controlling the population was fully recognized. Accordingly, at the same time as Snow was engaged in his investigations, William Farr of the Registrar-General's office in London was laying down the basis for the collection and analysis of births and deaths (Yach and Botha, 1986).

The conditions studied by epidemiologists always occur within a population, so epidemiology and demography form the two sides of the public health coin. Without epidemiology, the characteristics of the target problem cannot be defined, and without demography the magnitude of the problem cannot be calculated, since this is always relative to the size of the population and has different implications depending upon its characteristics.

Since their beginnings, epidemiology and demography have developed into sophisticated scientific specialities, and in investigating injuries employ two broad classes of procedure. First, injury surveillance systems use mortuaries and hospital emergency rooms to collect simple descriptive information on an on-going basis. Second, cross-sectional studies may be used. These studies, which may be performed in mortuaries, hospitals, and through community surveys, provide a snapshot of the injury problem for a particular time period.

In many high-income countries routine surveillance provides the data required to define the problem (Pollock, 1995), and frequent census counts provide sufficiently accurate demographic information for calculating the epidemiological indices used in the design and evaluation of prevention programmes. However, in South Africa (Butchart, 1996; Lerer, Matzopolous, and Bradshaw, 1995) and low-income countries more generally (Zwi et al., 1996), reliable demographic data is often lacking and injury surveillance is the exception rather than the norm. While hospital-based studies can be performed in such settings, they are of limited value because they are not designed to establish demographic information, and where injury victims use a geographically wide-spread variety of service providers, can be prohibitively expensive. Prevention workers in these settings must therefore rely upon population or community-based approaches for collecting injury prevention information, along the lines of the household survey method applied in the 'Three Neighbourhoods Safety Promotion Programme'.

3 The Three Neighbourhoods Safety Promotion Programme

Exemplifying the safe communities approach to injury prevention, the Three Neighbourhoods Safety Promotion Programme developed within the broader context of the Centre for Peace Action's (CPA) on-going injury and violence prevention activities (Seedat, 1995; Seedat et al., 1992).

3.1 The context of intervention

Initiated in 1990 as an outcome of the first hospital-based epidemiological study of injuries in Johannesburg (Butchart et al., 1992), the CPA is in Eldorado Park, historically a coloured suburb bordering the predominantly African townships of Soweto. According to the 1989 – 1990 epidemiological study, coloured residents of Eldorado Park manifested the highest injury incidence of all groups, and the highest rates of non-fatal violent injuries. Strong age and gender-related trends emerged for both incidence and causal profiles, the highest risk occurring among males aged fifteen to thirty, and among women in the age range fifteen to thirty-five. By age and cause, unintentional injuries dominated up to age five, while from fifteen until forty-five years of age violence accounted for the largest proportion of injuries (Butchart et al., 1992). For violent incidents (Butchart and Brown, 1991), men were equally likely to be attacked by strangers as by acquaintances, incidents usually involving sharp instruments and occurring most often in private homes and 'on the street'. In contrast, nearly 40 per cent of women were attacked by spouses and lovers, and a further 32 per cent by acquaintances. These attacks on women occurred most frequently in the home, some 50 per cent involving knives, 20 per cent fists and feet, and 15 per cent blunt instruments.

Figure 2 The Three Neighbourhoods survey: baseline neighbourhood injury profiles

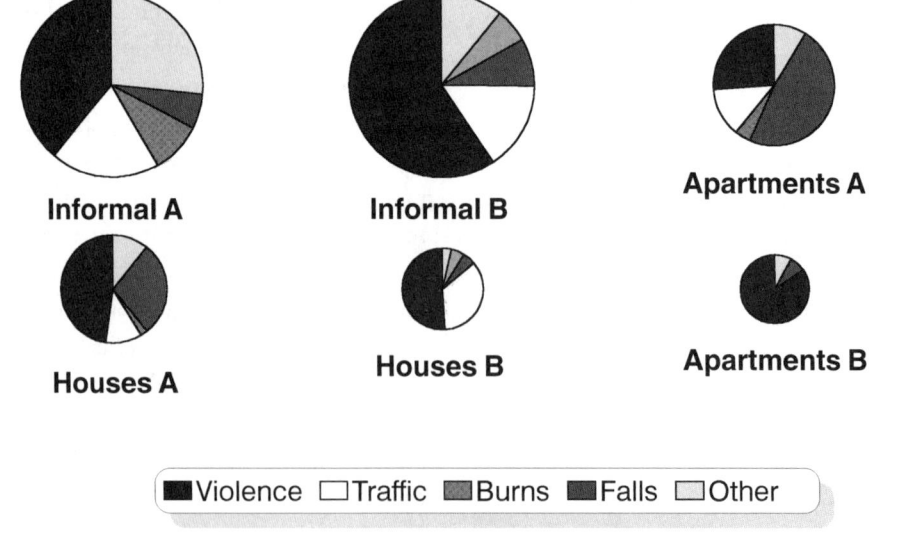

Informal A   Informal B   Apartments A

Houses A   Houses B   Apartments B

■Violence □Traffic ▨Burns ■Falls □Other

Selected findings for the Three Neighbourhoods survey

As shown in Figure 2 (see also Butchart, Kruger, and Nell, 1997), the incidence rate per 100 000 residents for the leading cause of injury in each neighbourhood was: Informal A: Violence: 8709/100 000 (n=87); Informal B: Traffic: 5381/100 000 (n=36), and violence 5231/100 000 (n=35); Apartments A: Household accidents : 4152/100000 (n=12); Apartments B: Violence : 2026/100 000 (n=11); Houses A : Violence : 3138/100 000 (n=22); Houses B : Violence 1897/100 000 (n=29). The injury mortality rate for the overall sample (N=4 729) was 381/100 000 (n=18), and for violent deaths 232/100 000 (n=11). Distribution of causes by age and gender followed the expected patterns. Alcohol use was a prominent risk factor, as were environmental factors including crowding and proximity to highways. The percentage of violent incidents reported to police ranged between 59 and 63 per cent in the informal settlements, to 44 and 62 per cent in the houses, and zero to 80 per cent in the apartment blocks. Just 68 per cent of cases were treated in hospital settings, the remainder using clinics, private doctors, and other treatment modes.

In addition to suggesting discrete injury prevention activities within each area, these findings constitute a natural experiment in injury prevention, suggesting that the formalization of housing and the community stabilization perhaps accompanying it can reduce the overall injury rate by 50 per cent or more.

This numeric data was complemented by detailed qualitative responses where respondents outlined the injury process, indicated what they believed to be the causes of each major injury category (i.e. violence, traffic, home, and other injuries), and said what they considered should be done to prevent these injuries (Butchart, Kruger, and Lekoba, 2000).

These and other findings were disseminated through meetings with community groups, local government and health sector agencies, the corporate sector, and international donor agencies, with the aim of securing multi-sectoral support for an injury and violence prevention programme. These efforts were successful and in 1990 the Centre opened with a small staff of professional psychologists and community residents. Over the last six years its prevention programmes have become increasingly consolidated and focused, and the CPA has achieved a stable presence in the communities it serves.

Despite succeeding as a service delivery organization, the Centre has been unable to evaluate the effects of its interventions at the population level. This is known as outcome evaluation (Berg et al., 1995; O'Donnell, Cohen, and Hausman, 1990) and requires at least two types of information for the target groups. First, demographic information about the background population, and second, data on the extent of the injury problem in the population prior to the intervention and at various points during and after it. In the CPA's case, none of this information was available from external sources. Estimates of the area's population size available in 1996 (Central Witwatersrand Metropolitan Chamber, 1994; Central Witwatersrand Regional Services Council, 1993) relied on 1991 census data that did not reflect the demographic changes that had occurred since then, and more detailed demographic information, including age distribution, income levels, and rooming density, was unavailable. Concerning the extent of injuries, while the 1989-1990 epidemiological study afforded sufficient detail to target the intervention at a macro-level, its data reflected the injury situation prior to the post-election transformations, and were therefore of no utility in mapping the area's contemporary injury profile.

Against the backdrop of these challenges the South African Medical Research Council tendered nationally in 1994 for project proposals aimed at researching the efficacy of community-based violence prevention initiatives. The Centre's proposal was successful, and just under ZAR 100 000 per year for three years was granted for the implementation of a population-based injury measurement and outcome evaluation programme, which soon became known as the Three Neighbourhoods Safety Promotion Programme.

3.2 Methods

To produce information that is useful for action, an epidemiological survey must at the outset specify what kinds of information it aims to get and what population it wishes to get it from. Following Berger and Mohan (1996), at least three elements must be specified: (1) the nature of the injuries to be studied (e.g., intentional, occupational); (2) the severity level of the injuries to be studied (e.g., deaths, medically treated, hospital admissions); and (3) the target population in terms of age, geographic location, occupation, and so on.

In the Three Neighbourhoods programme, the injuries to be studied were all injuries of whatever cause and severity occurring one calendar year prior to the interview. The intervention population was defined as all residents within the geographical boundaries of Eldorado Park, as demarcated on town council maps of the magisterial district. However, an absence of data on the demographic characteristics of this population meant that the survey itself had to provide such information. A first step therefore involved analysing the area's demographic and environmental characteristics in sufficient detail to permit selection of a survey sample representative of the different residential groups.

3.2.1 Demographic and environmental analysis

The aim of analysing the community's demographic and environmental characteristics was two-fold. First, because the area's total population was estimated to exceed 80 000, a sampling-based approach to injury measurement was required whereby findings for selected respondents could be generalized to the entire population. Second, because the distribution of injuries has repeatedly been shown to co-vary with changes in the socio-physical environment, the sampling procedure needed to be sensitive to

Table 2 Neighbourhood housing and density profile

	DWELLINGS	DENSITY (PEOPLE PER DWELLING)	POPULATION
Houses	9 750 (57.7%)	5.5	53 625
Apartments	2 399 (14.2%)	5	11 995
Informal	4 750 (28.1%)	3.25	16 250
TOTAL	16 899 (100%)	4.8	81 870

such differences.

Analysis commenced by mapping the dominant housing types, and during a drive-through survey a 1:2 500 town planning department street and block plan of the area was annotated to show the various types of residential areas. This revealed a total of five different residential areas, three of which accounted for some 85 per cent of all residents: (1) four-room council houses; (2) high-density council apartment blocks; and (3) informal settlements. To estimate the number of persons resident in each neighbourhood type, the average number of residents per house, apartment, and informal dwelling was established, and this figure multiplied by the total number of such dwellings in the community. The resultant demographic profile appears in Table 2.

3.2.2 Sampling

In many settings where epidemiological investigations are used to provide preventive information, the size of the target population is too large to investigate every individual within it. It is therefore necessary to select a number of people small enough to be interviewed with available resources but also able to represent the full population. This is called sampling, and is a crucial component of any survey, since if the sample is not representative of the full population the information produced cannot be generalized to everyone, and resources spent on the exercise will be wasted.

In the Three Neighbourhoods programme, type of housing was the most prominent distinguishing feature between sub-areas within the community. To investigate possible injury differences between similar neighbourhood types, two each of the dominant residential areas were strategically selected as survey sites. Sample size per area was calculated according to the proportion of township residents living in such accommodation. Because informal settlements accounted for the largest and most rapidly expanding sector, 46 percent of all sampled households were allocated to the two informal settlements. Low-cost housing estates were the next most prevalent residential type, and were allocated 40 per cent of the final sample. Corresponding to the approximately 18 per cent of residents in apartments, these were allocated 14 per cent of the final sample.

In each area, dwellings included in the survey were randomly selected from a computerized listing of the numbers of all dwellings in the area as recorded by pro-gramme staff. Initially, of the two areas per neighbourhood type, one was to have served as an intervention area, and one as a non-intervention control. Within this research design, intervention areas were over-sampled to ensure that at least 65 per cent of all dwellings were surveyed, as against the 41, 40, and 17 per cent sampled respectively in control areas. However, as the magnitude of the injury problem became apparent, the ethical imperative of responding to it led to abandonment of this experimental model. Table 3 shows the final sample.

Sampling problems were most pronounced in the informal settlements, where individual dwellings were repeatedly moved and renumbered as the residents and land use patterns changed. While this limits the possibility of returning to the same dwelling in subsequent surveys, the current research design is not person or dwelling specific. Instead, research is directed at neighbour-

Table 3 Total dwellings and sample sizes for intervention and control groups

	Initial designation *	Neighbour-hood	Neighbour-hood	Sampled dwellings (percentage)	Percentage of overall sample
Houses	Control	Houses A	300	124 (41%)	11.5%
	Experimental	Houses B	307	307 (100%)	28.5%
Apartments	Control	Apartments A	132	53 (40%)	4.9%
	Experimental	Apartments B	127	100 (79%)	9.3%
Informal	Control	Informal A	1016	174 (17%)	16.2%
	Experimental	Informal B	465	317 (68%)	29.6%
TOTAL			2347	1 075 (45.8%)	100%

* The ethical imperative of responding to the injury problem led to abandonment of this experimental design.

hoods as collectives, and is therefore interested in the dynamic monitoring of how injury patterns fluctuate with changes in the resident population.

3.2.3 Interviewer selection and training

Interviewers are the primary point of contact with respondents, and the validity of the data obtained from any survey is strongly dependent upon the reliability and integrity of the interviewers who collect it. Although safeguards can be built into the data recording process through design of the questionnaire, these cannot protect against the bias that can be introduced by interviewers. To get paid without in fact doing the work, interviewers may fake responses by filling out the questionnaires themselves. Others may soon become bored by the task, and in communicating this to respondents elicit poor quality answers, while in other cases interviewers may lack the perceptiveness and assertiveness needed to identify and probe for more information in sensitive areas. The haphazard selection and training of interviewers must therefore be avoided.

In the Three Neighbourhoods programme, concern for the personal safety of interviewers led to the decision that all interviews would be conducted by an interview team consisting of a man and a woman. Prospective interviewers were recruited from various neighbourhoods in Eldorado Park, with the exception of those to be surveyed, on the assumption that respondents would be reluctant to divulge sensitive information to people living in the same neighbourhoods as them.

During pilot testing, racial antagonism and threats of violence were encountered by African interviewers attempting to enter a coloured neighbourhood. Enquiries indicated that similarly hostile responses would be met by coloureds in the African areas. Symptomatic of the attitudinal violence that the programme aimed at preventing, it was initially proposed that this hostility should be overcome by working with community residents to facilitate the acceptance of different-race interviewers. Opinions were sought from community residents, and while most expressed acceptance of this proposal they also noted that their opinions were no guarantee that other residents would refrain from harassing different-race interviewers. To maximize interviewer safety the predominantly African residents in the informal settlements were thus interviewed by African field workers, and all other respondents by coloured field workers. Of twenty-two potential interviewers assessed, twelve were recruited for training.

Interviewer training consisted of four three-hour workshops spread over two weeks and interspersed with homework practice interviews. Training commenced by defining the concepts of injury and violence, describing the principles of the public health approach to prevention, and presenting an overview of the Three Neighbourhoods research design. Next, the concept of the information-gathering interview was explored through practical exercises, followed by discussion on the importance of randomizing individuals selected for interview in order to minimize respondent bias. The survey questionnaire was then reviewed question by question to identify points of possible misunderstanding and prepare a final draft. The last component of training involved trainees interviewing one another under supervision of the trainers, and then applying the questionnaire to family members and friends. These completed practice protocols were then reviewed with the trainers, and problem areas addressed through further coaching. Interviewers were paid on an hourly basis for the time spent at the training workshops and the interviews proper, which commenced three days after the final training session.

3.2.4 Ethical concerns and negotiating access to areas

Where epidemiological investigations involve information that could prejudice individuals, the investigator must ensure that all reasonable measures are in place to protect the integrity of the respondents and that the procedure is ethically acceptable.

Where investigations are conducted among university students, scholars, hospital patients, or other respondents within an institutional setting, the investigator is usually required to obtain ethical advice and consent to proceed from an ethical committee within the institution. In community settings, however, there are often no formally defined ethical committees, and the investigator must ensure the acceptability of the procedure by consulting with peers, and presenting the proposal to local leadership and residents for their consideration. In addition to meeting the ethical requirements of scientific investigation, this is a valuable way of generating interest in the programme and ensuring that interviewers

get access to residents of the area.

Efforts to have the Three Neighbourhoods programme reviewed by local leaders and residents commenced three months prior to beginning the survey itself. In the two informal settlements, local civic leaders were identified and informed of the rationale, aims, and methods of the survey. In both instances they communicated support for the programme, and suggested that project staff address public meetings describing it so as to encourage community participation. In the apartment blocks and housing areas it was more difficult to identify local leaders who enjoyed the common support of residents, and for all but one of these four areas permission was obtained from individual householders only. In the remaining case, an apartment block notorious for its gangland residents, permission was obtained through a local politician and church leader well-respected by the residents of this block.

Having obtained permission to access the areas and proceed with the survey, individual respondents were informed of its nature and aims when approached to be interviewed. They were assured of confidentiality, and explicitly requested to consent to being interviewed.

3.2.5 The questionnaire

The form used by interviewers to record information is critically important. First, the questionnaire determines the content of what will be recorded, and its questions must therefore be designed with careful attention to relevant empirical and theoretical information. Second, the length and layout of the questionnaire is crucial to determining the interviewers' level of involvement and the accuracy of what they record. Forms should always be as brief as possible, and the physical layout should make the mechanics of completing it as simple as possible. In addition, the form's design should address the needs of those who will process the information, such as the data punchers who must enter it into a computer.

The Three Neighbourhoods programme used an interviewer-administered questionnaire consisting of quantitative and qualitative items. This was designed to capture information in six areas: (1) demographic data for the respondent and all other household residents, with space for up to fifteen persons per dwelling; (2) information about the physical environment of the household (e.g., proximity to other dwellings, roads, number of rooms, type of dwelling, presence of street lights, security devices); (3) information about the neighbourhood psychosocial characteristics as perceived by individual respondents; (4) information about the perceived causes and suggested prevention strategies for injuries due to violence, transport, and other causes; (5) knowledge of other organizations active in the area; and (6) information about all injuries that the respondent could recall as having been suffered by him- or herself and other household members over the past year, with space for up to eight injuries per household. While many questions were quantitative, those concerning the injury incident and perceived causes and solutions were recorded as free text to enable the identification of unforeseen elements and capture data about the injury process.

The construction of individual questions and sub-scales was guided by reference to theoretical work on injury analysis, a review of questionnaires used in similar studies, and the experience of the community in question. Conceptually, the different data categories conformed to the four levels of 'community diagnosis' identified by Bjaras (1993) as needed for planning injury prevention programmes: (1) community demographic profile identifying who to target; (2) a health profile indicating the number and types of injuries; (3) a health risk profile detailing personal, product, and environmental risk factors for intervention; and (4) an organizational profile of the area that maps who does what and identifies prevention programme collaborators.

On completion of a first draft, the questionnaire was pilot tested (Butchart et al., 1996) on seventy households to include twenty-four from an informal settlement, twenty-seven apartments, and nineteen houses. The results were used to eliminate items that failed to provide useful data, revise the document's physical lay-out to increase ease of recording, and insert additional interviewer cues where these appeared necessary to improve response quality.

Once finalized, the questionnaire was translated into Afrikaans, and then back-translated to ensure accuracy. Because seven different African languages are spoken by the informal settlement residents, it was decided not to attempt translation of the questionnaire into an African language, but rather have interviewers translate the questions where necessary as they interviewed each respondent. The final questionnaire took approximately forty-five minutes to complete.

Respondents in the pilot study and the study proper were asked to evaluate their experience of being interviewed. Eighty five per cent described this as a positive experience that made them think in a new way about things concerning safety, and that made them feel good to know somebody cared enough to enquire into their situation. Qualitative responses suggested that the process of talking about daily struggles and problems was in itself therapeutic, one respondent saying 'it satisfied my soul', another 'it was good and very, very number one like toffee bar one', and a third that 'it is good and I clap hands for it because I hope you'll help us in the informal settlements'. Of the 15 per cent who experienced the interview negatively, 2 per cent said that it took too long and the remainder gave no reason.

3.3 Performing the survey

While good preparation is an important predictor of success for an epidemiological survey, it is equally important that the actual conduct of the interviews be closely monitored to ensure that sampling plans are followed and the information recorded by interviewers is accurate and reliable.

3.3.1 Selecting respondents and doing the interviews

The Three Neighbourhoods interview sample consisted of proxy respondents who answered for all persons resident in each household interviewed. Following the methodology used by Pick and Obermeyer (1996) in Cape Town informal settlements,

interviewers were instructed to interview the most senior female resident of each household, on the grounds that they were most likely to possess a comprehensive knowledge of all household members. This was not always possible, and the final sample showed that 63 per cent of the respondents were females (average age forty-seven). Where no response could be obtained from a household identified as part of the random sample, and to prevent interviewers from choosing replacement homes on the basis of convenience, they were instructed to try three further times before selecting as a replacement the house second to the left of the identified dwelling. The households where all residents were absent for work during weekdays were particularly difficult to interview, and to do so field workers returned to these dwellings on Saturday mornings.

To minimize the risk of violence to interviewers, interviews were conducted between 09h30 and 15h00. All interviewers were issued with prominent identity cards displaying their photographs, the Centre's official logo, and contact details for the study team. Respondents were presented at the time of interview with a simple 'safety information kit', both to encourage their participation and ensure that the interview was accompanied by at least a minimal level of safety awareness. Apart from three instances where field staff were verbally harassed, no threatening incidents were reported. Each team of two individuals completed an average of five questionnaires per day, and the first 200 protocols completed by each interviewer were screened by the survey co-ordinators and the interviewers given feedback as to the adequacy of their performance. Interviews commenced in May 1996 and were completed in early October 1996.

3.3.2 Data coding and analysis

After collection, survey information must be analysed, interpreted, and reported in a format appropriate to the target audiences. This requires transferring information from the questionnaires into an appropriate computer programme, checking this for accuracy and correcting errors, analysing it using statistical and qualitative techniques, and then writing up the results. Failure to adequately plan and budget for this step can result in survey data never being turned into useful information, and so this phase must always be addressed in the very earliest stages of planning.

Since most epidemiological surveys involve many respondents and many variables, the information entered into analysis should, wherever possible, be numeric to enable statistical analysis. Where qualitative data is recorded as free text, these can be turned into digital codes using appropriate methods of content analysis, and then analysed statistically. To reduce the coding load after interview completion, answers to most closed questions in the Three Neighbourhoods survey were coded during the interview by ticking a check box. All injury descriptions were coded after the interview by an experienced user of the tenth version of the *International Classification of Diseases* (ICD) (WHO, 1992).

Inter-rater reliability for the allocation of ICD codes was evaluated by having 20 per

Coding

For most diseases, including injuries, it is important that different studies apply a uniform system of coding so their findings can be compared. For all diseases, including injuries, the most widely used classification system is WHO's *International Statistical Classification of Diseases and Related Health Problems*, abbreviated as 'ICD' (WHO, 1992). The latest version is ICD-10, which was released in 1992.

Applied to injuries, ICD-10 requires the following information: first, a description of the type of injury and its site on the body (e.g., fracture of skull); second, a description of the external cause of injury, such as 'fall from roof of building' or 'stabbed in spine with bicycle spoke'; third, information about the victim's activity at the time of injury; and fourth, information about the injury setting. This information is usually recorded in narrative form, and then converted to a string of letters and numbers using the appropriate ICD code lists.

cent of all cases re-coded by an independent expert, which yielded a satisfactory level of agreement on 96 per cent of all cases.

Once coded, the data were entered into Microsoft's Access database. Free text fields were entered in slightly summarized form, but retaining the key content and process data. Analysis of the quantitative data was performed using SPSS, while the qualitative data were content analysed along the lines described in Krippendorf (1980).

Table 4 Total dwellings and sample sizes for intervention and control groups

Incidence	Informal A	Informal B	Houses A	Houses B	Apart-ments A	Apart-ments B	TOTAL
All Injury Incidence 95% CI	14 947 ±1 379	15 030 ±1 131	6 704 ±945	3 924 ±497	8 304 ±1623	2 394 ±656	8 331 ±402
Morbidity Incidence 95% CI	13 901 ±1 338	14 329 ±1 109	6 705 ±945	3 466 ±468	7 612 ±1560	2 394 ±656	7 845 ±391
Mortality Incidence 95% CI	1 046 ±393	701 ±264	0	457 ±173	692 ±488	0	486 ±101

Morbidity refers to all non-fatal injuries, while mortality refers to injuries resulting in death. The method is likely to have under-sampled the true number of injury cases due to the use of proxy respondents and recall bias.

3.3.3 Methodological strengths and weaknesses

No epidemiological survey can ever claim complete accuracy for the information it provides. Investigators must therefore critically interrogate their findings to identify sources of bias and inform end users about the strengths and weaknesses of the information. As well as assisting subsequent investigators to design better procedures, this ensures that applications flowing from the investigation are made with a clear understanding of how the predictive limitations of the data and data sources may reduce the effectiveness of interventions.

Table 4 shows the overall injury incidence rates for the six areas sampled in the Three Neighbourhoods study, and indicates alongside each rate the confidence interval. Confidence intervals show how much the reported rate may over- or underestimate

the 'true' incidence rate. In this case the incidence rates are likely to underestimate the true size of the problem. Many factors will have operated to determine this level of error, but among the more important to consider are those discussed below.

3.3.4 Proxy respondents

A major limitation of the Three Neighbourhoods method is its use of proxy respondents. Because such respondents could have been unaware of injuries sustained by co-residents, this may have led to a severe undercount of the events that actually occurred. It is reasonable to assume that such undercounting was particularly prevalent in respect of less severe injuries of low salience to the respondents, and injuries distant in time from the interview. Furthermore, respondents may have withheld information about injuries sustained in events associated with criminal activities owing to fears of legal retribution or revenge. Regarding the accuracy of respondent data about household co-residents, similar factors may have led to an undercount of the survey areas' population, particularly where it might have been believed that to divulge such information could result in negative consequences for the individuals concerned, as in the case of deportation of illegal immigrants.

3.3.5 Recall bias

Since the study aimed to generate injury information for a full year so as to reflect seasonal variations in the injury profile, the unit of recall was set at one year from the point of interview. When respondents had identified an event, interviewers were instructed to probe around the stated month and time of occurrence in an attempt to eliminate the over-inclusion of especially dramatic events. Accordingly, while the full count of injuries on survey completion was 579, 28 per cent (163) were found to have occurred more than one year before the interview, and for 4 per cent (22), respondents could not specify a date of occurrence. These cases were eliminated from the data set.

Beyond urging respondents to think about every injury that may have occurred, it was not possible to install a similar error checking method in respect of injuries that may not have been recalled (Mock et al., 1999). Some injury epidemiologists (e.g., Berger and Mohan, 1996) therefore suggest that the optimal recall period is 14 days, beyond which there may be under- or over-inclusion of injury events. To overcome this

limitation, it may therefore be appropriate in similar studies to commence with a two-week recall, and follow this with the one year recall.

3.3.6 Quality of injury information

Since data pertaining to the nature of injuries was collected from proxy respondents, it was not possible to obtain detailed information about injury severity, the precise combination of lesions that occurred in cases of multiple injury, or the projected level of disability. Some information about these areas was collected, and a coarse index of disability was provided by a question as to how the injury was treated, and whether it resulted in death, disability, or full recovery. It was not, however, the main aim of the survey to generate such information, and this limitation was adequately compensated for by the detailed data pertaining to external causes and risk factors required for the design and implementation of primary prevention programmes.

3.3.7 Cross-validation

Related to the limitations attaching to the use of proxy respondents and recall bias, is the lack of a technique to triangulate recorded injury information with collateral data sources. For instance, an index of reliability could have been obtained for hospital-treated injuries by cross-checking reports against hospital treatment data, and for injuries reported to the police by cross-checking against police records. While it was beyond the logistical scope of the present survey to perform such triangulation, it is recommended that, where possible, similar studies should attempt to do so.

3.3.8 Sampling and generalizability

It was hoped that by sampling the six strategically selected examples of neighbourhood type, findings from the study could be generalized to all such neighbourhoods in the township. The results, however, suggested that variations between neighbourhoods in the injury and risk profile were too great to permit such generalization. Most often, these variations seemed to reflect physical environmental features, such as proximity to highways, and socio-cultural factors, such as gangs, that were unevenly distributed across different neighbourhoods, despite their geographical proximity. However, insofar as the method appears to identify precisely these local-level variations, the generalizability limitation is perhaps as much a strength as it is a weakness.

3.4   Methodological strengths

3.4.1 The population-based approach

The main strengths of the Three Neighbourhoods methodology are two-fold. They pertain on the one hand to the limitations of service-based approaches in respect of the epidemiological and risk-factor data they produce, and on the other hand, to the ubiquitous difficulties entailed in establishing incidence rates where accurate demographics are lacking.

Previous South African epidemiological studies of injury have depended for their denominator data upon injury victims who report to hospitals, emergency treatment clinics, and private doctors (Bass, Albertyn, and Melis, 1995; Brown and Nell, 1991; Butchart et al., 1992; Van der Spuy, 1993). While convenient, the data produced by these service-based approaches may be biased by the pattern of service use within the population of interest, such that they identify less the actual injury pattern than the tendency of certain people with particular kinds of injury to use certain services. Further, service-based methodologies are not designed to identify injuries of insufficient severity to warrant formal treatment, which, especially in respect of injuries due to violence, may serve as important markers of more severe psychosocial dysfunction and therefore important indicators for intervention.

The greatest advantage of the population-based approach is therefore its potential to identify all injuries, and data from the present study would suggest that 5 per cent presented to private practitioners, 68 per cent to state clinics or hospitals, and 27 per cent outside such settings. The population-based approach can thus serve to identify disparities between actual and ideal hospital case loads, and inform approaches to minimizing these disparities by extending appropriate levels of care to injury victims who may have required but could not obtain formal treatment.

As Table 5 shows, similar reasoning applies in respect of the disparity between actual instances of violent injury and those reported to the police. In line with findings for the United States (National Committee for Injury Prevention and Control, 1989) and the United Kingdom (Shepherd et al.,

Table 5 Patterns of violence-related injury reporting in a township sample

		Reported to SAPS	Not reported to SAPS	Reported to SAPS unknown	Incidence of violence in this sample
	A. Mortality	11 (100%)	–		233 per 100 000 (11 per 4729)
M O R B I D I T Y	B. Medically treated and admitted to hospital	60 (70.6%)	25 (29.4%)	1	1 819 per 100 000 (86 per 4729)
	C. Medically treated (GP, clinic, or hospital)	28 (45.9%)	33 (54.1%)	1	1 311 per 100 000 (62 per 4729)
	D. No treatment or treated at home	7 [a] (36.8%)	12 [a] (63.2%)	3	465 per 100 000 (22 per 4729
	E. Treatment unknown	9	9	5	
	F. Total violence injuries	104 (56.8%)	79 (43.2%)	10	4 081 per 100 000 (193 per 4729)

a: violence to be reported.

1990), the present study suggests that, according to severity, the proportion of violent injuries reported to the police ranged from a 100 per cent high in the case of fatalities, to a 37 per cent low for cases treated at home.

Concerning the epidemiological limitations imposed by absent or inaccurate demographic data, the present methodology provides a means of bypassing this block to injury measurement, which is of especially great concern where the aim is to measure intervention outcome in fast-changing populations. By no means a novel strategy, a similar approach to the production of disease information and demographic data was deployed by Kark and others at the Polela experimental health initiative in the 1940s

and 1950s (Kark, 1944; Union of South Africa, 1941), and in recent years has been refined by the international agency Community Information, Empowerment, Transparency (CIET) (Andersson, 1995).

3.4.2 Quantitative and qualitative data

The combination of quantitative and qualitative information elicited by the survey meant that discrete injury events could be located within the psycho-social context of respondents' ideas and perceptions of risk, strategies for prevention, and sense of community (Robinson and Wilkinson, 1995). This psycho-social context is an important determinant of people's spontaneous actions towards injury, and of their readiness to accept or reject prevention strategies designed purely on the basis of quantitative data. Accordingly, the survey's findings allow for intervention designs that are shaped by the 'objective' reality of injuries and keyed to their 'subjective' meanings for the target population (Butchart, Kruger, and Lekoba, 2000). Most importantly, this allows for the identification of erroneous beliefs and information deficits, which can then be rectified through appropriate educational and awareness-raising campaigns.

Use of local residents as interviewers achieved the desired end of increasing rapport between respondents and the survey team. Interviewers were frequently drawn into conversations about social and other issues beyond the scope of the injury focus, and were able to complement the formal data with a rich store of anecdotes and informal observations. On completion of the baseline survey, all interviewers were presented with a certificate detailing the number of hours of training they had received and the nature of their work with the programme. This coincided with commencement of the October 1996 national census, and as a result of their employment in the Three Neighbourhoods programme, four interviewers obtained temporary employment as census workers.

The primary aim of epidemiological investigations is to produce information for preventive action. Because interventions always involve people with differing levels of expertise and influence, the information must be communicated in as many different ways as are necessary to 'speak' to different user groups. For example, while an illiterate resident will benefit from a simple oral or graphic display of the main causes of burns, a very different level of information would be needed to convince a municipality that they should invest in electrifying an area so as to prevent burns.

Analysis of the specific causes for the different categories of injury identified in the Three Neighbourhoods programme indicated three distinct levels of intervention target: (1) injury causes that can be removed by residents themselves (e.g., cleaning private yards, public roadways, and paths to remove pieces of broken glass, zinc, or wire that can cut the feet); (2) injury causes that can be prevented by providing training and education for residents (e.g., training about general safety and first aid); and (3) injury causes that can be prevented through environmental changes that cannot be achieved by residents acting on their own (e.g., traffic calming measures, provision of electricity and housing, access to public telephones). Corresponding to these target levels were three main application strategies.

Level one procedures involved using the data to stimulate injury prevention activities by residents themselves. This was done by convening public meetings in each neighbourhood at which the quantitative and qualitative injury information for each neighbourhood were set out as poster displays. These displays were broken down into in sub-sections detailing each of the major sub-causes of injury (e.g., transport, violence, burns). Following a general introduction to the programme, participants discussed the displays and possible intervention strategies with programme staff.

Level two interventions used the information gained from the survey and during feedback sessions to provide appropriate training to local residents as a means of empowering their injury prevention capacity. For instance, residents in the informal areas viewed the provision of better daycare for young children and infants as an important way of keeping them away from hazards such as poisons in their homes, strangers, and motor vehicles on the peripheral roads. Accordingly, a group of women were trained in how to operate a crèche. In order to reduce paraffin poisoning, an on-going programme was initiated involving the distribution of childproof bottle tops and safe containers, provided by the Paraffin Safety Association of South Africa.

At the third level of implementation, the survey data and concrete, geographically specific safety promotion recommendations were fed upward to local government. To secure their involvement in safety promotion, and as a criterion for designation as a WHO Safe Community, local government was required to sign a commitment to investing in a safer metropolitan structure using evidence-based strategies within a multi-disciplinary, intersectoral approach. As of November 1998, this had found concrete expression in the construction of a pedestrian bridge over the four-lane traffic highway separating Informal Settlement B from schools and shops in the formal housing areas. While of low prevention value compared with interventions such as building of shops and schools in Informal B, which would remove all need to cross the highway, the bridge is nonetheless an important symbol that steps towards safety can be made through evidence-led community-oriented public health interventions.

The four Es of injury control

The many possible strategies for injury prevention can be summarized into four abstract intervention categories. These are not mutually exclusive, and interventions often involve components from all four of the 'injury prevention Es'.

The first E refers to engineering, and involves changing the basic structure or function of injury-causing products to make them safer (e.g., making the base of paraffin lamps more stable so that they will not topple over). The second E concerns environmental modifications, such as improving the night-time lighting of streets, or modifying roads to prevent motor cars from exceeding a certain speed. The third E involves education, such as teaching parents how to store poisons in the home, or raising awareness about commonly occurring risk factors. The fourth E refers to enforcement, and refers to all interventions that involve the application of safety laws, such as laws to prevent the carrying of guns in public, drunk driving, and safety standards in respect of buildings.

Application of the survey data was thus radiated into and around the target population at all levels, from the individual and the neighbourhood, to advocacy and lobbying at the level of the local authorities directly responsible for policies and practices that influence structural and environmental factors.

4 Conclusion: the way ahead

The first household-based epidemiological survey of injuries in South Africa, the Three Neighbourhoods methodology complements the existing array of hospital and mortuary-based injury observation mechanisms, which have to date been the exclusive source of South African injury information. While certainly containing its own very obvious limitations, the present methodology offers one approach to gathering the demographic and epidemiological information without which effective injury prevention activities cannot be implemented. In areas where there is no surveillance and there are no demographic data, the method may thus be of some utility in helping to build an injury prevention response, and can be generalized to the preventive understanding of many other problems faced by community psychologists and public health practitioners.

Beyond its safety promotion implications, this case study also suggests the prevention potential produced by the synergy of public health and community psychology. With its emphasis on careful problem definition through quantitative and qualitative analysis, public health dovetails with community psychology's process orientation and preoccupation with the intangible yet important psychological, social, cultural, and political objects that are its main concern. Without community psychology, public health lacks the social technologies needed to convert its analytic products into effective and empowering interventions; without public health, the rhetoric of community psychology often appears hollow, its actions vague and lacking in clear direction.

Together, though, the two disciplines forge a potent machinery for change in which the rigour of public health is given a human face by the imagination of community psychology.

Exercises

1 Public health is driven by a clear and explicit set of values and ideals. For instance, the World Health Organization (WHO, 1997) notes that democratic values upholding individual autonomy and equity in relation to gender, culture, and power should be promoted, while safety promotion's defining interest is to reduce the amount and severity of injury in the target population. Accordingly, public health advocates that where communal values and behavioural norms infringe these principles, efforts should be made to change them in a morally better and more health-promoting direction. While not inevitable, this means that public health interventions must often conflict with the ideas and values of the target population.

   How should such conflict be dealt with, and in resolving such disagreements, whose reality should be prioritized: that produced through epidemiological investigation, or that sustained by the shared social reality of community residents?

2 What are all the possible reasons for doing research to measure the size of psychosocial problems in any given community? Consider the different

uses of a once-off approach as opposed to multiple measures over a period of time.

3 Considering that many communities are statistically illiterate, how could you creatively adapt your feedback mechanisms to fit into the normal ways of communication and dialogue in various areas? Remember that one of the functions of this feedback is to mobilize and enable the community to address issues that are within its power to address and at the same time to avoid creating false expectations about issues that are near to impossible to deal with in a short time frame and with limited resources.

References

AD HOC COMMITTEE ON HEALTH RESEARCH RELATING TO FUTURE INTERVENTION OPTIONS. (1996). *Investing in health research and development.* Geneva: WHO. (Document TDR/Gen/96.1).

ANDERSSON, N. (1995). *Four essays on evidence-based planning.* New York: CIET International.

ANNEST, J. L. and MALLONEE, S. (1995). Data needs for injury prevention. In *Proceedings of the International Collaborative Effort on Injury Statistics, Volume 1* (pp. 29-1 to 29-3). Hyattsville: US Department of Health and Human Services.

BASS, D. H., ALBERTYN, R., AND MELIS, J. (1995). Child pedestrian injuries in the Cape Metropolitan area. *South African Medical Journal,* 85, 96-99.

BERG, L., ABERG, A., SCHELP, L., and SVANSTRÖM, L. (1995). Data needs for evaluation of injury prevention programmes: Experiences from Sweden. In *Proceedings of the International Collaborative Effort on Injury*

Statistics, Volume 1 (pp. 19-1 to 19-5). Hyattsville: US Department of Health and Human Services.

BERGER, L. R. and MOHAN, D. (1996). *Injury Control: A global view.* Delhi: Oxford University Press.

BJARAS, G. (1993). The potential of community diagnosis as a tool in planning an intervention programme aimed at preventing injuries. *Accident Analysis and Prevention,* 25, 3-10.

BROWN, D. S. O. and NELL, V. (1991). The epidemiology of traumatic brain injury in Johannesburg. I. Methodological issues in a developing country context. *Social Science and Medicine,* 33, 283-287.

BUTCHART, A. (1996). Violence prevention in Gauteng: The public health approach. *Acta Criminologica,* 9(2), 5-15.

BUTCHART, A. and BROWN, D. S. O. (1991). Non-fatal injuries due to interpersonal violence in Johannesburg-Soweto: Incidence, determinants and consequences. *Forensic Science International,* 52; 35-51.

BUTCHART, A., KRUGER, J., and LEKOBA, R. (2000). Perception of injury causes and solutions in a Johannesburg township: Implications for prevention. *Social Science and Medicine,* 50, 331-334.

BUTCHART, A., KRUGER, J., LEKOBA, R., and SMITH, D. (1996). Evaluating injury prevention outcome in a developing country context: Lessons from a community-based violence prevention programme. *Urbanisation and Health Newsletter,* 29, 28-42.

BUTCHART, A., KRUGER, J., and NELL, V. (1997). Neighbourhood safety: A township violence and injury profile. *Indicator Crime and Conflict,* 9(Winter), 11-15.

BUTCHART, A., NELL, V., YACH, D., BROWN, D. S. O., ANDERSON, A., RADEBE, B., and JOHNSON, K. (1992). *The epidemiology of non-fatal injuries due to external causes in Johannesburg-Soweto.* Health Psychology Unit and Medical Research Council Technical Report 92/2. Tygerberg: Medical Research Council.

BUTCHART, A., NELL, V., YACH, D., BROWN, D. S. O., JOHNSON, K., and RADEBE, B. (1991). The epidemiology of non-fatal trauma in

Johannesburg-Soweto. I. Methodology and materials. *South African Medical Journal*, 78, 466–471.

BUTCHART, A., PEDEN, M., BASS, D., DU TOIT, N., and LERER, L. (1996). Injury in South Africa. In S. N. Forjuoh, A. B. Zwi, and C. Romer (Eds.), *Injury Control in Africa*. Proceedings of a round table session and associated meetings held at the Third International Conference on Injury Prevention and Control, Melbourne, Australia (pp. 13–18). Pittsburgh, PA: University of Pittsburgh.

CENTRAL WITWATERSRAND METROPOLITAN CHAMBER. (1994). *Population Figure Study*. Johannesburg: CWMC.

CENTRAL WITWATERSRAND REGIONAL SERVICES COUNCIL. (1993). *Population of the CWRSC area*. Johannesburg: CWRSC.

ENGEL, U. and THOMSEN, L. K. (1992). Safety effects of speed reducing measures in Danish residential areas. *Accident Analysis and Prevention*, 24, 17–28.

FARRINGTON, D. P. (1993). *Success stories in the prevention of adolescent aggression and youth violence*. Plenary presentation to the Second World Injury Prevention and Control Conference, Atlanta, GA, March 1993.

GAINER, P. S., WEBSTER, D. W., and CHAMPION, H. R. (1993). A youth violence prevention program. *Archives of Surgery*, 128, 303–308.

KARK, S. L. (1944). A health unit as family doctor and health advisor. *South African Medical Journal*, 18, 39–46.

KAROLINSKA INSTITUTE. (1992). *Research on community safety promotion*. Sundbyberg, Sweden: Karolinska Institute.

KRIPPENDORF, K. (1980). *Content analysis: An introduction to its methodology*. London: Sage.

LAIRD, M., SYROPOULOS, M., and BLACK, S. (1996). *Aggression and violence: The challenge for Detroit schools*. Lions – Quest International.

LANGLEY, J. D. (1988). The need to discontinue the use of the term 'accident' when referring to unintentional injury events. *Accident Analysis and Prevention*, 20(1), 1–8.

LAST, J. (1988). *A dictionary of epidemiology* (2nd ed.). New York: Oxford University Press.

LERER, L. B., MATZOPOLOUS, R., and BRADSHAW, D. (1995). *A profile of violence and injury mortality in the Cape Town metropole 1994*. Tygerberg: South African Medical Research Council.

LILIENFELD, A. M. and LILIENFELD, D. E. (1980). *Foundations of epidemiology* (2nd ed.). New York: Oxford University Press.

LINDQVIST, K. (1993). *Towards community-based injury prevention: The Motala model*. Linkoping: Department of Community Medicine, Linkoping University.

LINDQVIST, K. (1989). Epidemiology of accidents in a Swedish municipality. *Accident Analysis and Prevention*, 21, 33–43.

MCDOWALL, D., LOFTIN, C, and WIERSEMA, B. (1992). A comparative study of the preventive effects of mandatory sentencing laws for gun crimes. *The Journal of Criminal Law and Criminology*, 83, 378–394.

MOCK, C., ACHEAMPONG, F., ADJEI, S., and KOEPSELL, T. (1999). The effect of recall on estimation of incidence rates for injury in Ghana. *International Journal of Epidemiology*, 28, 750–755.

NATIONAL COMMITTEE FOR INJURY PREVENTION AND CONTROL. (1989). Injury prevention: Meeting the challenge. *American Journal of Preventive Medicine*, 5(3), 1–303.

O'DONNELL, L., COHEN, S., and HAUSMAN, A. (1990). *The evaluation of community-based violence prevention programs*. Atlanta: Education Development.

PICK, W. and OBERMEYER, C. M. (1996). Urbanisation, household composition and reproductive health of women. *Social Science and Medicine*, 43, 1431–1441.

POLLOCK, D. A. (1995). Trauma registries and public health surveillance of injuries. In *Proceedings of the International Collaborative Effort on Injury Statistics, Volume 1* (pp. 11–1 to 11–6). Hyattsville: US Department of Health and Human Services.

ROBINSON, D. and WILKINSON, D. (1995). Sense of community in a remote mining town:

American Journal of Community Psychology, 23, 137–148.

ROSENBERG, M. L. and FENLEY, M. A. (Eds.). (1991). *Violence in America: A public health approach*. New York: Oxford University Press.

SEEDAT, M. (1995). Creating safe communities in the context of reconstruction and development: The Centre for Peace Action. *Psychosocial Research and Practice*, 2, 27–32.

SEEDAT, M., TERRE BLANCHE, M., BUTCHART, A., and NELL, V. (1992). Violence prevention through community development: The Centre for Peace Action model. *Critical Health*, 41, 59–64.

SHEPHERD, T. P., SHOPLAND, M., PEARCE, N. X., and SCULLY, C. (1990). Pattern, severity and aetiology of injuries in victims of assault. *Journal of the Royal Society of Medicine*, 83, 75–78.

SVANSTRÖM, K. and SVANSTRÖM, L. (1989). *A safe community: How to prevent accidents at the local level*. Prepared for the WHO travelling seminar on community safety, Sweden – Thailand, 1989. Sundbyberg, Sweden: Authors.

UNION OF SOUTH AFRICA. (1941). *Department of Public Health. Report for the year ended 30th June, 1941*. Pretoria: The Government Printer.

VAN DER SPUY, J. (1993). Trauma research: A perspective. *Trauma Review*, 1(1), 1.

VICTORIAN HEALTH PROMOTION FOUNDATION. (1996). *VicHealth Annual Report 1996*. Carlton: Victorian Health Promotion Foundation.

WORLD HEALTH ORGANIZATION. (1989). *Manifesto for safe communities*. Geneva: WHO.

WORLD HEALTH ORGANIZATION. (1992). *International statistical classification of diseases and related health problems*. Geneva: WHO.

WORLD HEALTH ORGANIZATION. (1997). *Health for all in the 21st century*. Geneva: WHO.

YACH, D. and BOTHA, J. L. (1986). Epidemiological research methods. Part I. Why epidemiology? *South African Medical Journal*, 70, 267–269.

YTTERSTAD, B. (1995). The Harstad injury prevention study: Prevention of burns in small children by a community-based intervention. *Burns*, 21, 259–266.

YTTERSTAD, B. and WASMUTH, H. H. (1995). The Harstad injury prevention study: Evaluation of hospital-based injury recording and community-based intervention for traffic injury prevention. *Accident Analysis and Prevention*, 27, 111–123.

ZWI, A., FORJUOH, S., MURUGUSAMPILLAY, S., ODERO, W., and WATTS, C. (1996). Injuries in developing countries: Policy response needed now. *Transactions of the Royal Society of Tropical Medicine and Hygiene*, 90, 593–595.

12

Dealing with injury control and safety promotion in complex environments

Dinesh Mohan

Study objectives

After studying this chapter you should have a clear understanding of:

- why safety promotion programmes are not very effective if we depend only on education-type intervention strategies;
- the concept of injuries as a community health problem;
- the reason why all individuals cannot be careful all the time;
- differences in high-income and low-income communities for promotion of safety;
- why safety promotion programmes and policies have to deal with more complex situations in low-income communities;
- the need to develop self-sustaining and forgiving environments that help people behave in safer ways;
- why simple transfer of technology from high-income to low- income communities is not always successful, unless all the socio-economic issues are taken into account.

1 Introduction

Morbidity and mortality due to injuries have always existed in the past but their recognition as a public health problem is a phenomenon of the mid-twentieth century. Policy makers and safety professionals in every country find it very difficult to institute changes that actually result in a dramatic decrease in fatalities due to injuries. Past experience shows that individuals do not follow all the instructions given to them to promote safety. Attempts to educate people regarding safety are also not very effective and wide variations are found between people's knowledge and their actual behaviour (Robertson, 1983). This is particularly true for those situations where we cannot select the people who will be involved in a particular activity, for example, where almost everyone in the population is involved in domestic chores, in road use, and working in offices, factories, or on farms. It is not possible to select people who will always be careful in performing these activities. While some control can be exercised in licensing drivers of motor vehicles, almost no control is possible in selection of pedestrians and bicyclists. At the work place, only some very specialized jobs allow careful selection and monitoring. This makes it very difficult to promote safety by relying on improvements in individual behaviour and makes injury control a very complex process. This is illustrated below by using road traffic as an example.

Almost all the people in the school-going and working-age groups have to be on the road at least twice a day in every country of the world. This forces many individuals to use the road even when they are not adequately equipped to do so. These situations would include individuals with any of the following problems:

- Those who cannot concentrate on the road because they have suffered a personal tragedy recently, including death of a loved one, loss of a job, failure in an important examination, or monetary loss.
- Those who are disturbed because of problems in personal relationships with a spouse, parent, sibling, or close friend.
- Persons taking medication or drugs that alter behaviour and perceptual abilities, or those who are under the influence of alcohol.

- Children whose cognitive and locomotion abilities make it difficult for them to understand or follow instructions given to them.
- Elderly people whose motor and cognitive functions are impaired.
- Disabled persons who have to be a part of regular traffic if they have to earn a living.
- All psychologically disturbed persons who may not be able to function as desired on the road, but who cannot be singled out from participation in traffic.

If we add up the total number of individuals who could be included in the above categories on any given day it would amount to a significant proportion of people on the road. These individuals cannot always be identified or prevented from using the road space. At the same time it is also a fact that their presence on the road is not out of choice.

In our modern ways of living we have to use products and do things at places and at times that are determined by someone else or by society at large. The same holds true for activities at the work-place or even at home. Therefore, we have a societal responsibility to design our products and environment so that people find it easy and convenient to behave in a safe manner. The systems must be such that they are safe not only for normal people but also for those individuals who might belong to any of the groups listed above. These kinds of designs, rules, and regulations would reduce the probability of people hurting one another or themselves even when they make mistakes. Such systems are very often referred to as forgiving systems.

This approach has been accepted and used in most of the successful health improvement programmes in the past (Haddon, Suchman, and Klein, 1964). We have not waited for everyone to be educated or for each one of them to start behaving ideally to control diseases like polio, smallpox, malaria, or cholera. These diseases have been controlled because we have improved our environmental conditions; we purify water at source or give a one-time immunization, often mandated by law, to every individual in the population.

For control of diseases we usually like to understand the factors associated with the spread of the disease by employing the science of epidemiology, obtain recognition of the disease as a problem in society, and then get the government, societal groups, and individuals to do things that would help in the reduction of the problem. Some diseases are easier to control than others owing to the specific roles that the economy, environment, and individuals play in the spread of the disease. However, we never depend upon improving the behaviour of individuals as the main tactic for disease control.

This chapter presents an analysis of the complexities involved in safety promotion considering morbidity and mortality due to injury as a health problem.

2 Injury as a disease

We have to assume that most human beings would try to prevent the occurrence of an episode of ill-health if they are able to do so. If a disease is endemic in a population, then some or all of the following conditions may be present:

- Lack of knowledge regarding the causal factors associated with the disease.
- Absence of remedial measures.
- Inability of the society to control environmental conditions.
- Political and economic factors making it difficult for individuals to take the correct decisions.
- Presence of intrinsically hazardous designs of products and the environment.

The control of a health problem involves an understanding of the phenomenon to a certain extent and at the same time the provision of means to individuals and societies to be able to do something about it. Certain principles of public health need to be understood so that the same can be applied to the control of injuries. These principles are:

1 *There is no fundamental difference between injuries and the occurrence of any other disease.* When we go to a doctor with a complaint of ill-health the doctor does not spend a great deal of time trying to fix blame on individuals on why the problem may have occurred in the first place. The police department is usually not involved in trying to solve the problem. Law-makers, police departments, and others usually get involved if the treatment given is wrong, if some public health authorities have not been doing their jobs properly, or if the problem is so serious and widespread that societal intervention is necessary. We have understood for a long time that we should not treat the victims as criminals for contracting a disease if we want

Table 1 Comparative epidemiology of malaria and skull fracture as sustained by an unhelmeted motorcyclist crashing into a tree (Mohan, 1983)

PATHOLOGICAL CONDITION	HOST	AGENT	VECTOR/ VEHICLE	INTERACTION
Malaria	Human	Plas-modium vivax	Mosquito	Bite
Skull fracture	Human	Mechanical energy	Motorcycle	Crash

to solve the problem. This approach has helped us in improving our health status through the centuries. The same approach has to be adopted for dealing with injuries as a controllable disease.

2 *Injury can be defined as a disease that results from an acute exposure of the human body to transfer of energy from the environment around it.* There are no basic scientific distinctions between injury and disease (adapted from Haddon and Baker, 1981). When fluid collects in the brain due to a disease one may die or be disabled permanently if the problem is not controlled. The cause of death due to a head impact with the road in a motorcycle crash could be similar vis-à-vis, cerebro-vascular oedema. While the immediate cause of death or disability would be the same in both cases, most of us would use different approaches in trying to solve the two problems. The similarities in injuries and other diseases as health issues are illustrated in Table 1.

3 *Accidents and injuries are not acts of God.* It is a vital first step to realize that the occurrence and outcome of events that may cause injury are predictable and subject to human control. We are able to predict the situations under which the probability of road crashes, is likely to increase and where designs of vehicles and the road environment could result in severe injuries during a crash. Often an injury can be prevented even where an accident cannot. We may not be able to prevent all motorcycle crashes but in the event of a motorcycle crash, the occurrence and severity of head injury depend on whether or not a helmet was used and on the quality of the helmet.

Even the so-called natural disasters need not really be natural. If they were, then the effects of floods and earthquakes would be the same in the rich and poor countries. It is rare to see thousands killed and made homeless due to floods or earthquakes in high-income communities (HICs). But such disasters

246

are relatively common in low-income communities (LICs). Within the LICs, the poorest are more adversely affected by floods and storms than those who are relatively richer. How a physical event influences human beings is very largely influenced by human beings themselves. Even the occurrence of the physical event itself is very often a result of human activity.

For example, floods may be caused by deforestation, faulty design of dams, or blocking up of drainage in cities. The actions of human beings and how they organize their societies have a great deal to do with whether or not accidents and disasters take place and how these events affect us. We can design our environment and products so that the incidence and effects of accidents and disasters are minimized.

4   *All injuries cannot be prevented.* Most efforts to reduce injuries are termed accident prevention campaigns. We should be clear that accident *prevention* is just one aspect – and not always the most rewarding one – of a much larger range of countermeasures used in effective injury control programmes. It is important that all programmes also include measures of reducing injury severity if an accident does occur, as well as well-designed systems for emergency care, treatment, and rehabilitation after the accident. This is because making mistakes is very normal in activities that involve a vast majority of persons from a given population. It is normal for professional drivers to be distracted during some periods of their long driving hours;

it is normal for executives at work to be day-dreaming at some point in the day; it is normal for a young person to take more risks than an elderly person; and it is normal for children to do the unexpected and hurt themselves as pedestrians or bicycle riders. In short, we will never eliminate carelessness, absent-mindedness, and even neglect in day-to-day activity. However, by designing our products and environment to be more tolerant of these normal variations in human performance, we can minimize the number of resulting accidents and injuries.

In many areas of public health we understand this very well. We know that drinking-water should be purified at its source. It is unreasonable to expect everyone to boil water before drinking it. Those societies that depend upon individuals to purify their own drinking-water suffer from much higher rates of communicable diseases than those who purify water at source. Ironically, it is quite common to produce a product or environment that is likely to cause injury, warn the user to be careful, and then blame the user if a mishap occurs. We would never tolerate a person who introduced cholera germs in the city water supply and then educated every citizen to boil water before drinking it with the argument that those who knowingly do not do so would then be responsible for getting sick. This is the argument we all too often use when dealing with matters concerning safety. We put in place hazardous roads, vehicles, and driving rules and then expect road users to be safe by behaving in some ideal manner.

247

Once we are clear that injury control activities involve the same principles as any other public health problem, then we can institute policies and programmes for institutionalizing safety promotion. However, most models of safety promotion and community action have their origins in the HICS and it is important to understand the differences between HICS and LICS before we can become effective policy makers in our own environments.

3 Differences and similarities between high-income and low-income communities[1]

Injury control policies have been put in place in many HICS over the past two decades (in this chapter the terms HICS and LICS are used interchangeably both for countries and communities). This is partly because of the realization that deaths due to injuries occur at relatively younger ages compared with those due to cardio-vascular diseases and cancer. The years of life lost due to injuries are obviously more than those due to diseases occurring in the later years of life. Studies have shown that years of potential life lost due to injury mortality in HICS are much greater than those due to any other disease (Berger and Mohan, 1996; Injury Control, 1988; Murray and Lopez, 1996).

The recognition of this problem led to the evolution of major programmes in injury prevention, education, development of safer designs of products and the environment, institution of safety standards and regula-

tions, and enforcement of the same (Bonnie, Fulco, and Liverman, 1999; Strategies for Accident Prevention, 1988; Van Beeck, 1998). Injury rates in most activities were seen to decline significantly in the 1960s and 1970s. However, in many sectors, the decline in the 1980s was seen to be much less than those in the 1970s. This was one of the many reasons why health professionals started questioning the adequacy of the top-down approach in safety promotion. It was claimed that much better results could be obtained if total community involvement was elicited for injury control programmes. It is argued that such an approach would make it easier for a community to pay attention to problems the community itself identified as important. If the community initiated actions for installations of safer designs and stricter enforcement of regulations, then the efforts were more likely to succeed.

The effectiveness of some of these methods have been demonstrated in Western Europe in the 1980s and 1990s (Schelp, 1987).

However, the successes demonstrated in reducing the burden of injury in HICS has not been replicated in most LICS. The incidence and rate of accidental injury and death continue to increase in most sectors of activity in LICS. It is important for us to understand the differences and similarities between HICS and LICS so that practical safety programmes can be put in place in the latter also.

3.1 Characteristics of high-income countries

The following factors played an important role in instituting safety programmes and policies in HICS:

1 *Decline of mortality due to infections and contagious diseases.* This made the community more aware of injuries as a health problem and therefore gave support to injury control initiatives as a priority.

2 *Development of a middle-class society.* By the mid 1980s a significant majority of Europeans had incomes that would define them as middle class. At the same time an equalization process took place, which made most professionals equals. This meant that policemen, school teachers, doctors, nurses, lawyers, and university professors could sit around a table and actually communicate and respect each other as equals. Co-operation between various interest groups, law enforcers, policy makers, and policy implementers then became more possible. These processes resulted in conglomerations of people, which could be called communities in a real sense. Most countermeasures for injury control benefit large proportions of the community. It can also be assumed that particular countermeasures would not harm some sections of the population, since there are less conflicts of interest by different class categories.

3 *Acquisition of decision-making powers by local governments.* Over time local communities have been able to acquire decision-making powers over most aspects of community life, owing to national governments' inclination to decentralize policies that relate closely to the citizens' well-being. This gives them the confidence to attempt changes.

4 *Establishment of institutions and organizations with a high degree of expertise.* This makes it possible for reasonably accurate and reliable data to be collected. This data can then be used for policy-making purposes with support from most sections of society.

5 *Laws can be enforced.* Because of the relatively egalitarian structure of society it is assumed that most laws would affect most people in a similar manner. Since the law enforcers belong to the same social strata as the general public it becomes possible to enforce laws more efficiently and more uniformly.

6 *Availability of safer technologies.* Most technologies are developed and their designs controlled by the wider society where they are needed. The technologies are more in tune with the needs of the community and can be changed if necessary.

7 *Safety standards can be enforced.* Since most production is centralized, it is possible to make standards and enforce them.

3.2 Characteristics of low-income countries

In most LICS at the present time many of these conditions are not met.

1 *Heterogeneity.* The post-war period has witnessed the emergence of a very large number of independent nation-states in Africa and Asia. Most of these nation-states had never existed as in their present form. In many of the countries of these two continents the national boundaries have been drawn quite

arbitrarily. Because of the manner in which these countries came into existence, most of them have very mixed populations. These populations may differ in religions, languages, common law, and social customs, and may not have shared values. The urban areas in these countries house people with very diverse backgrounds and so there may be very little homogeneity. In many cities in LICs people live in developments characterized by ethnic and religions bonds.

2 *Inadequate public health facilities*. Most LICs have not been able to institutionalize twentieth-century levels of hygiene and public health. Infant mortality and maternal mortality indices remain much higher than those in HICs. In addition, infections, contagious diseases, and other health problems due to malnutrition, air and water contamination, parasites, mosquitoes, and unsafe work conditions dominate the attention of the public and policy makers. Under such circumstances it becomes very difficult to arrive at a consensus to consider injuries as an important public health problem.

3 *Hierarchical societies*. Most LICs have not been able to achieve high enough levels of economic growth over the past four decades. Low economic growth combined with non-egalitarian tendencies result in very low levels of upward mobility. The poorer sections of society remain dominant in terms of proportions of the population, but they have little influence on setting the policy agenda. Within institutions the hierarchy also gets to be embedded in all

functional details. Teachers, nurses, and policemen occupy low social status as far as decision making is concerned. They hardly ever get to sit at the same table where bureaucrats and experts discuss policies and make decisions.

4 *Inadequate control over technology*. Most LICs import almost all the technological products and processes from HICs. Even aid projects ensure movement of technology from the donor to the receiver. Very often this technology is old or less expensive, and therefore, more hazardous. Local communities have almost no control over the choice of these technologies. For example, when a highway project is executed, the design and construction are done by people who belong to the metropolis of that country, aided by experts from multilateral or bilateral international agencies and multinational corporations. The local community can hardly influence the execution of these projects except in the form of protests to halt the construction or change the location of the highway. Most of the time they do not have the expertise or the power to influence design. In addition, the local community may not possess the expertise to evaluate the hazards implicit in the designs of products or technologies being put in place.

5 *Increase of complexity in social and technological systems*. Over the past few decades standardization and homogenization of technologies have resulted in the reduction of complexity in many sectors in HICs. The roads have become identical in layout and design, vehicles

have become similar, the variety of vehicles has been reduced, school designs for most sections of the population are becoming similar, technologies used in houses are similar, and the labour component in industry and farming has been reduced. This reduction in complexity has made it somewhat easier to institute safety countermeasures.

On the other hand, in most LICs, both social structures and technologies include a great deal of variety, which leads to more complex systems. The most modern vehicles share the same road space with non-motorized transport, modern gadgets are used in a traditional kitchen, inadequately trained labour is forced to handle high-energy chemicals and equipment, and mechanized systems co-exist with labour-intensive ways of living. These issues concerning increasing complexity in LICs are discussed in the next section.

4 The consequences of increasingly complex systems in low-income countries

Systems that have unfamiliar feedback loops, many potential interactions, indirect or inferential information sources, and that require limited understanding of some processes are considered to be more complex than those with the opposite characteristics (Perrow, 1984). The characteristics described in the previous section show that LICs tend to have more complex social and technological

environments than those present in HICs. The most important issue to be understood regarding increasingly complex systems in LICs is that these societies face new problems that are different from the ones prevalent in HICs today. They also have little precedence in the past of the HICs. It is not usually possible to find solutions from the past of the HICs and transfer these old solutions to LICs of today.

The complexity in the socio-political domain is a result of centralized decision-making systems of nation-states and local government bodies not being able to accommodate the interests of the poorer sections of society. This happens at times because the individuals who make decisions are insulated from the daily lives and concerns of the disadvantaged communities. Ease in international travel and instantaneous communication links between the élite groups around the world tend to unify their interests and concerns. In the earlier centuries and the first few decades of the twentieth century there was greater conflict between the élite groups across nation-states than there exists today. This interaction and solidarity between richer sections of society in different communities and the conflicts between the poor sections within and across communities occur at the expense of the interests of the latter.

The interests of the poor communities can also be in direct conflict with the interests of the richer ones. Providing safety at the work-place to prevent a small number of injuries and deaths may reduce the profits of the owner and the shareholders of the company. Slowing down of traffic and providing a larger number of safer pedestrian crossings annoy car owners. Providing low-rise housing for low-income groups takes away expensive land for making larger houses for the richer ones.

These problems are further compounded by the fact that global information exchange makes poor people more aware of the latest happenings all over the world and raises their expectations for fair play. This results in greater conflict in society, making governance more difficult. In such situations it is not easy to promote safety programmes for the benefit of the disadvantaged sections of society through widespread consultations.

Known countermeasures for safety demand the use of the *latest* technologies, which may or may not be suitable for the problem at hand. For example, the incidence of home fires has been controlled in some HICs by the requirement that smoke alarms be installed in all homes (Residential Fire Safety Systems, 1997). However, these technologies are expensive and cannot be used by most households in LICs. A large proportion of families in LICs still do all their cooking on stoves using wood or coal. In such a situation the use of smoke detectors would be useless. To solve the problem of home fires in LICs innovative technologies or safety systems need to be developed, but most LICs do not have the financial base or the institutional structure to design and manufacture such new technologies. So communities end up trying out one unsuccessful solution after another. This promotes a feeling of helplessness, powerlessness, and lack of trust in the policy makers – not an ideal situation for community action.

What needs to be understood is that the theoretical base of injury control counter-measures may have international applicability but the actual physical solutions may not. There is clearly a *poverty of theory* among injury control professionals for handling the situation in LICs. For example, most road safety measures instituted in HICs have centered on the automobile and the automobile occupant. Road and intersection designs are based only on car, bus, and truck movement. The roads in LICs are dominated by motorcycles, human-powered vehicles, pedestrians carrying loads, and locally designed vehicles. No traffic flow models and computer programmes are able to accommodate this mix.

It is possible that even if all the solutions developed in HICs were put in place on the roads of LICs, the decrease in fatality rates would not be of the same magnitude as experienced in the HICs (Mohan and Tiwari, 1998).

Another example of the above is the role of expressways in intercity travel. When an expressway is built through the countryside, it divides the landscape into separate zones. People from one side of the expressway cannot go to the other side of the expressway easily on foot or on a bicycle. In HICs this does not pose a serious problem as most people possess motorized transport. However, in LICs the countryside may be heavily populated on both sides of the expressway by people of low incomes who need to interact with one another. They need to cross the expressway carrying or pulling heavy loads. In such a situation it is inconvenient to go long distances to cross the expressway at designated over- or under-passes. They end up breaking the fences and crossing the expressway at locations convenient to them. This makes the expressway much more hazardous for everyone concerned. But the decision makers associated with highway construction come from a different stratum of society who are only concerned with increasing the flow of intercity motor traffic and who see the villagers as impediments to progress. This is another example showing the conflict inherent among different communities and the difficulties encountered in promoting a safer environment for everyone.

5 Problems in data collection

Reliable data forms the basis of determining priorities for initiating action for developing safer communities. Our experience suggests that data collection procedures and the establishment of surveillance systems involve much more than just the existence of good forms, professionals, and computer packages. The people who collect and analyse data should have an understanding of the problem consistent with scientific facts. When this is not present, they see events according to their own pre-conceived notions (Tiwari, 1996). When setting up a surveillance system for recording details on injuries, the data collector must know that assigning *fault* should not be the main objective of data collection. The process of forging synergy between science and community perspectives takes time and seems to begin only when the community starts believing that injuries are indeed a health problem like any other disease.

The data collectors must also believe

that their efforts will result in changes. In LICs, the data collectors are very often at the lowest rung of the scientific social order. They do not really believe that their efforts will benefit their own community and the respondents share the same belief. This makes it very difficult to have on-going and regular data-collection systems of much integrity.

Thus, when a group in the LICs wants to start a safety promotion programme, it has a very difficult time in obtaining useful data. The community needs to invent and innovate to develop systems that would provide the necessary data. This obviously means that the community efforts have to be very specialized, specific, and self-sustaining.

6 Cost-effective methods of evaluating safety and injury control measures

The discussion above has highlighted some differences between HICs and LICs for professionals interested in injury control and safety promotion. In this section a brief description is given of some selected projects on injury control in India.

Areas of work include assessment of injuries in farming, fireworks burns, and road traffic. The approach adopted was to assess the magnitude of the problem by obtaining fatality and severe injury data, since these are generally reliable. This data was supplemented by small and focused studies of patients in hospitals, well-designed household surveys, and existing data from institutions and newspaper clipping services. The data so obtained was then compared and estimates made for deaths and injuries from different causes and associated factors. In addition, ratios between deaths and injuries could be estimated for each situation. The understanding obtained by such methods is adequate for instituting initial safety policies and injury countermeasures. A summary of these studies is given in the following sections.

6.1 Agriculture-related accidents and injuries in North India

This study was conducted to determine the epidemiology of factors associated with agriculture-related injuries and to understand the reliability of data obtained by a system of appointing informants in villages (Kumar, Mohan, and Mahajan, 1998; Mohan et al., 1989; Varghese and Mohan, 1990). The study was conducted in two phases. In the first phase an in-depth epidemiological survey was conducted by house-to-house bi-weekly visits to 3 500 homes in nine villages for a period of one year. The second phase was implemented in thirty villages comprising a population of 72 000 persons. Informants were appointed in all the villages to keep a record of agriculture- and transportation-related injuries. Research assistants visited the villages periodically to collect details on the reported injuries.

In HICs such information is usually obtained from hospitals, insurance, and other surveillance systems. In some cases telephone surveys are done to obtain data on a population-based sample. These methods could not be used in the above

study because most of the injuries sustained by inhabitants of these villages were not reported to any hospital or recorded by anyone. Most of the households in these villages do not possess a telephone either. In such a situation the data had to be obtained by training educated village youths in the collection and recording of data.

A total of 928 agriculture- and transportation-related injuries were recorded in the household survey and 551 in the study based on reporters. In the first phase almost all injuries were recorded, whereas in the second one only the more severe injuries were reported. In the first phase it was possible to get information on all injuries because all homes were visited every two weeks. The families were able to remember all injury events because of the frequency of visits and reported them when questioned by the surveyors. In the second phase the total number of injuries recorded was much fewer than the total in the first phase, though the population surveyed in the latter was larger. The second phase survey was conducted to get details from a larger sample of severe injury data.

These surveys were able to establish the role of injuries as a health problem in rural areas. The data revealed that there were 87 injuries per year per 1 000 persons in the villages studied. Moderate to severe agriculture-related injuries had a rate of 3 per 1 000 and, overall, agriculture-related injuries constituted 14 per cent of all episodes of ill-health. The data also helped in understanding the role of various implements and equipment that were associated with the injuries. The differences between HICs and LICs in the use of tractors are summarized below.

The details of all tractor-related injuries were recorded as a part of the larger study. In the period of two years, 76 cases of tractor-related injuries were identified, which included 5 fatalities. Farming activities resulted in 49 per cent of the injuries, transportation 43 per cent, and playing with equipment 8 per cent. Collisions with other road users resulted in 30 per cent of the injuries. Only 11 per cent of the injuries resulted from roll-over accidents. These patterns are related to the non-farming functions for which tractors are employed in India (e.g., power source and transportation). Tractor-related injuries in India have a very different pattern from that observed in highly industrialized countries. Safety-related countermeasures will have to be developed taking into account the India-specific use patterns of tractors.

6.2   Bicycle injuries in Delhi

Users of non-motorized transport constitute a significant proportion of the road users in all cities of India (Mohan and Tiwari, 1998). However, there are very few studies or reports that help us understand the incidence of road traffic injuries involving the non-motorized road users or the factors associated with these accidents. This discussion is based on two studies conducted on fatal and non-fatal bicycle crashes in Delhi. In the first study fatal and non-fatal crash reports of bicycle crashes were obtained from the Delhi Police for detailed analysis (Tiwari, 1993). The second study was done at the Neurosurgery Department of a premier referral hospital in Delhi, where details of all patients admitted with head injuries were

recorded (Mohan and Bawa, 1985).

The data indicate that: (1) the pattern of bicycle crashes are different from those experienced in highly motorized countries. These differences include locations of crashes, age groups of those injured, and types of vehicles impacting bicyclists; (2) there is a major difference in epidemiological details of fatal and non-fatal crashes. These differences are mainly in the proportions injured at intersections and mid-blocks and in the types of vehicles involved in crashes; (3) bicyclists comprised 14 per cent of all road traffic fatalities and 66 per cent of these crashes involved buses and trucks and 5 per cent cars; (4) buses and trucks were involved in 32 per cent of non-fatal crashes, and cars in 24 per cent. This shows that bus and truck crashes result in a higher proportion of fatalities than cars at similar velocities.

The motivations for bicycle use and issues concerning safety and convenience in Delhi are very different from those prevalent in HICs. These results can be used to optimize mobility levels in Delhi taking into account environment and safety implications. Provision of bicycle facilities and bicycle-friendly design policies, like segregated lanes and traffic calming, not only ensures safety for bicyclists but also increases overall mobility. Our study also shows that bus transport can be made more efficient only after segregated bicycle lanes are provided on arterial roads. To ensure safety of bicyclists in mixed traffic conditions it is also necessary to give attention to standards for safer bus and truck fronts. If such measures are instituted, safer and increased mobility would have a positive impact on economic activities in Delhi.

6.3 Fireworks injuries in India

Many people sustain burns when playing with fireworks during *Diwali*, the Hindu festival of lights. Two major hospitals in Delhi were selected every year from 1983 to 1986 and our observers were placed at the registration desks, where the burn victims reported on *Diwali* night. All types of fireworks available in Delhi were on display so that patients could indicate which ones had caused the injuries. Data were collected on patients' personal details, the incident, the fireworks involved, and first aid. A survey of 300 households in Delhi was also undertaken after the festival to determine the exposure rates of people using fireworks. In 1985 similar studies were conducted in Bombay, Pune, and Rohtak, and in 1986 a household survey was implemented in 2 400 rural homes.

The data collected from all the hospitals showed that the conical fountain, the roman candle, was involved with burns more than any other single firework (48 to 65 per cent of all cases) and a majority of the victims were young adults. Only 4 to 6 per cent of the victims used cold water as first aid. The household surveys indicated that 2 to 3 per cent of the families reported fireworks-related mishaps. This data suggest that about 100 000 persons suffer minor to major fireworks-related burns in two days and about 50 to 100 persons die due to burns in India.

The results of these studies have been widely reported in the Indian press, documentaries on the subject have been made and broadcast on TV, and public interest advertisements have also been broadcast, repeatedly warning of the hazards of fireworks and educating people about the use of cold water as first aid for burns. Later studies have indicated that use of cold water on burns as first aid has increased to almost 50 per cent among patients reporting to hospitals. However, the effect on the use of fireworks has been less pronounced. It appears that the proportion of persons injured by roman candles may have decreased by about 20 to 30 per cent, but it is difficult to estimate whether the total number injured has decreased or not as the exposure data is almost impossible to estimate.

The few examples given above show that it is possible to get a first-level understanding of injury events in a society even if sophisticated data recording and surveillance systems are not in place in the LIC. Very often the results showed that the injury prevalence and the factors associated with the injuries were at variance with the popular perceptions in the community or even among the professionals (Mohan and Tiwari, 1998; Mohan and Varghese, 1990). The results also showed that though the injury problem can be as much of a health burden in the LICs as in the HICs, the distribution of the injuries and the technologies and products involved can be very different.

7 Conclusion

We must not get preoccupied with determining a single cause of an injury. Most injuries are caused as a result of a number of events taking place together. Sometimes a factor contributing to an injury would be present because of a decision made long before the accident.

Prevention is not the only thing one aims for. Planning and designing is also done to reduce the severity of injuries if an accident does occur and also to provide adequate treatment of injuries if present.

The best form of protection is that in which people are safe automatically and do not need to take protective measures actively. This is particularly true for low-income communities where the creation of safety promotion institutions may be a difficult task. The situation in LICs is much more complex socially and technologically than that in the HICs and many problems of the former are not faced by the latter. Safety initiatives in LICs will have to develop their own political and social agenda. Much more work needs to be done on how such initiatives should be started. Future initiatives would have to consider the following:

- Installation of community consumer protection courts and community insurance schemes.
- Development of rapid data-gathering and assessment techniques.
- Starting with smaller initiatives.
- Greater involvement of labour organizations and other interest groups.
- Sharing of knowledge about inexpensive countermeasures worldwide.
- Integration of safe community activities with wider health promotion activities.

Exercises

1 Why has it become important for society at large to provide for safer designs and environment and not depend on individuals to behave more 'safely'? What are the moral, legal, and societal issues involved?

2 If we consider the occurrence of injuries as a *public health* problem, then the civil society and the state have to be involved in controlling the problem. Select an infectious disease and a serious injury problem involving your community and make a list of the past and possible future measures that would help to control the problems. What are the similarities and differences in the two approaches? Would less or more state involvement make a difference?

3 Why is it more difficult for poorer societies to control injuries than rich ones at present? What kinds of changes would make it possible for life to be safer in societies that do not have high incomes by international standards? You can include technical, administrative, political, and legal issues in your list.

4 What are the different ways in which you can define 'complexity'? For each of these definitions compare the situation of a safety issue in a rich and poor community by assigning levels of complexity to each group. Are there any issues that crop up that you had not thought of before? What are the lessons for the future?

Notes

1 In this chapter we have discussed the differences in injury control issues as a health problem in HICs and LICs. We have also maintained that the problem may be more complex in HICs. This is not to leave one with the impression that problems in LICs are unsolvable owing to low incomes, lack of educational levels, and differences in behaviour. On the other hand, we have tried to concentrate on the fact that international knowledge will have to be used in more ingenious ways to set up safety promotion systems in LICs, and a great deal of innovation is necessary in the societal and technological domains. More of the same will not do. We can take encouragement from the fact that in some low-income countries like China, Cuba, and Sri-Lanka, infant and maternal mortality rates have been reduced drastically, infectious diseases have been controlled, and nutrition levels have improved considerably. This has been achieved by improving the social, environmental, and public health conditions without waiting for income levels to reach those of the HICs. Similar approaches will have to be followed for injury control, and we believe that this is feasible.

References

BERGER, L. R. and MOHAN, D. (1996). *Injury control: A global view.* Delhi: Oxford University Press.

BONNIE, R. J., FULCO, C.E., and LIVERMAN, C. T. (Eds.). (1999). *Reducing the burden of injury: Advancing prevention and treatment.* Washington, DC: National Academy Press.

HADDON, W. and BAKER, S. P. (1981). Injury control. In D. W. Clark and B. MacMahon (Eds.), *Preventive and community medicine* (pp. 109–140). Boston: Little-Brown.

HADDON, W., SUCHMAN, E.A., and KLEIN, D. (1964). *Accident research: Methods and approaches.* New York: Harper & Row.

INJURY CONTROL (1988). *A review of the status and progress of the injury control program at the centres for disease control.* Washington, DC: National Academy Press.

KUMAR, A, MOHAN, D., and MAHAJAN, P. (1998). Tractor related injuries in North India. *Accident Analysis and Prevention,* 30(1), 53–60.

MOHAN D. (1983). Basic principles of injury control. In G. J. Wintemute (Ed.), *Injury prevention in developing countries* (pp. 119–140). Geneva: WHO.

MOHAN, D. and BAWA, P. S. (1985). An analysis of road traffic fatalities in Delhi, India. *Accident Analysis and Prevention,* 17(1), 33–45.

MOHAN, D., KUMAR, A., PATEL, R., and QADEER, I. (1989). Injuries in agricultural activities. *Indian Journal of Rural Development,* 1(1), 71–80.

MOHAN, D. and TIWARI, G. (1998). Traffic safety in low-income countries: Issues and concerns regarding technology transfer from high income countries. In *Reflections on the transfer of traffic safety knowledge to motorising nations* (pp. 27–56). Vermont South: Global Traffic Safety Trust.

MOHAN, D. and VARGHESE, M. (1990). Fireworks cast a shadow on India's festival of lights. *World Health Forum,* 11, 323–326.

MURRAY, C. J. L. and LOPEZ, A. D. (Eds.). (1996). *The global burden of disease.* Cambridge, MA: Harvard University Press.

PERROW, C. (1984). *Normal accidents.* USA: Basic Books.

RESIDENTIAL FIRE SAFETY SYSTEMS. (1997). *Building Code of Australia (BCA),* No. 07 (Replacement 1). Melbourne: Building Control Commission.

ROBERTSON, L. S. (1983). *Injuries: Causes, control strategies and public policy.* Lexington, MA: Lexington Books.

SCHELP, L. (1987). *Epidemiology as a basis for evaluation of a community intervention programme on accidents.* Sundbyberg, Sweden: Department of Social Medicine, Karolinska Institute.

STRATEGIES FOR ACCIDENT PREVENTION. (1988). *Report of a colloquium of the Medical Royal Colleges of the UK.* London: Her Majesty's Stationery Office.

TIWARI, G. (1996). Analysis of data collection

systems in Asian countries. In *The Proceedings of the Second Conference on Asian Road Safety* (pp. 105–118), Beijing, China.

TIWARI, G. (1993) Analysis of traffic crashes involving pedestrians and bicyclists in Delhi. In *Proceedings of the 2nd World Conference on Injury Control* (p. 121), Atlanta, USA.

VAN BEECK, E. (1998). *Injuries: A continuous challenge for public health.* Ph.D. thesis (published), Erasmus University, Rotterdam, The Netherlands.

VARGHESE, M. and MOHAN, D. (1990). Occupational injuries among agricultural workers in rural Haryana, India. *Journal of Occupational Accidents,* **12**, 237–244.

13 Community psychology and the problem of policing in countries in transition

Victor Nell

Study objectives

By the end of this chapter you should be able to:

- grasp the fragility of civil order in the modern state;
- understand why crime spirals out of control in countries in transition;
- ask whether the public health approach to violence prevention, which has achieved so much success in high-income countries, is appropriate for low-income countries and for societies in transition;
- examine the foundations of police accountability and ask what accountability means, and how it is applied in order to maintain a police force at top efficiency;
- understand why in weak states the police are virtually a law (or an anti-law!) to themselves, why strong states have police forces that are accountable

to the people they serve, and how civil society control of the police can be achieved and maintained;
- understand the role of civil society in helping South Africa climb back out of anarchy to order; and
- decide whether community psychology has a part to play in this process.

1 Introduction: the kind of world we live in

In *American Pastoral* (1997), Philip Roth tells what has become of the beloved Newark of his childhood, a well-ordered, family-centred, industrial city producing the torrent of manufactured goods that made America wealthy:

> Used to be the city where they manufactured everything. Now it's the car-theft capital of the world . . . . Forty

cars stolen in Newark every twenty-four hours. That's the statistic. Something, isn't it? And they're murder weapons – once they're stolen, they're flying missiles. The target is anybody in the street – old people, toddlers, doesn't matter . . . . They ram cop cars in broad daylight. Front end collisions. To explode the air bags. Doughnuting. Heard of doughnuting? Doing doughnuts? You haven't heard about this? This is what they steal the cars for. Top speed, they slam on the brakes, yank the emergency brake, twist the steering wheel, and the car starts spinning. Wheeling the car in circles at tremendous speed. Killing pedestrians means nothing to them. Killing motorists means nothing to them. Killing themselves means nothing to them. The skid marks are enough to frighten you. They killed a woman right out in front of our place, the same week my car was stolen. Doing a doughnut. I witnessed this. I was leaving for the day. Tremendous speed. The car groaning. Ungodly screeching. It was terrifying. Made my blood run cold. Just driving her own car out of 2nd Street and this woman, a young black woman, gets it. Mother of three kids. Two days later it's one of my own employees. A black guy. But they don't care. Black, white, they'll kill anyone. Fellow named Clark Tyler, my shipping guy – all he's doing is pulling out of our lot to go home. Twelve hours of surgery, four months in hospital. Permanent disability. Head injuries, internal in-juries, broken pelvis, broken shoulder, fractured spine. A high speed chase, crazy kid in a stolen car and the cops are chasing him, and the kid plows right into him, crushes the driver's side door, and that's it for Clark. Eighty miles an hour down Central Avenue. The car thief is 12 years old. To see over the wheel he has to roll up the seat mats to sit on. Six months in Jamesburg and he's back behind the wheel of another stolen car (pp. 25-26).

Throughout the world, in both high- and low-income countries, the failure of modernization – its hopes of a better life for all, of leisure and health and prosperity – has led to a breakdown of civil ordering and to massive crime. Residents of Washington, DC, in the United States tell of streets teeming with aggressive beggars and crazed kids; J. K. Galbraith (1992) writes of the 'golden ghettos' in Manila in the Philippines, which are 'distributed over that poverty-ridden metropolis, each with its own impenetrable fence and stern security force' (p.172). There the wealthy, as in Nairobi and Johannesburg, barricade themselves to keep the desperate and increasingly violent poor at bay.

In Johannesburg and Cape Town, as in Newark, New Jersey, people kill as easily as they breathe – to steal a car, snatch a wallet, or for no reason at all except the thrill of killing. I wrote the first draft of this piece on 2 January 1998: during New Year revelry that year, flat-dwellers in Hillbrow, Johannesburg, hurled bricks and bottles from upper-floor balconies into the crowds below. A year later, the violence in this inner-city slum escalated to an automatic weapon attack on an armoured police vehicle, two murders, and four shootings.

1.1 The collapse of *frith*

What these incidents in these many different settings have in common is a breakdown of the ancient notion of *frith*, a now obsolete Old English word from the same root as 'friend', meaning peace, or freedom from molestation (Shearing, 1992). In medieval England, *frith guilds* maintained the peace. Community safety is nothing more or less than *frith*: metaphorically, the purpose of community policing and community police forums is the resurrection of the *frith guild* as a primary mechanism for injury and violence prevention (Nell and Seedat, 1993).

The origins of *frith* are many and varied. Families teach children to love and protect their brothers and sisters, and as they mature, to extend this caring to their friends and to all other living creatures. Many social mechanisms – schools, churches, youth clubs – reinforce and extend these messages of protection, teaching us that the living body is sacred and untouchable. When no disciplinary authority is present, it is only these fragile inhibitory forces that prevent crime on the streets and violence in the home.

For community psychologists, the first question is why these forces are so fragile. Part of the answer is that the kind of world we live in is a world in which the thrill of risk-taking, and especially of antinomian risk-taking – the kind that breaks the law and thereby offers the added thrill of defying authority – far outweighs the sober and rational virtues of good citizenship. The emotions arise in the palaeomammalian circuits of the limbic system, and are so primitive that they have no language. Rational thought cannot touch an emotion.

The result is that hate and violence well up from the primitive brain structures we share with the most ancient of the mammals, whereas compassion and respect for the sanctity of the human body are the hard-won fruits of civilization – a thin veneer that holds society together. Compassion and respect for life are frontal lobe virtues that depend on rationality and language. They are weaker and slower than the emotions.

In the kind of world we live in, the primitive emotions will triumph whenever social systems break down in times of revolution and transition. On the one hand, these systems teach children to be compassionate. On the other, they put in place the external sanctions – police, courts, prisons – that maintain the rule of law.

1.1.1 Embedded policing: a Disneyland story

In *Policing for a new South Africa*, Brogden and Shearing (1993) argue for the notion of networked or embedded policing that derives from Foucault's dictum that there is no focal point to modern power, but an endless network of power relations. For example, Shearing and Stenning's paper, *From the Panopticon to Disneyworld*, first published in 1984 and frequently reprinted, poses an engaging question: Why is it that in Disneyworld, where there is no visible security presence, crime is unknown, although hundreds of thousands of people are packed tightly together in slowly moving queues under conditions of great frustration – a situation that lends itself to pickpocketing, mugging, and worse?

The simple answer is that surveillance – policing – is embedded in the corporate and organizational structure of Disneyworld. Every Mickey Mouse, Donald Duck, food server, and cleaner is a repository of public order:

> We invite you to come with us on a guided tour of this modern police facility in which discipline and control are, like many of the characters one sees about, in costume (Shearing and Stenning, 1984).

On a visit to Disneyworld, Shearing's daughter developed a blister on her heel, took off her shoes, and within ten paces was approached by a character costumed like a police officer in the Bahamas, with white pith helmet and white gloves, who told her that walking barefoot was not permitted 'for the safety of visitors'. When the young lady protested that her foot's safety required barefootedness, he replied that he would be compelled to escort her and her father out of the complex unless she put on her shoes again.

1.2 An explanatory political history

What is the role of South African community psychology and the South African non-governmental organization (NGO) movement in this complex set of interactions between civil ordering, based in the family and the

community (as illustrated by the Disneyland story); anarchic disorder in which human lives are snuffed out with laughter, like candles on a child's birthday cake (as in Roth's account of the decay of Newark); and coercion – the forceful prevention of violence by armed police? What are the most useful things students can learn from the community psychology literature, pass on to the NGOs they work with, and offer the new South African Police Service, struggling to assert its authority against rampant crime?

These are fundamental questions in today's South Africa, and to answer them systematically we will need to trace the separate but intertwined historical and political threads that were enumerated in the study objectives section at the beginning of this chapter.

2 The collapse of policing in countries in transition

There are two settings in which effective policing is taken for granted – in repressive police states and in democracies with well-developed accountability mechanisms. In countries that do not fall into one of these categories, policing is typically ineffective and corrupt. Moreover, when a police state or a well-functioning democracy collapses, policing is one of the first victims of disorder.

2.1 Police fragility

Though many other systems crumble in times of transition, the police are the most fragile of the state's ordering mechanisms, and the first victims of the rot of corruption. Police use the same methods – violence and subterfuge – as the criminals they fight, and they rely on intimate contact with criminals to get the information they need to make arrests. When authority is eroded, police are drawn like magnets into the willing arms of their former adversaries. Only the tightest accountability mechanisms can prevent a transitional society's police force from sinking into corruption and becoming implicated in smuggling, poaching, and well-planned violent crime.

A related aspect of police fragility is the sheer burden of work. It is one thing to expect police efficiency from a homicide squad dealing with 90 deaths a year in a city of a million people – the rate to be expected in a typical US city where the homicide rate is 9 per 100 000 population per annum (p.a.). It is quite another to have such expectations in Johannesburg, where at the current incidence of nearly 90 per 100 000 p.a. there are some 2 700 murders a year in a conurbation of some 2 million people. I recall a telling picture in the Johannesburg *Star* in about 1996 showing two detectives at the Protea police station in Soweto looking at the camera, almost hidden behind high piles of murder dockets. Under such conditions, police officers lose all hope of systematic case-by-case detection and can do no more than shuffle files from one side of their desk to another.

2.2   Crime prevention and state security

At a community policing workshop that our Health Psychology Unit[1] conducted in Soweto in 1994, a senior police officer was asked why crime prevention was so poor. 'We don't have enough vehicles to patrol the streets,' he said. He was challenged by a former political activist, now a member of a community policing forum, who asked him: 'What happened to all those yellow cars that used to chase us around Soweto?'

One answer is that they have been 'borrowed' for private use by senior officers, crashed, or otherwise written off – but now, there is no budget to replace these vehicles. In a broad-based democracy, competing demands for health and education have as strong a voice as the Minister of Police. But a police state will spend enormous sums of money on its security apparatus, and ensure that the security police attracts not only the most brutal men, but also the brightest and most competent. From the 1960s to the unbanning of the ANC in 1992, the best promotion route in the police was through the security police.

Indirectly, state terror keeps crime in check. Any security apparatus operates through a dense network of informers. The information that flows in is not only about politics – it's about robbery and car theft and drug dealing. All these criminal activities are either nipped in the bud by the security branch, or used for its own ends: 'You guys can carry on stealing cars or selling drugs as long as you tell us all about Dr Motlana and the Committee of 10.[2] If not, we'll wipe you out.' So, in a perverse way, this system controls and manages crime.

When the security system disintegrates, the informer network dissolves, and the crime checks that were in place are lifted. Under apartheid or Stalinism, the forensic

Table 1: Homicide and suicide rates† for some high- and low-income countries

	HOMICIDE	SUICIDE		HOMICIDE	SUICIDE
Switzerland	1,1	22,4	Ex-USSR	6,4	22,3
England	0,7	8,2	S. Africa	85,1*	Not given*
France	5,2	22,0·	Mexico	26,5	3,0
Ex-GDR	2,8	16,1	Ecuador	13,7	5,4
USA	8,2	13,1	Puerto Rico	16,0	10,2

† Rates are per 100 000 population per annum
SOURCES: *Brits (1995). All other data from Bourbeau (1993)

and investigative skills that form the foundation of effective policing are redundant and wither away. Who needs an efficient fingerprinting system if there are a dozen informers for every suspect, and if 'confessions' can be extracted by torture?

But when an authoritarian regime begins to crumble – under F. W. de Klerk or Gorbachev – the state security system disintegrates. The bright and brutal lords of the security police shred their files and run for cover. They become the heads of the security firms for which the disintegration of the police force has produced the appetite. The price one has to pay for moving from terror to freedom, like lifting the lid off a pressure cooker, is that crime boils over, feeding on itself and escalating in endless spirals of greed and power. It may be argued that Johannesburg has become the murder

capital of the world, and criminal gangs run Moscow because, among other reasons, state security systems have disintegrated. International homicide data (Table 1) bears out these assertions.

The homicide rate in South Africa is some eighty times higher than in Switzerland, England, and France, and ten times that of the United States. In the low-income countries of the southern hemisphere, the problem is especially acute. For example, the homicide rate in Colombia increased by 50 per cent from 1972 to 1982, and tripled between 1983 and 1992 (Pan American Health Organization, 1983). The WHO Collaborating Centre for Injury Prevention in Cali reports that 92 per cent of criminal acts are immune from prosecution. A similar situation prevails in South Africa, which is both a developing and a transitional

Table 2: Reported crimes of violence

	1991	1993	1995	Percentage difference between 1993 and 1995
Homicide	17 812	19 584	18 983	+3,8
Assault	270 437	293 340	348 173	+9,4
Robbery	68 907	87 083	102 809	+6,4
Rape	22 749	27 039	36 888	+15,3

SOURCE: Smit and Cilliers, 1997, citing SA Police Service Crime Statistics, 1996, p. 2

society, where alongside a collapse in state policing, the murder rate has increased from 56 per 100 000 in 1992 (Butchart, Seedat, and Nell, in press) to 85 per 100 000 in 1994 (Brits, 1995). The data in Table 2 confirm this escalation.

Nor, as noted above, can these problems of social order be solved by putting more police with more guns onto the streets (Brogden and Shearing, 1993). In 1991, South Africa had 84 776 police (South African Police, 1992) for a population of some 27 million in that year. This yields a density of 1:318 – a ratio that is 12 percent better than the German federal average of 1:356 (data cited in Nell, 1993). If the full authorized SAP establishment in that year of 89 021 police had been recruited, the police-population ratio in South Africa would have become 1:303, 17 per cent better than the German federal average.

Despite this relatively high police density, criminality in South Africa far outstripped that in Germany for precisely these underlying social order factors.

2.3 Transformation and crime in former East Germany

The reunification of Germany in October 1990 provides another case study of a society in transition, with striking parallels to South Africa. I visited Schwerin, the capital of the former East German state of Mecklenburg-Pomeranz, two years after reunification. Prosecutors and police officers there – all of them from former West Germany – told me that local people were losing faith in the ability of the police to protect them. Crime was increasing and the clearance rate declining. The grand explosion of freedom in the East had led to particular problems in the new states. Professional gangsters from West Germany and from Russia had begun moving into the new states because they knew the police there were not very effective. Despite their new uniforms, perceptions of the police were tainted with memories of denunciations they had made to the Communist Party. The police had become too insecure and afraid to be sufficiently forceful. Moreover, with the increase in crime, police were becoming overworked, with up to thirty cases a day coming to one criminal investigation unit.

The underlying reason for this escalation of lawlessness was that the former East German security police, the Stasi (Staatssicherheitpolizei), which had employed some 600 000 people throughout East Germany, had been dissolved, together with its network of informers. Stasi collaborators had penetrated every branch of East German society. They were unpaid, but would receive an occasional cash bonus and many favours such as better apartments and opportunities for themselves and their children to study.

Because security throughout the former German Democratic Republic (GDR) was so tight, these collaborators would by and large have been unknown. However, the Stasi maintained a huge system of files. In terms of the unification treaty, a federal law opening the Stasi files to inspection came into effect: this entitled individuals to inspect their own files and determine who had informed on them – the file might also contain the co-operation contract signed between the informer and the Stasi. Sometimes the informers were friends or even members of their own family (sources cited in Nell, 1993).

Figure 1: Homicide and purposeful injury in the European Union (EU), central and eastern European countries, excluding the former USSR (CEE), and Newly Independent States (NIS). All per 100 000

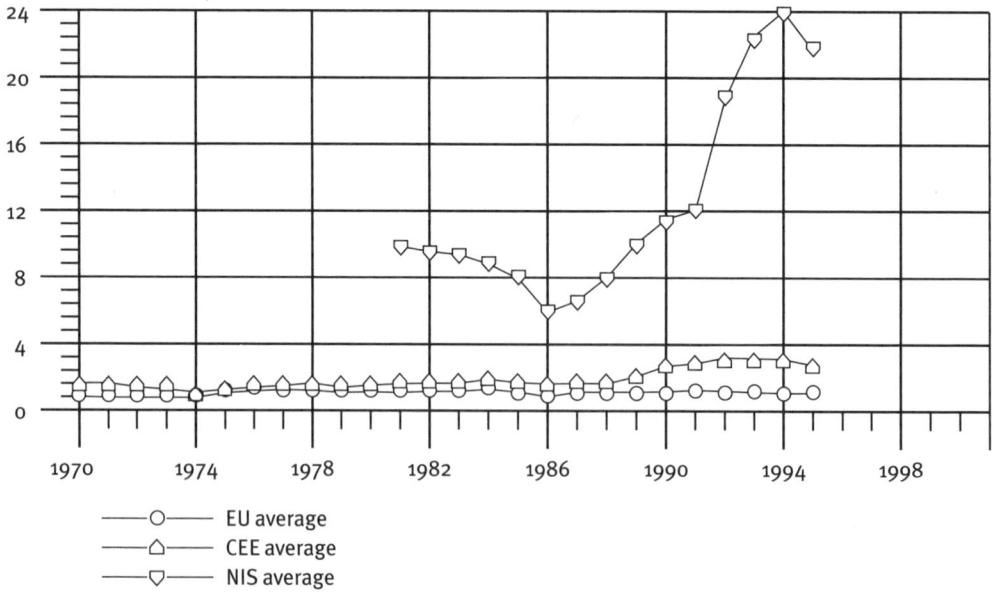

Figure 2: Motor vehicle traffic accidents in the European Union (EU), central and eastern European countries, excluding the former USSR (CEE), and Newly Independent States (NIS). All per 100 000

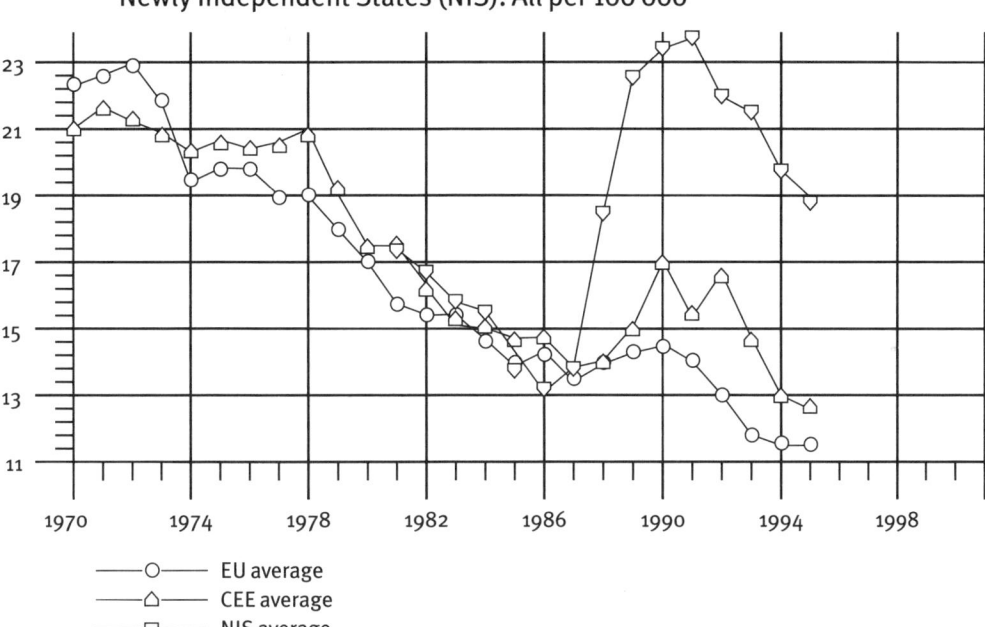

Data assembled by the Department of Social Medicine at the Karolinska Institute in Stockholm give striking confirmation of the high social costs of transition. Figure 1 shows that in the ten years from 1987, homicide and interpersonal violence rates declined marginally in the countries of the European Union (EU), which are by and large models of stability and accountable policing, but have risen in the newly independent states of the former Soviet Union (NIS) from a 1986 low of 6 deaths and violent injuries per 100 000 population a year to 24 per 100 000 a year in 1995. The number of traffic-related injuries, like homicides, is also an indicator of police efficiency, and here the comparison between the EU and the former Soviet Union is even more striking. Figure 2 shows that as the number of traffic accidents per 1 000 population declined in the EU in the 1990-1995 period, it increased sharply in the NIS countries.

2.4 Public responses to police incompetence

The easiest response to police incompetence is to abandon the police as useless and turn instead to private policing. The specific response is class-dependent. The rich turn to paid private security services[3]; the poor turn to vigilantism and people's courts that mete out rough but instantaneous justice (Schärf, 1989); the criminal and the disaffected murder or torture those who oppose them. All three categories effectively bypass the police, further weakening an already weak state by subverting two pillars of

269

orderly government – the state's monopoly of coercion held by its police and army, and its exclusive control of the criminal justice system. Popular justice also further demoralizes the police, who are drawn into unpopular, no-win confrontations with vigilante groups that enjoy wide grass-roots support, as with 'People against Gangsterism and Drugs' (PAGAD), which originated in South Africa's Western Cape region and then spread like wildfire to other areas – this rapidity itself showing the depth of popular contempt for the police. When, in the name of the rule of law, the police are compelled to confront such groups, whether they are nationally prominent, like PAGAD, or quite obscure, such as the 'judges' of a local people's court, they are seen to be 'taking sides' with drug dealers and rapists, and their precarious credibility with local communities is further undermined.

Among the wealthy, private policing proliferates, so that additional armed nodes of violence rather than ordering spring up. This again weakens the state's grip on public order. Electric fences, surveillance cameras, mechanized gates, and armed guards unmistakably proclaim to the world that the the state has lost its ability to protect its citizens and highlight the depth of the social divide between the vulnerable poor and the well-protected rich, though the protection lasts only as long as they remain behind the walls.

Finally, as hysteria at escalating crime increases, raucous demands for harsher punishment are made, and in particular for the death penalty. What the public outcry overlooks is that 'you've got to catch 'em before you can hang 'em', and the problem

with the criminal justice system is not the severity of the penalties but that so few criminals are brought to court to be punished. The point is nicely illustrated by the South African traffic safety data. Since 1993, there have been draconian penalties for drunk driving – the legal blood alcohol limit was halved from 0,15 to 0,08 – but the prosecution rate for drunk driving has not gone up by as much as a single percentage point (Van der Spuy, 1997).

3 The public health approach to violence prevention may be unhealthy for low-income countries

In Chapter 11 on public health and community psychology, Butchart and Kruger define public health as the identification of all points at which an exchange of matter, energy, and information occurs between individuals and their environment, and the macro-management of these exchanges to promote well-being in its widest sense. As a result of this inclusiveness, the range of analytic-intervention skills this approach can mobilize is unprecedented, making it the most powerful currently available modality for injury and violence prevention. The case studies they cite are ample demonstration of this capability.

In the international violence prevention community, the superiority of the public health approach to other competing models of violence prevention – including stricter policing – is accepted as a truism. For example, after describing the psychodynamic, demographic-sociological, behaviourist-social learning, and criminal justice models of violence prevention, Butchart and Nell (1996) conclude that these approaches have achieved only limited success, and that in response to this preventive failure, public health principles and methods have over the last fifteen years shown the greatest promise:

> Fundamental to the public health approach is the recognition of violence as a major contributor to premature death, disability, physical injuries and psychological morbidity, including post-traumatic stress disorder and family dysfunction. Central to this vision is a shift in the social response to violence: from a reactive stance imposed after the event and informed by the criminal justice concepts of retribution, deterrence and incapacitation, to a response aimed at changing the social, behavioural and environmental factors that cause violence (Butchart and Nell, 1996).

These are stirring words. However, critical analysis of the politics of violence prevention in low-income countries and transitional settings shows that, despite the power of the public health approach, its premature adoption in countries without a strong accountability culture can be a significant setback for violence prevention.

This is because the public health approach takes for granted that policing has already produced the best possible results. In Germany, for example, with a clearance rate of over 92 per cent for homicide, further gains

in this area obviously require the new methods and insights that can be offered by a radically new paradigm. But if the clearance rate for homicide is 10 per cent or even 50 per cent, public hysteria develops. People cast around wildly for a magic bullet that will make life safe again, the police are caught up in this panic of helplessness, becoming even less efficient. The most obvious solution to the problem is ignored – which is to ensure that the police are able and willing to do their job at an acceptable level of efficiency, following the internationally tested methods described in Sections 4, 5, and 6 below. This is the prime task of civil society, community psychologists, and NGOs, and any alternatives that divert public and political attention from the police should be avoided.

The founder of the Blockwatch system in Johannesburg, Clive Keenan, begins his recruiting meetings with the statement, 'Ladies and Gentlemen, the lie of the century is that crime does not pay. Crime does pay!' Indeed, the psychological rewards of criminality bear thinking about. For a poor kid from the slums of Johannesburg or Bogota, an entry to the world of car hijacking or drugs brings instantaneous and immensely powerful rewards – greater wealth than years of honest labour, the admiration of women, who for good evolutionary reasons are drawn to powerful rather than good-looking men. Crime is a violent business, and violence, at every level of the social hierarchy, brings the power to terrorize and coerce, with the feelings of triumphant dominance that are linked to such power, together of course with the awe and respect of their peers.

On a lighter note, you may recall Woody Allen's interview with the prison governor in *Take the money and run*. This kindly gentleman asks Mr Allen what his career plans are, to which he replies, 'Sir, after much thought I have decided to devote myself to a life of crime.' And why not? – crime is a brilliant and instantaneous solution to the existential problems of marginalization and powerlessness.

In this light, the political foolhardiness of moving violence from the criminal justice to the public health arena is that in settings in which the payoff from crime is higher than the risk of punishment (as it will be for any clearance rate below 50 per cent), the public health approach cannot succeed, and its adoption as the principle method of violence prevention is a strategic mistake. It lets the police off the hook and reduces pressure on the minister to get the police house in order.

Psychologists in particular need to be deeply suspicious of political initiatives that individualize and medicalize a larger social problem. The international politics of mental health – a problem that is in principle no different from the problem of violence – gives some striking insights into the ways in which governments and international government agencies, such as the United Nations and its specialized programmes, are able to evade their responsibilities by making believe that a huge social problem is no more than a 'health' problem (Nell, 1996). Like 'complete mental, physical and social wellbeing,' in the words of the 1978 Alma-Ata Declaration, violence prevention requires very large government expenditure, directed in the first instance at adequate social security, the regeneration of decaying inner cities, and the elimination of the huge informal settlements that are evidence, in all the low-income countries, of the failure of modernization.

But taxation politics and international fiscal constraints make it very difficult even for a populist government to embark on the necessary social revolution. So in Los Angeles, Washington, DC, and the Johannesburg metropole, violence prevention workers are compelled to accept an infrastructure that breeds violence, and to bootstrap under-resourced communities up the mountain of violence containment.

At the same time, and in parallel with the massive political task of re-establishing police efficiency and accountability, local and limited public health initiatives must also be pursued. These interventions are described in the violence prevention literature – for example, establishing activity centres that offer attractive alternatives to gang membership, or teaching primary school children that their bodies are private and inviolable. These softer options are immediately accessible to grass-roots and community-based NGOs – they are readily doable, under local control, improve life quality at the local level, and can be pursued while the larger battle for the restoration of *frith* continues on the national stage.

4 The foundations of police accountability

'Accountability' has become one of the catchwords of the new South Africa – but what does it actually mean? Accountability is a legal duty imposed on an individual to give account of his or actions – or failure to act – to a superior authority, which might be a public service commission or a supervisor. The higher authority is in turn empowered to take disciplinary steps against that person if the actions in question have been irregular or insufficient (Crane, 1977; Greer, 1978).

There are two main areas in which the police have to be accountable to the public: they must give account of their efficiency, and of their good conduct.

4.1 Achieving police efficiency

4.1.1 Informal quotas

How does a tough-minded local police chief make sure that his officers are delivering the goods? A couple of years ago, to learn more about police efficiency mechanisms in the United States, I visited the International Association of Chiefs of Police in Arlington, Virginia. I talked there with Bill Krueger, a veteran of twenty-seven years in the Michigan State Police Highway Patrol (citations in Nell, 1993).

In his years in Michigan, he ran a tough informal quota system to ensure that there was constant vigorous enforcement. Krueger says, 'You don't expect a patrol car to cover much more than 20 miles in an hour. It's slow work. You do a vehicle assist, give the guy a jump start or a drink of water, you check out rest areas for criminal activity, you check a stopped car without a driver and call for a tow, you work your radar. So at the end of the day you look at the guy's event sheet and you expect to see that he's covered

about 160 miles. If he's working traffic on an expressway, you'd expect him to come in with 10 to 20 tickets, about two-thirds for speeding and the rest for other violations. If you stop 10 cars, you should have at least one licence violation.'

As head of the Michigan Highway Patrol, Krueger says that he would have expected a patrolman to produce an average of ten tickets a day. In a heavily populated urban area, the expectation would be nearer twenty – but, adds Krueger, 'if he'd pulled into the parking lot of the Giant Muffler[4] Company and given out 20 citations, I'd also bend his ear. It's the moving offences that kill people, not noisy mufflers.'

He continues, 'If a cop averaged 10 citations across the week, I'd question that. If he didn't come up to average, he'd get a day off' – which doesn't mean vacation, but a day's work without pay, which is a disciplinary measure the patrol sergeant can impose.

Krueger notes that there is no separate traffic police force in America. Instead, half of most city police forces, and two-thirds of the state police, are designated for traffic duties. But Krueger emphasized that any other police officer will cut into whatever he or she or is doing to give citations for speeding or reckless driving. On the day I interviewed Krueger, there was a front-page picture in the *New York Times* of a huge homicide squad detective in the Bronx glaring at a motorist who had jumped a red light, and giving him a ticket. Traffic enforcement is beneath no one's dignity.

Krueger makes a final point: 'You don't get enforcement unless there's community pressure. Your chief of police must be taking strain. He's got to have the community on his back. That's when he really works his men.'

4.1.2 Formal measurement: clearance rates as the key to measuring police efficiency

Public service effectiveness auditing, which must be distinguished from the narrower discipline of financial auditing, is a recognized academic discipline, widely applied in countries with a strong accountability culture. For programmes that are publicly funded, public service audits are required by law. For example, Lyndon Johnson's Executive Order of 1964 required the withdrawal of federal funding from institutions that were in breach of affirmative action policies, and elaborate audit procedures were set up to monitor compliance (for citations, see Nell and Van Staden, 1988).

In Canada, police audits are carried out by trained federal auditors from the office of the Auditor-General, assisted by seasoned police officers on the Auditor-General's staff. In the United Kingdom (UK), the audit office reports to the House of Commons or to its select committees, which may summon the Commissioner to answer questions that arise (Nell, 1993, Part 4).

In all strong democracies, the primary police audit statistic is the clearance rate: a cleared case is defined as one for which the police have delivered a completed file to the public prosecutor, setting the judicial process in motion. The *clearance rate* is the number of cleared cases divided by the total number of cases reported to the police in that particular category.[5] Suppose, for example, that in the Johannesburg metro-

politan area, 1 000 murders were reported to the police. Of these – again by way of example – 100 dockets went missing (an all-too-frequent occurrence in apartheid South Africa, and one that continues unabated if the suspect has friends in high places), in another 200 cases the complainant failed to identify the suspect at an identity parade, and in a further 600 cases, witnesses went missing or forensic evidence was lacking, so that, in the course of 1997, 100 cases were handed to the Attorney-General for prosecution. The clearance rate is thus 100/1 000 x 100 = 10 per cent.

Criminal statistics for the Federal Republic of Germany are published annually in Bonn. These figures are assembled by requiring each local police organization to send its statistics, collected in a standardized fashion, to the state capital, which collates the information at that level and then sends them through to the Federal Ministry of Interior.

For the Federal Republic a total of 4 752 275 criminal cases were reported in 1991, of which 2 155 386 were cleared, for an overall clearance rate of 45,4 per cent. For crimes against life, including murder, manslaughter, and sexual murders, the clearance rate was 92,2 per cent, and for robbery, assault, kidnapping, and hijacking, the rate was 80,9 per cent, though for sexual crimes, the rate was 63,4 per cent. For lesser crimes, clearance rates decline – for thefts of vehicles and other property it is 13,5 per cent, though for fraud it is 87,1 per cent (citations in Nell, 1993).

In South Africa, and probably in most of the low-income countries, such figures are not published. What might they show if they were? A senior official in the Gauteng Department of Safety and Security speculated in conversation with staff of our unit that for crimes against the person, the current clearance rate is probably less than 10 per cent. Ordinary people's perceptions of the police suggest that this appalling estimate is correct. Asked if he had reported an assault to the police, a Centre for Peace Action worker, looking surprised, said: 'Everyone knows the police are useless.'

4.1.3 How NGOs can audit police efficiency

If clearance rates are the key to measuring police efficiency, what happens if the key is missing? In countries in transition, this will very likely be the case. A police force that has traditionally been centralized and authoritarian will not take kindly to the idea that its efficiency should be measured. Also, putting in place a new nation-wide surveillance system to produce local and regional clearance rates is a daunting task – and one that will be very expensive. So the resistance of the police to this new measure will be welcomed by an embattled Minister of Police and a cash-strapped central government.

If police efficiency at the local level is to be measured, NGOs will have to do it themselves. Fortunately, a powerful tool with built-in feedback mechanisms is available from an increasing number of NGOs that have been trained in this method. This is the service delivery survey (SDS) developed by CIET[6], an international NGO that has been commissioned by the World Bank, the United Nations High Commission on Refugees, and other agencies to conduct service delivery surveys in Nicaragua, Mali, Tanzania, Bosnia, Afghanistan, South Africa, and other countries.

In summary, a typical survey begins by identifying a pocket of problems the client organization – in this case, the client might be a community policing forum – wants researched. The objectives are clarified with the client and the service provider – for example, the local police station. A useful tool in developing a set of focus items that are likely to matter most to the community and the police is the community policing charter (see Section 4.2.4).

A questionnaire is then developed, field-tested, and applied to households in the catchment area. For epidemiological purposes, the population of these households becomes the denominator, so that the incidence of violent crimes for the community can be calculated, together with the percentage of these crimes that have been reported to the police, and the percentage that have come to trial. This latter figure is a guide to the local clearance rate.

At the heart of the SDS method is the conviction that measurement alone makes no difference; only if the results become a topic of discussion between clients and service providers will action steps emerge from the collated data, which can then be implemented.

There are great benefits both to the police and to communities in following this or a similar method, since the log-jam caused by a slow-moving central government and a recalcitrant police service is bypassed, and change can begin at the local level.

4.2 Maintaining police discipline

4.2.1 A German police view

The German penal code lays down that the supervisor is responsible for the actions of officers. So, if I witnessed a misdemeanour, I would report this to the Public Prosecutor, who would direct police officers to investigate the complaint. If the offence was minor, the police officer would be reprimanded. For major offences, the police officer is immediately suspended from duty, and the regional president orders a full investigation, making use of special civil service investigating units. An irregularity such as a death in a police cell results in an investigation by the state criminal authority – which is disliked in police stations because of the authority it has.

4.2.2 A German public prosecutor's view

A public prosecutor at the Frankfurt-on-Main State Court (Mr Wolfgang Schaüdensteiner, personal communication, 3 October 1992) described his duties and powers in investigating police misconduct by telling me the following story:

> Yesterday afternoon an attorney called me about a client, a black man, a Moroccan, who had been accused by the police of being a drug dealer. There's an open drug market in Frankfurt, you can watch them from my office window. The client said the police had beaten him. I asked the attorney if any injuries were visible. He replied that there were none, but I nonetheless asked him to see a doctor, and if there was any evidence of injuries, to have these photographed. I did not ask for an identity

parade immediately that afternoon, because late on a Friday afternoon it is difficult to find six or eight people who look similar to the accused. I asked the attorney to have his client open a file with me on Monday by making a statement to me at my office. In less serious cases, I will delegate taking the statement to a police officer, but in this case I did it myself.

If the police deny wrongdoing, I will nonetheless lay a charge, and leave it to the judge to decide. My job as State Prosecutor is to find evidence both against the accused and for him or her. It is to find the truth, not to prove guilt. When I give an order to a policeman in Darmstadt or Wiesbaden to investigate police misconduct, I know they will do it well and not favour the accused policeman. Also, there's a special department in the Frankfurt police that deals with accusations against the police.

If there's a serious case, and I believe the police might not have the ability to investigate the problem fully, I'll call for forensic examinations by experts that are available – medical experts from the university, fingerprint and other resources outside the police, and so on. Nobody asks how much it will cost because the state is obliged to pay, whether it costs DM 5 000 or DM 500 000.

What I want you to understand is that I don't need the police in order to do an investigation.

4.2.3 Using London's community policing forums to enforce good conduct

The Police and Criminal Evidence Act of 1984 makes the Commissioner of Police responsible for making arrangements to 'obtain the views of the people in that area about matters concerning the policing of the area and for obtaining their cooperation with the police in preventing crime in the area.' For each of London's cities (London and Westminster) and its forty municipalities, there is a Police and Community Consultative Committee.

The senior local police officer submits a list of people representative of the community's political and organizational structures for approval by the Commissioner. A group will typically have thirty to forty members. The Chief Superintendent for the area presents an annual policy statement on how the area is to be policed, which is considered by the group's policy subcommittee. Other subcommittees would, for example, deal with traffic, race attacks, or lay visitors. However, the consultative committees have only partially achieved their objectives in resolving conflicts between police and particular sections of the public. One reason is that these committees attract participation from people who are already well disposed to the police and seldom include representatives of hostile groups. Another is that many committees have become 'talking shops', with little resulting action.

Nonetheless, the London community policing forums have real teeth. For example, police forces are required to submit to oversight of detention in police cells by lay visitors recruited from the community. For instance, in Camden, London, 200 people responded to an advertisement by the Consultative Committee for Lay Visitors, of whom twenty were selected. These individuals are independent of the police and 'may visit police stations unannounced at any time of the day and night and expect to gain immediate entry.'

Once inside the police station, lay visitors can expect 'to have access to those places where suspects are detained; talk to suspects, in private, about how they are being treated in police custody and whether they have been able to exercise their rights; with suspects' consent examine custody records; and receive explanations from senior officers for police failure to comply with their legal obligations.'

Lay visitors' main weapon is publicity, and hence the potential for causing embarrassment, since they may choose at any time to make a public statement about what they found. Local police must also publicly state their standards of service to the Committee, and these must be publicly accepted. Examples might be a written commitment by the police to matters such as:

- Answering all telephone calls within thirty seconds.
- Response time of one hour to a burglary and ten minutes to a 'real emergency', defined jointly by the consultative committee and the police.
- A meaningful reply to every letter within fourteen days.
- A specified minimum number of uniformed officers on duty at a given time at any given place that has been defined as a trouble spot.

A monitoring group designated by the consultative committee would have the right to check continually on the implementation of these provisions.

4.2.4 Community policing defined

What does 'community policing' mean? Is it another clever slogan that exploits the popularity and political correctness of the term 'community'? Has community policing begun when the police are smiling and friendly? Or does it have a hard operational meaning?

In the first place, community policing means community participation in the determination of police priorities and methods in visible and effective ways.

Second, community policing means local policing. The unit of analysis is a single police station and the demarcated geographical area it serves. In this context, 'the police' are the personnel of the local police station and 'the community' is the population of the geographic area in question.

Third, community policing means competent, effective policing carried out by disciplined, professional personnel – policing that produces visible crime prevention and detection, and statistically measurable results.

Fourth, it is transparent and accountable policing. What the police do, and how they do it, must always be lawful, open to public scrutiny, and subject to accountability provisions.

In the present South African context, how might one set about achieving community policing that is participatory, effective, transparent, and accountable? The most powerful mechanism towards achieving this end is to tell communities what they can

reasonably expect of their local police station, and to convince police, in one way or another, that compliance with these expectations, though burdensome, will produce many benefits for the police themselves.

The draft community policing charter, presented below, sets out these expectations in simple and readily attainable form. It deals with two sets of expectations: What the community can expect of the police, and what the police can expect of the community. This draft is in immediately usable form; the final version will always be the product of local negotiations.

The charter describes a bottom-up method at a local level toward the achievement of accountable local policing. There are also important top-down strategies, which compel police compliance with the terms of the community policing charter by giving state teeth to its provisions. But these require the full co-operation of the Minister of Safety and Security and the Commissioner of Police, and are not the province of this document.

The bottom-up method described below, leading to the establishment of a community-police accountability forum (CPAF), is a powerful method of achieving local police reform, because it sets in motion the community consultation and mobilisation processes that are necessary first steps for the establishment of credible local policing – which is where policing happens and where it is most meaningful.

4.2.4.1 The community policing charter: what the community can expect of the police

Every community has the right to nine deliverables from its local police station.

278

These are:

1 *Emergency response times*

A cornerstone of effective policing is rapid police response to emergency calls, to which vehicles of the local police station are usually able to respond more rapidly than a centralized flying squad.

A response has two components. The first is the efficient handling of telephone or walk-in reports of life-threatening emergencies by experienced and well-disciplined police, who will at once state whether or not the police will be dispatched to the scene.

The second component is that police should arrive at the scene of such emergencies – assaults, brawls, rape, domestic violence, robberies, or housebreaking in progress – within a designated time. Certain other situations, even though not in themselves life threatening, such as a sighting of a person wanted by the police for a violent crime, must be designated as full emergencies. In the London Metropolitan Police Service, many police and community consultative groups have written undertakings from the police that designated emergency telephone numbers will be answered within, for example, thirty seconds, and that police will be at the scene of an emergency within a maximum of ten minutes.

Non-emergency response times for arrival at the scene of a burglary, an accident, or the aftermath of a violent confrontation should also be negotiated. In London, the maximum allowable delay is about an hour.

2 *Complaint management*

The ideal toward which policing strives is that every crime reported to the police will be fully investigated and cleared by charge. In working step by step toward this ideal, there must be clear initial agreement between the community and the police on which categories of complaint will be investigated with maximum vigour; these categories will be defined by each community in the light of its own experience and, at regular three- or six-month intervals, as the effects of more efficient policing become evident, this definition will be broadened to include further and progresssively less serious categories of crime that are perceived by the community as important to them.

A helpful strategy is for the community to agree with the police that offences perceived as unimportant by the community receive a minimum of police attention. However, the police are obliged to write to the person laying the complaint that the crime has been recorded, giving the case number, and that if any further information becomes available, he or she will be notified, but that the crime as reported does not warrant a full police investigation. And if a complaint has been investigated with no good result, the complainant will be notified by letter of the closure of the file.

The problem of lost dockets, which for years plagued the freedom struggle in South Africa, and is still used by lazy or incompetent detectives to terminate an investigation they dislike, must be addressed. The community-police accountability forum must insist that if a docket is lost, the case must at once acquire investigative priority and the contents of the docket reconstructed through re-investigation; the loss of the docket must be recognized as a serious failure of police competence and investigated by the station commissioner.

A full written apology and explanation, together with a statement that disciplinary steps have been taken, should then be addressed to the complainant.

3 Victim management

Victims of violence – especially sexual violence – are also psychologically traumatized. Competent disposition of such cases has five elements.

First, police response to the initial call must be immediate to prevent further injury to the victim.

Second, victims must be rapidly processed through the charge procedure, including the necessary medical examinations, accompanied at all times by personnel with specialist training in dealing with the victims of violence so as to minimize psychological trauma. Since a police station is an inappropriate environment for the dedicated processing of the victims of sexual and child abuse, each participating police station should acquire a safe house, the location of which is known only to designated police. The safe house is staffed by female civilian members of the police service with appropriate training, usually at no cost to the police through community-based NGOs or university departments of social work or psychology.

The safe house also provides forensic advantages, because the victim's clothing or person cannot be contaminated by contact with the assailant, which may happen if both parties are processed through the same police station.

Third, appropriate community-based agencies, such as counselling services, shelters for abused women, and legal resource services, should at once be advised of the incident in order to assist victims.

Fourth, victim safety requires full information on assailant disposition. The policeman or -woman assigned to the case bears responsibility for keeping the victim informed of developments such as the arrest of the assailant, his or her release on bail, or escape from police custody.

Maximum police resources must be made available for the clearance by charge of all crimes against the person – both for the sake of the victim and of society itself. Violence that goes unpunished sets in motion a vicious cycle of police demoralization and hopelessness, leading to increasing anarchy and reduced life quality.

4 Witness protection

Witnesses to crimes of violence, especially gang violence, have reason to fear for their lives if they come forward to give evidence. The community-police accountability forum should lay great stress on the need for an adequate witness protection plan – however, this requires greater resources than a single police station can muster. The witness protection plan will therefore also need the top-down political pressure described in Section 6 in the text. Protection of the witness should begin at the first contact of the witness with the police, continuing through identity parades and court appearances; protection for defined categories of crime should continue for a defined period even after a conviction has been secured.

5 Crime and clearance rate reporting

There is only one internationally accepted yardstick by which the effectiveness of a police force can be judged by the public it serves, and that is the regular publication of clearance rates by category of crime and by geographic area. Such statistics should be published within thirty days of the end of each quarterly reporting period, publicly displayed in the police station, and released to the press. By accumulating these figures and reporting the clearance rate by category, the community and the police themselves know how effectively the basic police function of crime detection is being performed.

Many South African police stations already produce monthly crime statistics by category, for example, how many cases of rape, housebreaking and theft, and hijack or theft of motor vehicles were reported to the police. Unfortunately, the number of prosecutions is never published, so that the figures are meaningless in terms of community safety. A suburb with ten rapes and convictions in all ten cases is likely to be much safer than one with only two rapes and no convictions!

6 Treatment of suspects

Police violence against suspects feeds into the national cycle of violence in South Africa. Respect for the law can only become a credible social value if the police themselves are seen at all times to respect the law, and to abhor violence in their own ranks as much as among the public. The rights of suspects to lawful treatment must therefore be upheld. They must be advised of their rights. Interrogations must be tape recorded using sealed recorders under the control of the audit officer and take place in designated areas that are at all times accessible to lay visitors (see below).

7 Lay visitors

As soon as possible after its establishment, the community-police accountability forum (CPAF) (see Section 4.2.4.3) should call for applications for lay visitors from among its members. Those appointed will be issued with picture identity cards by the police, and empowered to visit the police station at any hour of the day or night.

Immediately on arrival of a lay visitor at the police station, he or she will have access to all premises in the police station, including cells, interrogation areas, storage areas, living quarters, and any other premises available to the police.

8 Complaints review committee

The community-police accountability forum should as soon as possible set up a three-person complaints review committee made up of the station commissioner, the chairperson of the CPAF, and a third person who is a practising or retired advocate or judge, and acceptable to both parties, who should chair the committee.

The duties of the committee will be to resolve matters relating to the implementation of the charter that are in dispute between the CPAF and the police, and to deal at local level with complaints about the conduct of individual police.

For non-critical infringements of the charter, suitable action will be recommended to the station commissioner. If there appear to have been breaches of the law, the committee must ensure that the matter is handed over to the Attorney-General.

9 Accuracy and completeness of police records

The necessary audit and reporting functions

cannot be discharged without a commitment by the station commissioner and all personnel to the maintenance of complete and accurate primary records of all police activities, including occurrence books, vehicle log books, and dockets. Day-by-day monitoring of these records is the responsibility of the audit officer, with ultimate responsibility resting with the station commissioner.

4.2.4.2 The community policing charter continued: what the police can expect of the community

Once the police have by authority of the Commissioner of Police signed the charter, and all its elements are in place, the CPAF undertakes:

- To inform the community through press statements and public report-back of the extent of police co-operation with the community policing charter.
- To report frankly and fairly to the community of police progress toward meeting the charter, on obstacles to its fulfilment, and on the practical steps taken to address these obstacles, at all times giving due weight to police strengths and not only weaknesses.

Once there has been significant measurable progress towards attaining the objectives set out in the charter, the CPAF can in turn take the following steps toward the restoration of trust between the local police and the community:

- To advocate for improved community co-operation with the police in laying and pressing charges, and giving evidence, on the understanding that an

effective witness protection programme is in force.
- To institute a neighbourhood watch system.
- To speak out to the community, within the limits of the evidence, for the credibility of the station commissioner and his or her personnel.

4.2.4.3 The community-police accountability forum and community-based monitoring mechanisms

In demanding effective policing, communities must concede that policing is always and necessarily a deeply political activity through which a society imposes consensual standards of socially acceptable behaviour. Social norms change ahead of the law, and an essential aspect of policing is discretionary enforcement. Some laws are vigorously applied, while police will turn a blind eye to the breach of others. Police-community liaison must be directed to regulating the scope and nature of this discretion, rather than a false striving to 'depoliticize' policing. At best, the law the police uphold, and the way they do so, will conform to widely held local notions of natural justice and equity. At worst, the police may be constrained to enforce laws that lack local legitimacy. Community monitoring mechanisms will ensure they do so impartially and with least force.

Specific oversight and monitoring structures that can be instituted by the community, even without a formal police commitment to accountability monitoring, are described below. These measures would have the effect of involving representative community bodies, constituted as a community accountability forum, in a constructive dialogue with the police, aimed at more effective local policing, and in securing local police cooperation in this enterprise. The outcome of the collaboration might be voluntary police participation in the forum, which would then be renamed the community-police accountability forum.

1 Establishing the community accountability forum

The process by which the twenty- to thirty-person community accountability forum (the forum) is constituted should ensure representation for numerically significant constituents of civil society in the community – schools, churches, business, industry, and NGOs. A first step is to review the community policing charter, modify it as needed for the community in question, and then negotiate its acceptance by the personnel of the local police station – bearing in mind, despite the frustrations that may arise, that for better or for worse, this is the only police force we have, and only it has the capability to deal effectively with crime.

2 Structuring the forum

Monthly meetings of the community accountability forum should be advertised so as to invite the public and the press, held after working hours to encourage community attendance, and held at locations so selected that, in the course of a cycle of six or twelve months, the forum will have met in each of the geographic areas or suburbs of the community. At its first meeting, the forum should elect an executive and what-

ever working committees it wishes – but one of these should be a monitoring liaison group, whose job it would be to oversee the community monitoring described in the next section, and the appropriate dissemination of the information it gathers.

3 The monitoring liaison group

Community mobilization for more effective local policing brings the realization that good policing is a right, not a privilege – releasing hitherto untapped energies in the community. 'How NGOs can audit police efficiency' (Section 4.1.3 above) describes a powerful monitoring method that needs the help of a skilled NGO. This section sets out a supplementary method that is totally bottom-up and helps develop the community's own resilience. A first step in this bottom-up mobilisation is to set up monitoring structures in the community that gather information about the public and visible aspects of policing – patrols, response times, arrests, prosecutions – that are readily accessible to community surveillance, and crucial to the well-being of ordinary citizens, who are entitled to expect good service from the police. These structures are put in place by the forum's monitoring liaison group, chosen from among its most prominent and respected members. This group will publicly advertise its intention of interviewing persons in the community with direct personal knowledge of police response times, complaint and victim management, and the treatment of witnesses. These informants would, for example, be people who have reported an assault, rape, housebreaking, or theft to the police, as victims or as witnesses.

In order to ensure that as many incidents as possible are reported to the group, and that as much detail as possible is presented about police response and victim management, the monitoring liaison group should appoint area monitors drawn from among its own members, whose task it is to set up an information network by suburb, street, and block. By means of circulars, public meetings, and house meetings, this network will encourage every individual who has had an encounter with the police to be present at the next advertised meeting of the monitoring liaison group, in order to convey information on that encounter to the group. To ensure that information is publicly tested, area monitors should not themselves record this information, but ensure that it is passed on to the group as a whole at a formal meeting. In order to compile statistics that reflect the here-and-now quality of policing, all recorded incidents must have taken place during the previous thirty days; only exceptionally will incidents falling outside this time frame be recorded. Some three to six months into the experiment, by which time the monitoring liaison group should be functioning with a steady flow of informants, the station commissioner should be formally invited to attend meetings of the group. Thereafter, the charter should be formally adopted by the CPAF, the station commissioner, and his or her personnel.

5 Achieving civil society control of the police

Strong states have a strong civil society, and weak states do not. The difference between a strong state and a weak one, writes Joel Migdal (1988, p.13), is that the leaders of strong states are able 'to use the agencies of the state to get people in the society to do what they want them to do.' The two paradoxes of the weak state, on the other hand, are that the actual operations of state agencies differ radically from those conceived 'by their founders and creators in the capital city', and, secondly, that the top leaders of weak states, 'strange as it may seem ... have persistently and consciously undermined their own state agencies.'

I would add a further element to Migdal's definition: the sense of individual worth and control over one's own destiny is more fully developed in strong societies. So, if an individual or an organization wants their elected representative to get something changed, they do not plead – they demand, and they do not take no for an answer.[7] In other words, the democratic process persists beyond the ballot box, and politicians experience the full power of their supporters *after* the election more than before. Voters demand that the person they elected deliver the new factories, safer parks, and lower taxes they were promised – and make it very clear to the MP or congressman or -woman that, if not, their votes will go to someone else next time.

This is what makes policing work in the Western democracies. The local police chief is either an elected official who will not get re-elected unless he or she delivers what voters want, or a political appointee answerable to a mayor whose own re-election depends on public satisfaction with the efficiency of the local police service. Local residents use their votes to force politicians to deliver safer communities, and the politicians in turn ensure that their chiefs of police run a tight ship.

In the United States, local control of policing has been taken to its logical conclusion, truly making the police the servants of the people – sometimes good servants, sometimes bad[8], but always within the reach of the democratic process and civil society pressure. For example, in Stamford, Connecticut, a city of some 105 000, the mayor presents the city legislature with the names of persons he or she proposes as members of the police commission. This commission in turn appoints the police chief, who gets a salary of some $90 000 p.a. – a figure to make South African police officers weep with envy – and has a force of some 150 police under him or her (many American cities have had female police chiefs). Since the mayor is directly elected, and the police chief is seen as his or her appointment and therefore his or her responsibility, he or she has a direct interest in ensuring that this person runs a tight ship and that the city's orderliness is seen to be under control. If not, the mayor has the power to ensure that the chief steps down.

In the Third Reich, as under all totalitarian regimes, police structure had been centralized. But this system sat poorly with the postwar occupation forces. The province of North Rhine-Westphalia, for example, became a British occupation zone in 1945, and as an experiment a state police structure

was set up with a chief constable appointed by the local mayor on a regional basis. In 1956, the present provincial-regional-local police structure was adopted (citations in Nell, 1993).

The province is divided into five regions, with each region subdivided into districts. The big cities in the state such as Dusseldorf and Köln are 'free city districts'. In the Dusseldorf region, for example, there are five districts or counties and ten free cities. At the head of the regional government system is the regional president (Regierungspräsident); within the region, each district or county has at the head of its police force either an Oberkreisdirektor or a Polizeipräsident.

The five regions for which a Regierungspräsident is appointed are, in order of size, Dusseldorf (5,21 million), Köln (4,02 million), Arnsberg (3,73 million), Munster (2,47 million), and Detwold (1,89 million). At the district level, the Oberkreisdirektor and the Polizeipräsident are at the same administrative level; the difference is that the former has wide local government responsibilities, while the latter acts only on police matters.

This regional-local structure encourages a degree of regional loyalty, which is reinforced by the principle that the police in the local area are responsible for investigating a crime committed in that county and pursuing the criminal. For example, if a hostage is taken in the town of Glatbeek in Recklinghausen county, and the suspect flees to the state of Bremen, the county police in Recklinghausen would pursue this individual and would be in charge of his or her capture in the neighbouring state. Another aspect of local-regional co-operation arises with detective work. Since not every district has specialists, and will thus call on one of the sixteen detective divisions in the state, there are detailed regulations in the criminal law specifying for which crimes the higher levels of police must be called in.

The best hope for violence prevention in South Africa and other low-income countries is to expose the police to political pressure, which is the only means of compelling the police to do their job better. This in turn needs a transition from centralized policing – which politicians love – to locally managed policing – which politicians hate. The dangers of regionalization are outweighed by the benefits of politicians putting performance pressure on police chiefs, which in turn makes police chiefs make sure that their are delivering *frith* on the streets.

6 An action prospectus for community psychology

To borrow a famous slogan from the motor industry – 'Job One' for community psychologists, NGOs, and broader civil society in low-income countries and transitional settings is to ensure that the police are able and willing to do their job at an acceptable level of efficiency. It is 'Job One' because it will produce higher dividends than any other intervention in terms of violence reduction, injury prevention, the re-moralization of the police, and a new sense of hope in community policing forums.

6.1 What community-based NGOs can achieve – and what they cannot

Everyone knows the wisdom of the words, 'God give me the strength to change the things I can, the fortitude to accept those I cannot, and the wisdom to tell the difference.' There are some things about policing that communities and community-based NGOs cannot change – rooting out corruption, for example, or ensuring that the local police station publishes accurate clearance rate data. At this time in South Africa's history, it is impossible to predict whether a national alliance for regionalizing and democratizing the police will emerge. If it does, it will likely be an alliance between business interests and NGOs with national political clout, such as the Institute for Democracy in South Africa (formerly IDASA) or the Institute for Strategic Studies.

Meanwhile, sustainable community mobilization for better policing must aim at achievable goals – or fail. These goals are spelt out in the community policing charter, for example, rapid emergency response times, efficient complaint and victim management, correct treatment of suspects, and community monitoring of local crime clearance rates. The key instrument in achieving the achievable is the community policing forum (CPF) – or even better, as described in the charter, the community-police accountability forum (CPAF). However, the obstacles to making a CPF a hard-hitting and results-oriented body are formidable.

The first of these obstacles is that, however poorly they may be performing, the police remain a powerful social institution. Civilians entering a forum meeting to be confronted by uniformed men with guns and nightsticks are intimidated, and all too willing to accept the 'official' version of events as given by the station commissioner and his or her senior officers. Whereas in working democracies, community policing is a mechanism through which community representatives make demands of the police, the police in settings without an accountability culture use the CPF to make demands of the community. 'We can't prevent crime until the community cooperates fully with us', or, 'If you want us to be more efficient, why don't you raise the money to buy us a new patrol car?' The CPF is soon co-opted by the police, its more energetic members find better things to do, and the CPF becomes a talkshop instead of a powerful reformist instrument.

The second and even greater obstacle to an adversarial and therefore successful forum is that, from the highest levels of police management down to the station commissioner, the police are bitterly opposed to 'interference' and fault-finding from outside bodies. In Wachthuis in Pretoria – the national police headquarters – a senior police administrator told our unit's management, 'The one thing we don't need is more advice.'

At local level, an anecdote is instructive. In 1993, I attempted to set up a strong adversarial CPF in my home suburb in Johannesburg. Prior to the launch, the station commissioner gave a bitterly critical interview to the local newspaper (the substance was that people who should know better were busy setting up a 'complaint shop'), and at the launch meeting – which

was boycotted by the police – local residents who were still locked into the apartheid era asked angrily, 'Don't you know there's a war on out there and the boys in blue are our only protection? Why are you criticising them?' Needless to say, the new forum's few supporters took fright and abandoned the project.

Under these circumstances, successful CPF leaders are those able to remain courteous but adversarial, openly and clearly expressing displeasure with inadequate police performance, making their praise contingent on increasing police efficiency, and insisting on clearance rate publication as proof of these improvements.

6.2 The community psychology foundations of police reform

In determining the fit between this plan of action and the principles of community psychology, it is first necessary to consider the cost of crime at the individual, community, and national level. Very briefly, at the individual level, the burden is bodily injury resulting in temporary or permanent loss of income, coupled with psychological traumatization that undermines many aspects of life quality, the capacity to nurture spouse and children, and other aspects. At the community level, the lack of personal safety produces a fortress architecture of high walls, barred windows, and guard dogs, with a resultant loss of free-flowing interpersonal interactions and of recreation quality, while also undermining economic activity by direct and indirect losses to crime. At the regional and national level, crime-related injury burdens the hospital and mental health care systems, and impacts on economic productivity.

To the extent that police reform results in the pro-active prevention of crime, it has a good fit with the principles of the primary prevention of injury and psychopathology (Albee, 1986, 1999; Guernina, 1995; Kessler, Goldstone, and Joffe, 1992). Because it empowers communities by compelling the police service to respond to community pressure, it can be seen as an aspect of the social action model of community psychology (Seedat, Cloete, and Shochet, 1988).

Finally, effective policing activates several of the paradoxes to which Rappaport (1981) points: for example, it is necessarily intrusive, impacting negatively on individuals' right to live in freedom from interference – even if that interference is at the benign level of roadside driver alcohol testing. At this point in South Africa's history, there is no doubt that this intrusivenes would be widely welcomed; the question for community psychologists is whether, in the longer term, as South African society normalizes, the tension between freedom and effective surveillance can be contained.

7 Conclusion

What broad conclusions can students of community psychology draw from this analysis of the collapse of policing and its reconstruction? In my view, community psychology will be at its best if it positions itself as a *preventive* discipline that works at the causes of psychological distress rather than its symptoms. George Albee, the visionary leader of the primary prevention movement, writes:

> A hundred years hence, around the year 2100, the history of psychology will recognise a major intellectual breakthrough that occurred in the second half of the 20th century. It is the conclusive insight that most mental disorders are learned in a social context. They are NOT 'diseases like any other.' Mental disorders are problems in interpersonal (or intrapersonal) relations (Albee, 1999, p.30).

The primary business of community psychology is to change that context. In an earlier paper, *Toward a just society*, Albee identified the fundamental causes of psychopathology as:

- emotionally damaging infant and childhood experiences;
- poverty and degrading life experiences;
- powerlessness and low self-esteem;
- loneliness, social isolation, and social marginality (Albee, 1986, p. 891).

Within the helping professions, it is only community psychology that has the broad social sciences knowledge base, the political know-how, and the interpersonal skills to address all four of these root causes of psychological suffering by changing the social contexts in which they develop. One of the most basic of these contexts is the restoration of *frith* to the many South African communities that are traumatized by violent crime.

Exercises

1 This exercise is suitable for either individual or group work – though it is more fun in a group. Your task is to:

1.1 Describe your target community in terms of its leadership structures and relations with the local police.

1.2 Set up your own monitoring liaison group – even if it consists of only one monitor – and gather information over a two-week period from informants in the community, using as many as possible of the techniques suggested in the charter.

1.3 Request a meeting with the station commissioner of the local police station and review your findings with him or her.

1.4 Write up your project using the standard organization of a research paper – objectives of the study, subjects, procedure, results, discussion, and conclusions.

2 In your opinion, is police reform a legitimate field of activity for community psychologists – or would they do better to leave such work to politicians, police scientists, and other content area experts? Support your conclusion by a critical review of Section 6 of this chapter in the light of the cited papers of Albee (1986, 1999), Guernina (1995), Rappaport (1981), and Seedat, Cloete, and Shochet (1988).

Notes

1 The Health Psychology Unit was established in Johannesburg in 1986 as a University of South Africa research unit to carry out epidemiological research on injury and violence in South Africa. Initial funding came from the Human Sciences Research Council (in 1990, the Unit became a joint HSRC-UNISA research unit). In 1989, with Medical Research Council funding, the Eldorado Park Violence Prevention Project was launched, later renamed the Centre for Peace Action. In 1994, the Unit was designated a World Health Organization Collaborating Centre for Injury and Violence Prevention. In 1998, the Health Psychology Unit and its Centre for Peace Action, which had grown to a well-funded NGO with a staff of 35, became the University of South Africa's Institute for Social and Health Sciences.

2 A medical practitioner and community activist in Soweto in the years of the freedom struggle.

3 In *Policing for a new South Africa* (1993), Mike Brogden and Clifford Shearing review the spread of private policing in the high-income countries, and the conditions under which it produces legitimate nodes of safety and should therefore be encouraged.

4 American English for the silencer in a car's exhaust system.

5 The UK distinguishes between cases cleared by charge, as in Germany, namely, completed case files submitted to the judicial system for prosecution; and 'cleared otherwise', for example, a juvenile who cannot be charged, a prisoner already serving a term who confesses to a lesser crime, etc.

6 Community Information, Empowerment, Transparency. CIET began in Mexico in 1985 as *Centro de Investigacion de Enfermades Tropicales* (Centre for Tropical Disease Research) – hence the acronym, which has been adapted to reflect CIET's present focus on the measurement of social problems.

7 Linked to this is an axiom of modernist thought – that things are getting better all the time. Accordingly, to demand action for change is a historical as well as a political right.
8 As the Rodney King beating and movies like *Boyz 'n the Hood* show, despite these strong accountability safeguards, police harassment of African Americans continues to be a widespread failing of many American police departments.

References

ALBEE, G. W. (1999). Critique of psychotherapy in American society. In R. E. Ingram and C. R. Snyder (Eds.), *Handbook of psychological change: Psychotherapy processes and practices for the 21st century.* New York: Wiley.

ALBEE, G. W (1986). Toward a just society: Lessons from observations on the primary prevention of psychopathology. *American Psychologist,* 41, 891-897.

BOURBEAU, R. (1993). Comparative analysis of violent deaths in the developed countries and in some developing countries, 1985-1989. *World Health Statistics Quarterly, 46*(1), 4-31.

BRITS, K. N. (1995). The incidence of murder in Gauteng. In H. Conradie (Ed.), *Crime in Gauteng,* 1995. Pretoria: University of South Africa.

BROGDEN, M. and Shearing, C. D. (1993). *Policing for a new South Africa.* London: Routledge.

BUTCHART, A. and NELL, V. (1996). *Proposal for a global research and development initiative against violence.* Proposal submitted to the Final Meeting of the World Health Organization Ad Hoc Review on Health Research, Geneva, June 28.

BUTCHART, A., SEEDAT, M., and NELL, V. (in press) Violence in South Africa: Its definition and prevention as a public health problem. J. Seager and C. Parry (Eds.), *Urbanisation and health in South Africa.*

CRANE, E. G. (1977). *Legislative review of government programmes: Tools for accountability.* New York: Praeger.

GALBRAITH, J. K. (1992). *The culture of contentment.* London: Sinclair-Stevenson.

GREER, S. A. (1978). *Accountability in urban society: Public agencies under fire.* Urban affairs annual review, Vol. 15. Beverley Hills, CA: Sage.

GUERNINA, Z. (1995). Community and health psychology in practice: Professor George Albeew interviewed. *Journal of Community and Applied Social Psychology,* 5, 207-214.

KESSLER, M., GOLDSTONE, S. E., and JOFFE, J. M. (Eds.). (1992). *The present and future of prevention. In honor of George W. Albee.* Newbury Park, CA: Sage.

MIGDAL, J. S. (1988). *Strong societies and weak states.* Princeton: Princeton University Press.

NELL, V. (1993). *Toward community policing in South Africa.* University of South Africa Health Psychology Unit, Technical Report 93/1.

NELL, V. (1996). Critical psychology and the problem of mental health. *Journal of Primary Prevention,* 17, 117-132.

NELL, V. and SEEDAT, M. A. (1993). *Accountability foundation for South Africa: Working methods at local and national level.* Johannesburg: University of South Africa Health Psychology Unit, Technical Report 93/2.

NELL, V. and VAN STADEN, F. J. (1988). An affirmative action prospectus for South African universities, Part 1, Affirmative action in the United States and at the University of Zimbabwe. *South African Journal of Science,* 84, 19-22.

PAN AMERICAN HEALTH ORGANIZATION. (1983). *Violence and health.* Washington, DC: PAHO.

RAPPAPORT, J. (1981). In praise of paradox: A social policy of empowerment over prevention. *American Journal of Community Psychology,* 9, 1-21.

ROTH, P. (1997). *American pastoral.* Boston: Houghton Mifflin.

SCHÄRF, W. (1989). The role of people's courts in transitions. In H. Corder (Ed.), *Democracy and the judiciary.* Cape Town: IDASA.

SEEDAT, M., CLOETE, N., and SHOCHET, I. (1988). Community psychology: Panic or panacea? *Psychology in Society,* 11, 39-54.

SHEARING, C. D. and STENNING, P. C. (1984).

From the Panopticon to Disneyworld: The development of discipline. In A. N. Doob and E. L. Greenspan (Eds.), *Perspectives in criminal law: Essays in honour of John Ll. J. Edwards.* Toronto: Canada Law.

SHEARING, C. D. (1992). Conceptions of policing: The relationship between its public and private forms. In M. Tonry and N. Morris (Eds.), *Modern policing.* Chicago: University of Chicago Press.

SMIT B. F. and CILLIERS C. H. (1997). Violence and the criminal justice system. Unpublished paper, Department of Criminology. Pretoria: University of South Africa.

SOUTH AFRICAN POLICE (1992). *Annual report of the Commissioner of the South African Police, 1991.* (RP68/1992). Pretoria: South African Police.

VAN DER SPUY, J. (1997). *South African road traffic trauma: Toward prevention.* Address to the 6th International Safe Communities Conference, Johannesburg, 15-18 October 1997.

14 Gun violence as an issue of community psychology in contemporary South Africa

Jacklyn Cock

Study objectives

After studying this chapter you should have an understanding of:

- the incidence of gun violence in contemporary South Africa;
- the militarized context that framed the identities of those who engage in gun violence;
- the relationship between gun violence and contested social identities and meanings; and
- the challenges inherent in the solutions for containing gun violence.

1 Introduction

In contemporary South Africa there is a strong need for an indigenous community psychology that engages with contemporary issues of which the roots lie deep in the social structure. The incidence of gun violence in contemporary South Africa is such an issue. The main objective of the study on which this chapter is based was to demonstrate that those individuals who engage in gun violence are not atomized individuals; they exist in communities and contexts that have been shaped by our militarized past. The chapter argues that much gun violence is about contested social identities and meanings. The argument is based on material collected from both primary and secondary sources. The most important primary source is a series of eighty in-depth interviews. These interviews were conducted with key informants selected for their expert knowledge or experience of supply aspects of the proliferation of small arms in the southern African region, as well as in-depth interviews with informants from the diverse and overlapping social categories that create a demand for guns. The chapter also draws on participant observation through involvement in the organizations Gun Free South Africa and Ceasefire.

The solution to the problem of gun violence goes beyond individual therapy or state policy. It includes an indigenous anti-militarism and a transformative feminism that challenges our understanding of 'difference' and the relation of gender identities to violence and power.

The extent of gun violence illustrates the crisis in the contemporary South African social order. The gun is a symbol of our failure to build a secure society. At present in South Africa thirty-one people are killed with a firearm every day. (Personal communication, Sheena Duncan, chair of the Commission of Inquiry into the Central Firearms Register, 1998.) According to official sources guns were used in approximately 40 per cent of all murders and 79 per cent of all robberies in 1995. In 1995, 15 778 guns were reported stolen from or lost by private individuals. In 1996, this figure rose to 17 600, and this refers only to private licensed individuals. During 1997 there was no reliable information on the numbers missing from the SAPS and SANDF (Interview with Director of the SAPS Crime Management System January, 1997).

Clearly the level of violent crime and conflict linked to the proliferation of guns threaten the consolidation of democracy in South Africa. However, gun violence is not just an issue of public order, it is also a crucial health issue (Lerer et al., 1995) as well as a development issue, as it threatens to subvert the social stability that development requires.

I have chosen to write about the issue of gun violence, not only because of this threat, but also because of a number of problems in much of the existing social scientific literature.

2 The absence of social or community perspectives on guns, violence, and identity

The first such problem is that there seems to be a widespread conviction that violence in some form or another is ineluctably present in human affairs. In much of the current literature there is a tendency to see violence as either biologically determined (in the sense of being intrinsic to the human condition) or socially determined (in the sense of being an inevitable aspect of social change). This is expressed in Marx's (Keane, 1996, p.8) dictum that 'violence is the midwife of every old society pregnant with a new one' or, as Lenin stated it more crudely, 'you can't make an omelette without breaking eggs.' In addition, there is an intellectual trend to romanticize violence, a trend stretching from Sorel to Sartre and Fanon, who stressed the liberating and cathartic impact of the exercise of violence by colonial subjects.

In loose and expensive formulations that equate so-called 'structural violence' with injustice and inequality, social scientists have contributed to the contested nature of what we mean by 'violence', so that in scholarly discussions it often has no stable, consensual meaning. By contrast, gun violence is concrete and specific.

The second gap in much of the literature is that in discussions of violence there is a tendency to neglect the primary tools of violence, such as weapons and ammunition. There is no mention of guns in the three key published volumes of scholarship on violence in South Africa. Most surprising of all, in Ruth First's book, *The barrel of a gun*

(1970), there are important insights into the relation between militaries and political power in Africa, but no mention at all of the arms that are – at least in part – the material basis of that power.

The third gap is that the literature that does address these material vehicles of violence addresses questions of supply to the neglect of questions of demand. Guns are not value-neutral. We can hope to wean people off firearms only when we understand why people are attached to them. This requires a fresh approach to the problem of gun violence from psychologists, historians, and sociologists.

The final lacuna of concern is that most contemporary social scientists have avoided the study of violence, war, weaponry, and the military. One exception is Charles Tilly, who has argued for what he calls 'a renewed, expanded, sociology of war, one thoroughly grounded in history' (1991, p.1). This expanded approach to war suggests that the current global problem of gun violence is a social issue. Guns have become embedded in the identities of diverse social groupings.

In the post cold war world, armed violence and war is increasingly about contested identities, in the sense of different and antagonistic definitions of the self. Since 1989 there has been a shift away from war between states, involving major weapon systems such as tanks, aircraft, and warships, to intrastate war between internal groups, involving light weapons. These intrastate conflicts are part of a global relocation of power: 'Many of the new claimants to power within states are organised around issues of identity – whether of an ethnic, religious, tribal, or linguistic nature' (Klare, 1995, p.10).

3 A social perspective on identity

A social perspective on identity is central to my argument.

However, the concern with identity often involves a paralysing relativism and a retreat from political struggle. Lenin's question, 'What is to be done?' comes to be replaced by the question, 'Who am I?' (Bondi, 1993, p.84). These two questions are inextricably connected.

Identity is neither fixed and essentialist, nor completely fluid and shifting, but rather historically and socially constructed in changing processes of social interaction. Identity depends on a sense of difference that distinguishes 'us' from 'them'. All identities operate through exclusion. The lines of 'difference' imply the boundaries of identity.

It follows that collective identities are defined negatively, that is to say, against others. But as Hobsbawm (1996, p.41) has written, 'most collective identities are like shirts rather than skin, namely they are . . . optional, not inescapable.'

However, discussions of collective identities and difference need to be linked to an analysis of power relations; of how some social categories have the power to define difference as deficiency or as threat. Ignoring difference perpetuates these unequal power relations.

A crucial related question is how difference and identity are transformed into antagonism. Ignatieff (1994) reminds us that Freud once suggested that the smaller the real difference between two people the larger it loomed in their imaginations. He called this effect the narcissism of minor difference. According to Ignatieff (1994, p. 14):

> It's corollary must be that enemies need each other to remind themselves of who they really are. A Croat, thus, is someone who is not a Serb. A Serb is someone who is not a Croat. Without hatred of the other, there would be no clearly defined national self.

Edward Said (1988) connects the process of identity formation in modern society directly to violence. He writes: 'One belongs either to one group or to another; . . . one acts principally in support of a truimphalist identity or to protect an endangered one' (p. 54). He concludes that:

> while it would be a mistake to ascribe all the problems associated with random violence to . . . [a] maelstrom of escalating identity-demands, it would be an even graver mistake to ignore the process altogether (p. 58).

This chapter will argue that part of the solution to gun violence involves recasting the relation between guns and social identity. This is evident in relation to a particular weapon – the AK-47, the Kalashnikov assault rifle.

4 The AK-47: contested social meanings and identities

The Kalashnikov assault rifle is not just a gun; it is 'the most potent symbol of conflict and violence in the closing years of the 20th century' (Smith, 1996, p. 1). Since it first went into production in 1947, some 70 million AKs have been manufactured. It has been described as the most effective assault weapon in the world and has forever changed the way wars are fought .

What requires emphasis is that the AK is invested with powerful symbolic force. This is also true of other types of weaponry, for example, the tank, which is one of the twentieth century's most potent global symbols – a symbol of the repressive power of the authoritarian state. This is illustrated by events in Budapest in 1956, Prague in 1968, and Tiananmen Square in 1989. Similarly, the machine gun represents the power of the imperial armies, while the AK is an icon of the anti-establishment insurgent, the symbol of revolutionary resistance.

Especially during the apartheid era for many young, black South Africans the AK became a mythic icon, a 'marker' of group identity, and a kind of code to assert one's political allegiance, one that carried great significance for individuals. At this time the AK was an important ingredient in the state's portrayal of the African National Congress (ANC) as a demonic force. The extent of this demonization is suggested in a quotation from a police source warning of an African National Congress (ANC) action that would involve '7,000 local saboteurs and gorilla (sic) fighters' (South African Police Service, 1994).

Part of this process of demonization involved stressing the relationship between the ANC and the Union of Soviet Socialist Republics (USSR) – and the AK provided the link. The AK was the bearer, the material evidence of the 'communist onslaught'; it was constantly described as 'a Russian-made' weapon, and there were frequent references to 'Russian arms and ammunition' in the state-controlled media, as well as in displays of captured weapons. This was the evidence to support the apartheid regime's assertion that resistance to apartheid was not indigenous but inspired and supplied by the USSR. Thus, the identity of this gun marked the identity of the Russian demon-terrorist.

Ironically, supplies of thousands of AKs were an important part of the apartheid regime's destabilization activities. AKs were included in weapons that were supplied to rebel groups in Mozambique and in Angola, as well as to the Inkatha Freedom Party (Inkatha). For example, according to the Cameron Commission (1995) almost 40 000 AKs were purchased by the apartheid state between 1976 and 1986, specifically to be given to the main rebel group in Angola.

The AK is attractive for a number of reasons. Firstly, it is relatively cheap. At the time of writing this chapter an AK could be bought for less than $15 or for a blanket or a bag of maize in the neighbouring countries of Namibia, Angola, and Mozambique. In South Africa the going price could be as high as R1 500, so there are substantial profits to be made (Smith, 1996). Secondly, the AK is extremely robust; it has only sixteen moving parts, is easy to maintain, durable, and rarely breaks down. It is also easy to operate, which makes it particularly suitable for the increasing numbers of child soldiers in the world.

For all these reasons the AK is appealing to criminals and has also become a powerful symbol of criminal lawlessness; for terrorists

or revolutionaries and freedom fighters; these are the contested social identities that are condensed in the image of the AK-47. These contestations run deep. South Africa is not a consensual society and there are few shared maps of meaning. Current media accounts of gun violence involve fragments, or what Gramsci termed 'traces', of knowledge that have acquired the status of ordinary 'common sense' (Gramsci, 1971).

The AK is not the most commonly used weapon in violent crime compared with pistols and revolvers. For instance, high calibre automatic weapons such as AKs were used in only 6 per cent of the murders reported in 1995 (Interview with Director of the South African Police Service, Crime Management System, 1997.) Admittedly, this represents an increase from 1992 when less than 3 per cent of all murders were perpetrated with such guns. However, these figures would suggest that the author's impression of a focus on AKs in the contemporary South African media is an ideological hangover from the demonization of ANC guerrillas during the apartheid era.

This discussion of AKs, following Stuart Hall's (1978) analysis of mugging in British society, treats gun violence not as a uniform, undifferentiated phenomenon but as a relation – the relation between gun violence and the response to gun violence. In other words, the concern is with both the incidence of gun violence and the social reactions to it.

These social reactions reflect how our transition from authoritarian rule has produced a deep well of social anxiety as the familiar social identities and traditional practices have been disrupted and breached. One consequence of this social anxiety is as

Stuart Hall (1978) has written in a different context, the 'emergence of a predisposition to the use of "scapegoats" into which all disturbing experiences are condensed' (p. 157). In our context there are two categories of such scapegoats – the ex-combatant and the illegal immigrant. Much press coverage of gun violence reflects a sense of blame and indignation towards these social categories. In the vocabulary of social anxiety, ex-combatants and illegal immigrants are easy symbols of menace, social dislocation, and threat.

The policy solution generated by this anxiety – the tightening up of border security to block illegal immigration and prevent the smuggling of guns by Mozambican ex-combatants – is inadequate. Effective policy solutions have to include an understanding of how guns are invested with powerful social meanings and linked to contested social identities. The present romanticization of the AK and other firearms is, in part, the historical legacy of colonial conquest and revolutionary struggle in southern Africa, a process in which access to guns and land were the crucial themes.

This historical legacy includes antagonistic social identities and an ideology of militarism that regards violence as a legitimate solution to conflict and a crucial means of both obtaining and defending power. The material legacy of war includes a proliferation of small arms. Together these three elements form a lethal mix; guns provide the power to express social antagonisms in violent ways. The outcome of this legacy is that today the supply of guns is deeply embedded in the South African social and economic order.

5 The socially organized sources of gun supply

Discussions of the supply of small arms tend to be concerned exclusively with one source – cross-border smuggling of AK-47s by Mozambican ex-combatants. The issue is more complex. The supply of guns through the illegal arms trade is connected to many other social and economic activities, which include the trade in ivory, rhino horn, diamonds, teak, drugs, and even second-hand clothing. Our indigenous arms industry was built on linkages with most of South Africa's major manufacturing companies.

The majority of informants interviewed for this study who had licensed guns obtained them at prices of up to ZAR8 000, from licensed commercial gun dealers. Sometimes they did so on easy hire purchase terms of 10 per cent deposit and twelve months to pay. Most of these guns were imported, but small arms are also produced locally.

For example, the Denel subsidiary Lyttleton Engineering in Verwoerdburg (LIW), which produces the R4 and R5 automatic assault rifles, sells about 15 000 pistols a year to the civilian market. Another small pistol, the Vektor CPI 9 mm parabellum compact pistol, was available from local gun dealers for ZAR2 500 in early 1996. Numerous police informants stressed that this 9 mm pistol is one of the main weapons of violent crime.

As regards the illegal arms market, apart from smuggling across our porous borders, there are leaks from poorly controlled state armouries and security force personnel.

What this means is that the current proliferation of arms is not only a legacy of the apartheid regime. In several ways the post-apartheid state is encouraging this proliferation and thus paradoxically contributing to the erosion of its own authority. It is doing so through its support for the import and especially for the manufacture of small arms, through the encouragement of private gun ownership in the form of liberal licensing, and through the extensive arming of the security forces and weak control over their weaponry. Several informants maintained that security force personnel – especially poorly paid policemen – were themselves involved in the illegal arms trade.

The consequent proliferation of the means of violence is one of the most distinctive features of contemporary South African society. This 'diffusion' of arms suggests the dispersion and recirculation of arms through multiple channels to all levels of society. Consequently, the social categories involved with small arms include very different people; there is no homogeneous category of gun owners. But the argument of this chapter is that small arms are often the basis of a militarized identity that legitimates violence and thus is lethally connected to gender, ethnicity, race, and nationality.

6 The socially constructed demand for guns

The largest category of people who possess small arms are the 'security forces'. During the 1996 Defence Review process it was disclosed that the SANDF had a total inventory of almost a quarter of a million R1 rifles,

almost 200 000 R4 and R5 rifles, 17 000 pistols, and thousands of machine guns – and that excludes the so-called war reserves (Colonel Williams, the South African National Defence Force, Personal Communication, 14 March 1997).

The number of private security guards now outstrips the number of officers in the police force. This is a global trend. In the United States of America there are now seven times more individuals in private security firms than there are police officers. There are currently some 240 000 registered security guards in South Africa (Blecher, 1996). They have easy access to weaponry and less training than police officers. In one case firearm training involved a five-minute demonstration by a fellow worker (Blecher, 1996).

The number of licensed firearms in South Africa has increased dramatically since 1976 and at the time of writing this chapter, they numbered at 4,1 million. Licences are easily available and enforcement is minimal. One of the conditions is mental stability, which, according to one of my police informants, can be established easily in a ten-minute conversation! A number of informants maintained that there is a massive degree of police corruption in the processing of firearm licences, extending deep into the Central Firearm Register (Sheena Duncan, personal communication, 12 August 1998).

Increasing numbers of licensed firearms are landing up in criminal possession. Obtaining access to these criminal informants is one of the hardest parts of my current research. But analysing gun violence as a social phenomenon involves more than exploring individual biographies, motives, and meanings. Exploring gun violence as a social phenomenon also involves examining the diverse social practices built up around guns. Collectively these constitute a robust 'gun culture' in contemporary South Africa.

This gun culture is a set of highly heterogeneous resources that are used selectively by members of different social groups. Overall, this culture operates to provide a social sanction to the possession of guns, and much gun violence follows culturally defined repertoires of behaviour.

The values, social practices, and institutions that together constitute this gun culture include what Williams (1972) calls 'consumerist militarism'. It involves the normalization – and even glorification – of war, weaponry, military force, and violence through television, films, books, songs, dances, games, sports, and toys.

Toy guns are a significant component of this culture. A total of forty-eight different varieties of toy guns were on offer at a Johannesburg shop in December 1996; for ZAR120 you could buy a model of the American automatic assault rifle, the M-16. Significantly for the argument about difference and identity, this toy was advertised as an 'alien blaster'.

All of these cultural forms constitute a kind of 'banal militarism'. Banal militarism operates near the surface of social life. It is embedded in everyday activities and works through prosaic routines and rituals to make war, weaponry, and violence appear natural and inevitable.

Such banal militarism is exemplified in war games such as paintball, which has become increasingly popular among white South Africans since 1985. At its core, paintball simulates the sequence of killing.

One informant involved in this 'gun culture' spent much of his leisure time playing paintball, practising at shooting ranges, and cleaning and 'stroking' (his word) the twelve guns that he owned. This behaviour is chillingly reminiscent of that of the killer responsible for the Dunblane massacre in Scotland in 1996 in which a number of school children were shot.

This gun culture does not only operate to glamorize war and weaponry but also to 'normalize' these social practices. Part of this 'normalization' is the notion that private gun ownership is legitimate; it is a right, not a privilege.

This notion that private gun ownership is legitimate is linked to the belief that guns are an effective and necessary form of protection. Now, the gun combines two contradictory images – it is a means of both order and of violence; paradoxically, it is believed to provide protection from violence through the potential threat of violence. This has a powerful appeal in our context where, since the 1980s, there has been a 'privatization of security' as increasing numbers of citizens have lost confidence in the capacity of the state to protect them, and have come to rely on private security arrangements, and individual gun ownership.

A common theme articulated by many of my informants who had purchased guns for self-protection was a sense of being powerless. However, the power of the gun as protection is largely illusionary. According to numerous police sources, the great majority of crimes committed with firearms are committed with either legally owned weapons used for an illicit purpose, or weapons that have been stolen from their legal owners. It follows that the distinction between legal and illegal weapons is a dubious one. Guns are long-life commodities and their change of legal status does not affect their lethal power. The legal supply of small arms is generally the seedbed of illegal flows. The fact that over 17 000 licensed firearms probably fell into criminal hands in 1996 dramatizes the dangerously self-contradictory potential of guns as a means of individual protection.

There is reliable evidence, ironically from the United States of America, that people are safer without guns. Epidemiological research there has established that a gun in the home is 43 times more likely to kill a member of the household than to kill an intruder (Kellerman and Reay, 1986).

There are disturbing parallels between South Africa and the USA. The sociologist J. Gibson (1994) has identified a new, highly energized paramilitary culture in contemporary America, which he relates to a crisis of identity among American men. Many white male informants interviewed for my study articulated a lack of confidence in the government and the economy, and seemed uncertain of their future in relation to political change generally and affirmative action policies specifically.

Both white and black male informants are also troubled by changing gender relations. In our society there has been a reconfiguration of the discourse on gender since 1990 and women are presenting a challenge to customary male behaviour. Among diverse categories of men there seems to be different versions of a 'crisis of masculinity', which reflect a social dislocation and confusion about their gender identity.

Even though men may be 'the primary agents of violence in most societies' (Beinart, 1992, p. 473), violence is not an exclusively male practice. But for men violence is bound up with their identity. Guns are part of the dominant masculine code in many different cultures. This code frequently links guns to men's role as protectors and defenders (Cock, 1991).

To a diverse number of young South African men guns are a marker of status, and signal a particular style. For example, to many members of organized crime syndicates in the township of Soweto, near Johannesburg, ostentatiously displayed firearms indicate the status of being a 'big man' (Wardrop, 1996).

However, the style that guns signal is not restricted to political allegiance or criminal defiance. Guns are also a form of social display that can signal male affluence. As one of my informants from the community of Lenasia near Johannesburg expressed it: 'If you have a BMW, a cell phone and a glamorous woman you've got a lot; if you've got a gun as well, you've got everything.' According to one source, guns have even penetrated the Johannesburg clubbing scene (Webster, cited by Coetzer, 1997).

This militarized masculinity evokes an ambiguous response from women. In South Africa increasing numbers of women are purchasing guns, which could indicate that a male style is being homogenized and spread more widely. This is part of a global trend. The growing power of women within the USA gun lobby was illustrated last year with the election of a woman as the National

Rifle Association's first female president. She has a solution to gun violence: 'Instead of getting rid of all guns ... why not just get rid of all liberals' [who moan about gun violence] (Anthony Lewis, cited in *The New York Times*, 14 April 1996).

To some informants gun ownership among women represents an assertion of a feminist identity. A South African woman firearm trainer argues that 'we have come through the sexual revolution to be regarded as equals. We have lost the male protector. Women have to take responsibility for their own protection' (Kirt Stuart, cited in *The Saturday Star*, 2 November 1996). She advises on how 'women can carry guns for self defence and still look feminine, sexy and demure.'

Sixty years ago the French feminist Madeline Pelletier (in Scott, 1996, p. 137) insisted that 'girls were to be given a rigorous physical education that included learning to use a revolver .... The gun in a girl's (or woman's) hand was tangible evidence of her power, a phallic prosthesis that made her feel the equal of men.'

One of my female informants linked her gun ownership directly to her feminist identity as an independent woman. She maintained that owning a gun, which she wore tucked into the back of her jeans, made her feel powerful, self-reliant, and in-dependent.

This kind of thinking is partly a response to an increasing trend for women – in both the United States and South Africa – to be the victims of gun violence. Increasing numbers of the 36 000 rapes reported in 1996, as well as domestic violence generally, involved firearms (Interview with Director of the SAPS Crime Management System, January 1997).

The gendered nature of gun violence is significant, but gender, class, race, and ethnic identities are inseparable; they construct and reinforce each other. Much gun violence relates to deep-seated fears and insecurities that are grounded in racial and ethnic iden-tities, which are antagonistically defined.

At present, for many South Africans, ethnic identities are the strongest source of social cohesion. The mobilization of ethnic-ity by Inkatha to secure economic and poli-tical goals has deepened animosities along ethnic lines, and the supply of weaponry enables these animosities to be expressed in particularly lethal ways. Similarly, some right-wing Afrikaner groupings have mobi-lized around a politicized ethnicity, and have formed armed, paramilitary organiza-tions. The availability of guns encourages these militant political groups to engage in violent rather than democratic opposition.

Some of the worst non-state gun vio-lence in our history – such as the random killing of twenty-three black people by an Afrikaner man named Barend Strydom, in 1988 – is explicable partly in terms of this lethal mix of access to weaponry, gender identity, and racial antagonism. Barend Strydom maintained that racial difference defined the boundaries of human identity and humane treatment.

The contested notion of 'non-racialism' offers an alternative interpretation of differ-ence and identity and has been linked to an inclusive ANC nationalism, but nationalism also involves identities, which may legitimize violence, which guns potentially make lethal.

Nationalism as an ideology involves two

claims. Firstly, while men and women have many different identities, it is the imagined political community of the nation that provides them with a primary, fixed, and categorical form of belonging that trumps all other sorts of identities. Secondly, violence is justified in defence of one's nation against enemies. Of course there is a paradoxical relation here: nationalism is persuasive because it both legitimates violence and offers protection from violence. This relates to nationalism's two faces: the one of group identity, solidarity, and inclusion; the other of exclusion.

Until very recently the nation was the main vehicle of warfare. National identity involved the gender-specific obligation of military service and was the chief justification for participation in lethal combat. However, today, as Ignatieff (1994) has argued, an 'ethnic nationalism' is the main source of contemporary violence. It is what he calls a language of blood and belonging. He distinguishes it from civic nationalism, meaning a shared attachment to certain political institutions and laws. In contemporary South Africa this ethnic-nationalist identity is being challenged in the name of a more inclusive civic national identity, which defines a common citizenship.

What is less often contested is the connection between this civic nationalism and militarism. Even the most inclusive statement of a common South African identity – that of Thabo Mbeki marking the adoption of our constitution in May 1996 – involved him in invoking the militarist image of his identity as 'a foot soldier of a titanic African army, the ANC' (Craig Urquhart, cited in *The Star*, 17 May 1996).

This militarist imagery is partly a legacy of the apartheid era when citizenship involved national military service for white males, and blacks were denied access to weaponry, a denial that involved a denial of African manhood as well as citizenship (Hellman, 1943). This militarized citizenship and militarized masculinism will be very difficult to dislodge.

However, a statement from a former self-defence unit member points us to a crucial aspect of the solution to gun violence in South Africa – the forming of new, demilitarized social identities that are sources of affirmation. Now part of the Daveyton Peace Corps, this young man commented: 'I was really disappointed at not getting a gun when I first joined the Peace Corps in 1994.' He went on to say: 'After a while I realised that I did not need a gun . . . . I now know that the community needs and values us' (cited by Kirsten, 1996, p. 1).

7 Solutions to the problem of gun violence in South Africa: the forming of new social identities

The argument in this chapter is that as the supply of guns is socially organized, the demand for guns is socially constructed and embedded in various social practices and cultural forms. Guns are connected to various overlapping social identities, particularly those defined by gender, race, class, age, political affiliation, nationality, and ethnicity. All of these are strong representations of common interests and carry powerful mobilizing sentiments within them. They are all relational identities; they involve boundaries demarcating 'us' from 'them'; they mark lines of exclusion and difference, which perceptions of threat and access to weaponry make potentially lethal.

In political terms, gun violence is ultimately about the contestation of power invested in these identities. The relation between power and violence is an ambiguous one. The power that 'grows out of the barrel of a gun' is often the obverse of moral authority and political legitimacy. Paradoxically, the perpetrators of much criminal violence, such as robbery and car hijacking, belong to marginalized and powerless social groups to whom guns represent the power to enforce compliance.

The core of the argument put forward in this chapter is that a control policy that ignores the historically and socially constructed meanings attached to firearms will not be effective. We need to alter the allegiances and identities that underlie acts of gun violence.

Ex-combatants are only part of the problem; the failure to provide for the effective social integration of ex-combatants is only one symptom of our broader failure to build a common society and a new collective identity for South Africans. To do so requires confronting the legacy of war through an indigenous demilitarization movement that involves the kind of mass mobilization that marked the anti-apartheid struggle.

It is arguable that the social mobilization necessary to form such a demilitarization movement is particularly difficult in South Africa. During the process of 'élite-pacting' that marked our transition from authoritarian rule, an alliance of militarists from the various armed formations, but particularly the South African Defence Force (SADF) and Umkhonto we Sizwe (MK), was firmly established. No strong grass-roots anti-militarist movement emerged during the 1990-1994 period to challenge this alliance.

However, there is at present an embryonic demilitarization movement in organizations such as Gun Free South Africa and Ceasefire, though these are marked by a 'social shallowness', being extremely small, fragmented, and mainly white and middle-class.

Both organizations are involved in policy advocacy, which involves engaging with state structures and processes, such as the consultations around the 1996 Defence White Paper and the 1997 Defence Review. Both organizations are also committed to public education campaigns.

The Gun Free campaign was launched in September 1994 and encouraged people to hand in their guns in return for food vouchers, lottery tickets, and a letter of thanks from former President Mandela. Only 270 firearms – mainly white-owned and licensed – were handed in, but according to the co-ordinator of Gun Free, the campaign:

> raised public awareness about the proliferation of firearms in our society and made it an issue for public debate. It also placed the issue on the political agenda. The ANC December national conference adopted a resolution supporting Gun Free (Interview with Adel Kirsten, 1996).

Since 1994, the organization has grown and increasing numbers of public buildings have been persuaded to declare themselves 'gun-free zones' in which firearms are prohibited. Gun Free has extended its public education activities and lobbying of politicians. The organization maintains that its successes include the fact that the new constitution excluded the right to own firearms. This 'has ensured that gun ownership will remain a privilege rather than an entrenched right' (Adel Kirsten, cited in *The Star*, 14 May 1996).

The second significant grouping in the South African embryonic demilitarization movement is Ceasefire. This organization has been active in lobbying politicians for reductions in defence expenditure, and in protesting with placards and balloons against issues such as the production and export of the Rooivalk attack helicopter, and war games at the Lohatla infantry training school near Kimberley in the Northern Province. During 1997 it co-ordinated a national campaign for the banning of land-mines and the destruction of all existing stockpiles.

The two organizations' main concerns are the two most lethal and plentiful categories of light weapons dispersed through-out the region at present – anti-personnel landmines and firearms. Ceasefire has suc-cessfully conducted a campaign of stig-matization, emphasizing the long-lasting destructive and indiscriminate impact of landmines. One of the challenges of a de-militarization movement is to stigmatize firearms in a similar way.

Both organizations – in which women are a powerful presence – are connected with similar movements in other societies and are thus part of what Richard Falk (1992) has termed 'globalisation from below'.

Falk points to an emerging 'global civil society', which, he argues, is disseminating powerful new social identities as people challenge violence, war, and militarization as 'citizen-pilgrims'.

This identity of 'citizen-pilgrims' is similar to Martin Shaw's (1995) notion of 'active citizens'. Shaw adapts the notion of duty that conscription mobilized, and gives it an anti-militarist content:

Just as the citizen formerly owed a military duty to the state, the active side of post-military citizenship can be defined in terms of the citizen's duty towards peace ... 'active citizens' should be concerned with positively extending the demilitarisation the end of the Cold War has begun (Shaw, 1995, p. 187).

In reality, a limited process of state demili-tarization has been under way in South Africa for some years. However, it is a com-plex and uneven process and has had some contradictory consequences. For example, the increasing emphasis on arms exports is partly a response to the reduction in domestic defence procurement. Thus, paradoxically, state demilitarization is contributing to global militarization.

Policy solutions that are overtly statist ignore the plurality of institutions and social relations with which the state must engage. The process of demilitarization needs to go beyond the restructuring of state institu-tions in a much broader project of social transformation.

This transformation involves delinking guns and masculinity, a challenge posed most sharply by Virginia Woolf in the 1930s when she asked: 'How can we alter the crest and spur of the fighting cock?' Today many feminists are insisting on the need to form new gender identities. This is one theme in a transformative feminism that confronts the connections between the private and public spheres, questions our understanding of 'difference', and challenges the relation of gender identities to violence and power. There is an urgent need for psychologists and other social scientists to connect with these social movements, and engage with the crucial events and issues of our time.

8 Conclusion: gun violence and applied social science

To conclude, this chapter has tried to give a social-scientific perspective on a particular social problem – that of gun violence in contemporary South Africa. This perspective is extremely relevant to community psychology. Community psychology should point us to the causes of social problems, which lie deep in social structure and process and beyond individual expression. The solutions to social problems such as gun violence involve far-reaching social change. In contemporary South Africa we need to think imaginatively, which means a 'Utopian' dimension to problem solving. Richard Turner (1972) spoke of 'the necessity for utopian thinking', which, by emphasizing the social construction of existing arrangements, opens up the possibility of radical alternatives.

In the process of addressing the problem of gun violence there is the necessity for Utopian thinking. Weaponry and war are not fixed topographical features of the social landscape; armies are not essential to the existence of a nation-state, as the experience of Costa Rica and Panama demonstrates; and private gun ownership is not essential to citizenship.

Anchored in a conception of the social totality, community psychology is necessarily holistic, and necessarily informed by the interconnecting patterns that constitute our social life. This is the perspective that is strengthened by historical and theoretical frameworks as well as by research strategies for producing comparative material and reliable evidence about the social world. Drawing on these multiple streams, community psychology could engage more with problem solving to bring about a just and peaceful social order in South Africa.

Exercises

1 Name five factors that threaten your security.
2 Would you feel more secure and safer if you owned a gun? Give five reasons for your answer.
3 Interview someone you know who owns a gun. Try to find out why they obtained it, how they obtained it, how much it cost, where they keep it, whether they know how to use it, whether they have ever used it, under what circumstances they would use it, and how much they know about the problem of gun violence in South Africa.

4 How would you conceptualize the relation between guns and gender identity? Does the increasing purchase of firearms by women indicate that a militarist masculinity is being homogenized and spread.

5 Why does the social-scientific literature neglect the relation between guns, violence, and social identity?

6 What social and historical processes account for the proliferation of small arms throughout southern Africa? What are the most important consequences of this proliferation?

9 References

BEINART, W. (1992). Political and collective violence in southern African historiography. *Journal of Southern African Studies,* 18 (3), 455-486.

BLECHER, S. (1996). *Safety in security: A focus on the role of the private security industry and the potential for violence.* Unpublished paper compiled for the Network of Independent Monitors.

BONDI, S. (1993). Locating identity politics. In M. Keith and S. Pile (Eds.), *Place and the politics of identity.* (p.84-101). New York: Routledge.

CAMERON COMMISSION. (1995). Inquiry into alleged arms transactions between Armscor and one Eli Wazan and other related matters. First Report. Pretoria: Government Printer.

COCK, J. (1991). Colonels and cadres: Gender and militarisation in South Africa. Cape Town: Oxford University Press.

COETZER, J. (1997). Jacknife hurtle down the freeway of fame. *Music Africa,* 25, 10.

FALK, R. (1992). *Explorations at the edge of time.* Philadelphia: Temple University Press.

FIRST, R. (1970). *The barrel of a gun: Political power in Africa and the coup d'état.* Harmondsworth: Penguin.

GIBSON, J. (1994*). Warrior dreams, violence and manhood in post-Vietnam America.* New York: Hill & Wang.

GRAMSCI, A. (1971). *Selections from prison notebooks.* London: Lawrence & Wishart.

HALL ET AL., S. (1978). *Policing the crisis, mugging the state and law and order.* London: Macmillan.

HELLMAN, E. (1943). Non-Europeans in the army. *Race Relations,* X(2), 45-53.

HOBSBAWM, E. (1996). Identity politics and the left. *New Left Review,* 217, 38-47.

HOBSBAWM, E. (1994). *The age of extremes: A history of the world 1914–1991.* New York: Vintage Books.

IGNATIEFF, M. (1994). *Blood and belonging: Journeys into the new nationalism.* London: Vintage.

KEANE, J. (1996). *Reflections on violence.* London: Verso.

KELLERMAN, D. and REAY, D. (1986). Protection or peril? An analysis of firearm related deaths in the home. *New England Journal of Medicine,* 314(24), 314.

KIRSTEN, A. (1996). *The Peace Corps.* Unpublished report.

KIRSTEN, A. (1996, May 14). Gun free zones. *The Star.*

KLARE, M. (1995). *Light weapons arms trafficking and the world security environment of the 1990's.* Paper presented at UNIDIR Conference, Berlin.

LERER, L.B., MATZOPOLOUS, R., and BRADSHAW, D. (1995). *Profile of violence and injury: Mortality in the Cape Town Metropole 1994.* Tygerberg: South African Medical Research Council.

LEWIS, A. (1996, April 14). The gun issue. *The New York Times.*

ROTH, M. (1983). If you give us rights we will fight: Black involvement in the Second World War. *South African Historical Journal,* 15, 85-103.

SAID, E. (1988). Identity, negation and violence. *New Left Review,* 171, 46-62.

SCOTT, J. W. (1996). *Only paradoxes to offer: French feminists and the rights of man.* Cambridge: Harvard University Press.

SHAW, M. (1995). 'Partners in crime'? Crime,

political transition and changing forms of policing control. CPS Research Report No. 39.

SMITH, C. (1996). Light weapons and the international arms trade. In United Nations Institute for Disarmament Research, *Small arms management and peacekeeping in southern Africa.* (p. 1-60). Geneva: United Nations.

SOUTH AFRICAN POLICE SERVICE. (1994). *Annual report of the Commissioner of the South African Police.* RP 58\1994. Pretoria: SAP.

STUART, K. (1996, November 2). Packing a pistol in style. *The Sunday Star.*

TILLY, C. (1991). *War in history.* Centre for Studies of Social Change.

TURNER, R. (1972). *The eye of the needle.* Johannesburg: Ravan Press.

URQUHART, C. (1996, May 17). Our new constitution. *The Star.*

WARDROP, J. (1996). *Policing the cities: Soweto, syndicates and doing business.* Paper presented to the SAIIA conference, Johannesburg.

WILLIAMS, R. (1972). *Towards 2000.* Harmondsworth: Penguin.

WOOLF, V. (1973). *Three Guineas.* Harmondsworth, Penguin.

15

Consciousness-raising groups as an intervention strategy against gender oppression

Cheryl de la Rey

Study objectives

After studying this chapter you should have an understanding of:
- gender as a form of social inequality that impacts upon mental health and mental health service provision;
- the conciousness-raising empowerment approach to groupwork.

1 Introduction

The literature on the impact of social inequalities on mental health and mental health service provision has expanded in recent years. For example, in 1996, the *Journal of Community and Applied Social Psychology* devoted a special issue to the theme Social Inequalities and Mental Health: Implications for Service Provision. Jennie Williams (1996), the editor of this special issue, pointed out, however, that in spite of an increase in the volume of such literature, it still has a marginalized status within the overall field of mental health. Most mental health services continue to be dominated by individualistic models that ignore the impact of social oppression on the lives of people.

In this chapter I discuss gender as a form of social inequality that impacts upon mental health and mental health service provision. Although gender inequalities are not separate from other forms of inequalities such as race, class, sexuality, disability, and age, the particularities of gender as a social category demand close attention. Lessons from other countries in Africa, South America, and the former Soviet Union all show that gender relations have relative autonomy from other forms of inequality, since the overthrow of one form of oppression does not necessarily lead to liberation from gender oppression.

The central objective of this chapter is to present an empowerment model of groupwork that may be incorporated into community mental health programmes to successfully intervene in the arena of gender inequalities. This model combines the principles of consciousness raising within self-help groups. Various projects will be outlined to illustrate the model, but firstly a brief overview of the effects of gender inequalities on mental health is presented.

2 Gender and mental health

Debates about the effects of gender on mental health have revolved around two central questions: firstly, do women display higher rates of mental illness compared with men, and secondly, are there gender differences in types of mental illness and symptomology?

Discrepancies in mental health between women and men have been reported across various societies. Surveys of mental health statistics in North America and Britain generally show that women present with more pathology than men (Al-Issa, 1980; Walters 1993). There are fewer surveys from African countries, but some data from Africa contradicts the pattern found in Western countries. For example, Kisekka (1990) reported that studies of admission rates to psychiatric institutions show higher rates for men than women. One of the difficulties in interpreting these patterns stems from the lack of clarity on whether these statistics merely represent differences in help-seeking behaviour and in access to mental health services, rather than gender differences in pathology itself. Kisekka argued that in

African countries men's greater access to the formal economic sector gives them better access to psychiatric institutions and this may then explain the higher admission rates for men. In contrast, many African women show a greater orientation to traditional healers as a source of help, so they would not be reflected in the bio-medical statistics.

Gender-related variations in symptomology have been reported more consistently. Desjarlais et al. (1995) noted that across diverse societies and social contexts 'symptoms of depression and anxiety as well as unspecified psychiatric disorder and psychological distress are more prevalent among women, whereas substance disorders are more prevalent among men' (pp. 179-180). Sizable gender-related discrepancies in clinical depression have been frequently reported in the literature. The gender ratios of women to men vary between 6:1 to 2:1 (Brown and Harris; 1978; Gove, 1972). Data from Africa supports this overall pattern. There is generally a higher incidence of depression and psychosomatic disorders among women and a predominance of conduct disorders, alcoholism, and drug abuse among men.

If mental health is defined more broadly beyond the limitations of psychiatric disorder, the impact of gender inequalities becomes more pronounced and complex. Violence, sexuality, and reproduction are three issues that illustrate the complex interaction between gender and mental health. Estimates derived from studies in Britain suggest that between 1 in 3 and 1 in 10 women are sexually abused in childhood and that most perpetrators are male (Watson, Scott, and Ragalsky, 1996). A Cape Town-based organization, Research Centre aimed at Prevention of Child Abuse and Neglect (RAPCAN), estimated that 1 in 4 girl children and 1 in 5-8 boy children are subjected to child sexual abuse (Cassiem, S., personal communication, April 1998). After a long history of silence, the past ten years have seen a steady accumulation of research, which has documented the negative mental health consequences of child sexual abuse, rape, and battery. These consequences include an increased risk of attempted suicide, alcohol and drug abuse, depression, and women abusing their own children (Mercy et al., 1993).

The link between gender inequalities and mental health is also starkly evident in the reproductive sphere. Kisekka (1990) has argued that a primary source of stress for women in Africa, regardless of career and educational achievement, revolves around reproduction. She pointed to the significance of the internalized traditional value of having many children, together with the disproportionate family and child care responsibilities placed upon women as sources of stress.

Butler and Wintram (1991) offered a model for understanding the impact of gender inequalities on the lives of women. Based on their work with numerous rural and working-class women in Britain, they argued that fear, loneliness, and isolation lay at the root of many women's experiences: fear of violence or the threat of violence, isolation frequently caused by material constraints such as poverty, lack of transport or child care facilities, and loneliness that arises when the woman feels that she is a failure and that she is the cause of her problems. Recent research conducted within a community-based programme for teenage mothers pointed to the relevance of this model to the lives of South African women. De la Rey and Parekh (1996) reported that fear, loneliness, and isolation were three factors that seemed to permeate the lives of teenage women who had returned to school after unplanned pregnancies and childbirth.

3 Gender as an analytic concept

Gender inequalities affect not only the mental health of women but that of men too. Miller and Bell (1996) have drawn attention to the prevalence of men as a high-risk group for suicide, homicide, addictions, imprisonment, and morbidity. Very recent work such as that reported by Cavanagh and Cree (1996) has foregrounded the need to see male domination and power as complex and contradictory. This is perhaps best illustrated in interventions with violent men, which have shown how men can be traumatized themselves and at the same time inflict trauma on others. Hence an emphasis on gender analysis is not simply about seeing women as victims and men as perpetrators. It is far more complex.

Very often the concept gender is used narrowly and erroneously to include women only, while male-gendered experiences are ignored. Recent research on social constructions of masculinities (Connell, 1995; Segal, 1990) has drawn attention to the ways in which gender oppression also has negative consequences for men even though it privileges them as a group. Frye (1992) explained the differential impact of gender oppression as follows:

311

Barriers have different meanings to those on opposite sides of them, even though they are barriers to both . . . . A set of social and economic barriers and forces separating two groups may be felt, even painfully by both groups and yet may mean confinement to one and liberty and enlargement of opportunity to the other (p. 14).

Therefore, we need a conceptual understanding of gender that includes experiences of both women and men but with recognition that women are structurally and systemically oppressed in relation to men. Gender as a concept covers social constructions of individuals as feminine and masculine, as men and women, the relations between women and women, between men and men, and between women and men as gendered beings. Men and women are positioned in relation to one another in a group sense, and the power dynamics of this relationship are manifest in the structured inequality of access to material and social resources so that men have privileged access over women. As Maharaj (1994) suggests, the recognition that male privilege and domination over women are produced and maintained through socially constructed meanings and institutional arrangements gives rise to crucial questions about how we bring about the conditions for changing the status quo.

A critical component of social change is the reinterpretation of a social situation or a new way of seeing so that circumstances, which for a long time may have been accepted as normal, are then seen as producing disadvantage. The need for a critical understanding of the intricate and complex connections between institutional arrangements, social norms, and individual experiences has been recognized as fundamental to social action aimed at the eradication of inequalities. While social action is often presaged by individual advocates and activists, social change requires collectivity (Lewis, 1991). Such collectivity may take many forms; one such form is the small group.

4 Rationale for groupwork

Debate about the potential link between groupwork, empowerment, and social action has had a fairly long history in the social sciences. Shapiro (1991) reports that in North America early conceptualizations of the role of groupwork in social service provision saw groups as agents for social change. But with the ascendancy of individualism, groupwork theorists shifted away from an explicitly political approach to an almost exclusive emphasis on the personal and interpersonal dynamics of groups. According to Shapiro (1991), 'along the road the concept of the centrality of social action was lost. Even more important, the concept of the centrality of groups in social action and social change processes was lost as well' (p. 15).

However, with the development of community organization and community-oriented approaches to mental health, there has been a renewed emphasis on the politics of groupwork. The work of theorists such as Paolo Freire in South America and the impact of political movements such as feminism have contributed to shifts within the international literature on social service provision, in general, and groupwork in particular. Concepts such as consciousness raising, advocacy, and empowerment have become part of the language of mental health practitioners internationally. These three concepts are central to the model of groupwork presented in this chapter.

A consideration of the potential usefulness of groupwork is perhaps particularly appropriate in low- to middle-income countries like South Africa. Scarce resources and an immense need for mental health services in a context of transformation, which includes a shift from a history of oppression to emancipation for all citizens, renders groupwork particularly poignant. The significance of group-based experiential sharing is that the group experience through mutual exchange facilitates the recognition that the source of many problems is not located in the individual, but is the result of exploitation and discrimination (Brannon, 1996). However, as pointed out by Lewis (1991) and Shapiro (1991), the centrality of social action in groupwork has shifted in and out of focus over the years and not all models of groupwork have embraced an examination of the social structure as a source of individual problems.

5 A consciousness-raising empowerment approach to groupwork

The empowerment approach to groupwork explicitly addresses issues of oppression in

the lives of participants. While there are different theoretical strands in the literature on empowerment, common themes are easily identifiable. Gutierrez and Ortega (1991) have distinguished three levels of empowerment that feature in the literature:

- personal empowerment, which encourages the development of feelings of personal autonomy and self-efficacy;
- interpersonal empowerment, which comprises the dynamics of relationships between individuals; and
- political empowerment, which incorporates collective social action for the achievement of freedom from oppression.

It is imperative to note that with empowerment models these three levels are not seen as independent and separate from one another. Personal empowerment is crucial for interpersonal empowerment, and similarly, political empowerment is based on the other two levels. Individual change is seen as inseparable from social change. Therefore, all three levels are interwoven and interconnected.

Within an empowerment approach, the development of a critical consciousness is seen as crucial in the psychological process of changing the perception of one's own life experiences and in changing one's perception of society in general. One of the techniques for developing a critical consciousness is through a process of consciousness raising.

Consciousness-raising groups were a key strategy in the development of women's movements in various countries throughout the world. The basic idea was that women would meet in small groups where they felt

313

both safe and comfortable to explore issues of importance in their lives, but also to examine the connections between personal issues and political structures and processes. The well-known slogan 'the personal is political' was enacted through such groups. In speaking out about personal experiences in a collective, shared space, women realized that personal experiences were not isolated, individual events, but that similar experiences were shared by several other women. In this way a consciousness about the politics of the personal emerged. Out of these experiences, many strategies for social action aimed at social change were planned.

Consciousness-raising groups have not only been used in the women's movement, but also as an empowerment strategy in a variety of different contexts by researchers, mental health practitioners, and political activists. Gutierrez and Ortega (1991) conducted empirical research to investigate the influence of group interaction and group content on empowerment among Latino undergraduate students in the United States. They compared measures of different dimensions of empowerment over three types of intervention: an ethnic identity group, a consciousness-raising group, and a control group. The results showed that group interaction was a necessary and sufficient condition to increase interest in and intention to become more involved in activities related to the upliftment of the Latino community. Hence, we see that group interaction by itself is important. However, both group interaction and a critical consciousness component were necessary for individuals to make the linkages between their own situations and collective action strategies. Gutierrez and Ortega (1991)

therefore argued for the use of consciousness-raising groups as a means to better serve the needs of Latinos who, as a group, have a low mean level of education, a high rate of unemployment, and are overrepresented in the United States prison population.

Another arena in which consciousness raising has been used is in contexts of multicultural counselling. An example is the work of Parker (1988), who sought to contribute to the process of preparing counsellors and other professionals to work with numerical minority ethnic groups in the United States. In instances such as this the interpretation of consciousness raising differs from that which has been outlined in this chapter. Parker's (1988) interpretation centred on cultural knowledge acquisition in relation to self and others. Consequently, his approach consisted of techniques for self-exploration and awareness of attitudes toward own and other ethnic groups.

Therefore, although the concept of consciousness raising has been used in various contexts, political empowerment in the sense of liberation from oppression has not always been the goal. Similarly, groupwork has been used in many different ways for a variety of purposes. Taylor (1991) has argued that it has been in the women's movement that consciousness-raising groups have been most successful in meeting the twin goals of empowering individuals and promoting social change. Although her argument was based upon the women's movement in North America, consciousness-raising groups have been used for women's empowerment in other contexts. Some years earlier Browning (1987) wrote about the Zhensovety, women-only groups, in the then Union of Soviet

Socialist Republics. Whereas these groups were formed out of a very different set of circumstances to that in the United States, there were parallels in the aims in that these groups were intended to raise women's political activity, teach women political skills, and be sources of support. More recently, Mama (1995), a Nigerian psychologist, wrote of the significance of consciousness-raising groups for black women living in Britain during a period in which the political interests of black liberation and feminism were influential.

The principles of consciousness-raising women's groups have been successfully applied in the arena of mental health service provision. The work of Butler and Wintram (1991) is an approach that explicitly addresses gender oppression, the crux of this chapter. Consequently, it warrants more detailed description.

5.1 Feminist groupwork

Feminist groupwork as explicated by Butler and Wintram (1991) is grounded in the conviction that collectivity among women is central to the struggle to end gender oppression. Hence, they see women working together in groups as an exemplar of collectivity in dealing with the consequences of gender oppression on mental health. They argue that in the context of a group, women sharing their individual experiences can offer each other support, validation, and strength. Moreover, the contact and sharing that happens within the group is seen to be crucial in breaking down the hegemony of individualism, which constructs women's issues as individual pathology without making any

connections with structural and systemic oppression. In this way groups also permit the reconstruction of alternative personal realities that explicitly acknowledge the role of oppression in the lives of individuals.

Yet, Butler and Wintram (1991) take the concept of groupwork further in advancing the need for such groups to be community-based, to establish links with other groups, and to be ultimately self-sustaining without any professional involvement. Herein lies the potential relevance of this model to South Africa and other low- to middle-income contexts. Not only do we need a model that challenges oppression and promotes social change, we also need a model that is feasible given the constraints on resources.

Having outlined the philosophical and political underpinnings of the Butler and Wintram model, what about the processes and techniques used within the groups? While noting the importance of the practical details, these authors emphasize the centrality of paying attention to the broader goals, which they saw as 'providing a forum in which it was possible for women, whose identities are shaped in isolating and oppressive ways, to recognise themselves as members of a social group with the potential to alter their collective situation' (Butler and Wintram, 1991, p. 38). In realising these goals they highlight the two crucial phases of planning and preparation, and structuring the group programme.

The basic reasoning is that once a secure framework for groupwork has been developed, other practicalities may then be worked out jointly with the participants. Within these two phases a number of factors have to be considered, such as: the demand and need for groupwork; group size and membership; group programme and methods; and co-facilitation. Each of these dimensions will be discussed in relation to cases described below.

5.2 Key decisions and processes

5.2.1 The demand and need for groupwork

According to Butler and Wintram (1991) the opportunity for groupwork can come from many sources. However, there are basically two routes to be considered: does the demand come from the community or is the demand externally imposed by mental health agencies? The source of the demand can be an important factor in determining the success of the project. Home (1991) gives an account of a student in Australia who encouraged low-income mothers in a housing project to get together for mutual support and collective action. Although the need for such a group was obvious to the student, the women resisted her efforts and as a result the idea was abandoned. In a project in the KwaNcgolosi area of KwaZulu-Natal, South Africa (see box below), the idea of groupwork for teenage mothers was proposed by the researchers in response to a needs assessment study in which residents had identified teenage pregnancy as a social problem (De la Rey and Parekh, 1996). Therefore, in this case the nature of the problem vis-à-vis teenage pregnancy emerged from the community itself, but the decision to use groupwork came from the researchers.

Groupwork with teenage mothers

Context
The KwaNcgolosi area of KwaZulu-Natal, a semi-rural area about 40 km from Durban, South Africa.

Participants
Ten teenage mothers between the ages of fifteen and twenty-one whose babies were in the age range twelve to thirty-six months. All mothers were attending school and all ten were in their teens at the time of the birth.

Facilitators
Two black women who were both in their early twenties. The facilitator spoke Zulu as a first language and the co-facilitator was able to communicate in basic Zulu.

Group contact
The facilitators and the participants jointly agreed that:
- whatever was discussed within the group would remain confidential among the group members;
- no negative judgements would be made about each other;
- every attempt would be made to give each other positive feedback; and
- if at any time someone had negative feelings about the group she would talk about it.

Programme
Sessions were planned around the following themes:
- Introductions.
- Rapport building.
- Sexual behaviour before pregnancy.

- Discovery of pregnancy.
- Others' reactions to the pregnancy.
- Giving birth and the first three months.
- Life at present.
- Advice to others.

Training in group facilitation skills
A one-day training session for group participants included the following:
- What is a group?
- Why are groups useful?
- Characteristics of small groups, such as size and intimacy.
- Role and functions of a facilitator.
- Group process.

(Adapted from De la Rey and Parekh, 1996)

A crucial phase in a community-based project is that of negotiation and consultation with relevant persons and organizations. In the case of the KwaZulu-Natal project, before any groupwork was initiated there were consultations with the local community health workers to discuss the feasibility and the merits of the researchers' proposal. The project would not have been possible without the support of the local community, particularly key role players such as the community health workers. Indeed, access to potential participants was facilitated by one of the community health workers, a woman who had expressed specific interest in working in the project.

When women are the target group in a community-based programme, using existing structures and organizations to gain entry may not always be a useful strategy. Given the gendered organization of society, those in positions of power within local structures are usually men. Moreover, women who are most marginalized are often not part of any organized structures such as self-help groups, savings clubs, and religious groups. Clinics, where they exist, may be a good contact point since most women use a health service even if it is more often for their children rather than for themselves (Budlender, 1995). There are other advantages of a linkage between a clinic and the group or between a religious organization and a group. Women who are overburdened with work (income-producing work as well as child care, family, and household work) often do not feel a sense of entitlement toward spending time on their own issues, or they may have to seek permission from a male partner or father. In such instances, linkages with clinics and religious organizations serve a 'legitimating' function.

5.2.2 Group size and membership

The recommended size for groupwork is typically between six to ten participants, not counting facilitators. However, this may be extended up to twelve members. More than this tends to obstruct intimacy and equality in participation. Of central importance is that membership and participation must be voluntary.

Who qualifies for group membership? What are the criteria for any specific group? Here too the question of whether such groups can include men needs to be considered. Although the Butler and Wintram model of feminist groupwork was aimed at women only, gender (including women and men) is now widely accepted as a category of analysis, rather than an inclusion of women only. Therefore, we could pose the question of whether we should not have both men and women in consciousness-raising groups.

Lee (1994) used a consciousness-raising group approach for African-American men. The objective was to develop a liberatory masculine consciousness free from both the impact of racism in the United States and the oppression of women. Membership in this group was limited to black men only although there was heterogeneity in other characteristics such as age. In South Africa the Centre for Peace Action, a community-based violence prevention agency, used a similar approach in an empowerment pro-gramme for school-going boys between ten and fifteen years of age. Using positive role models, anecdotes, and drama, the boys reflected on gender-related norms and be-haviours with the aim of developing a positive identity (Williamson, 1997). Thus, conscious-ness-raising groups have been used with men to raise awareness of the linkages between hegemonic constructions of gender and oppression. But a strong argument has been presented against mixed-gender conscious-ness-raising groups. Given the history of male dominance, men's views are likely to dominate within mixed groups and the issues in the lives of women and men are likely to be different (Home, 1991). There-fore, even though the approach may be used for both genders, mixed groups are not always seen as appropriate.

Other criteria for group membership are typically set by the agency, organization, or practitioners who initiate the project. This,

of course, places the organizers in a position of relative power. Whether this may be avoided is a complex issue. Butler and Wintram's (1991) recommendations were found to work well in setting up the Kwa-Zulu-Natal group for teenage mothers. They advised that contact with potential participants be made before the group process begins to discuss expectations and provide sufficient information to enable individuals to decide for themselves whether the group will be useful or not. Heeding this advice, teenage mothers who were potentially in-terested were invited to a meeting to discuss the idea of forming a group for teenage mothers. Ten teenage mothers attended the preliminary meeting and all were keen to participate in the group.

5.2.3 Group programme and methods

A structured programme in relation to the objectives of the group must be planned. There is widespread agreement that partici-pants must be provided with a clear frame-work that meets their expectations, though the 'structure needs to be subtle without becoming obtrusive and an end in itself' (Butler and Wintram, 1991, p.42). The trend is that the programme structures each meeting around specific themes that tie into the overall objective, but there is flexibility in the details of the methods and techniques to be used. Butler and Wintram recount how they had planned a programme round the themes of women and stress, or women and health, but this had to be changed when the participants preferred a variety of topics. Similarly, the participants in the group for teenage mothers expressed a need for information on contraception. In response, an educational talk on contraception by a community health nurse was arranged; this had not been in the programme. Home (1991) makes the point that using a programme that suits members' needs, whatever those may be, is a critical factor in engaging the interests of participants.

It is typical for the introductory session to include a discussion on ground rules, which cover issues such as attendance, confidentiality, values, and participative style. Since sharing of personal experiences are part of the process, there is usually a contract of confidentiality, which attests that whatever is discussed within the group will remain confidential among the group members. Group practices within an empowerment model encourage equality, personal autonomy, mutual respect, and support. It is incumbent upon facilitators to do all they can to ensure that a safe, comfortable, and supportive environment is created.

Music, dance, poetry, and other creative exercises are frequently used to ensure that participants have a positive experience. Lee (1994) used jazz, soul, and rhythm and blues music to explore representations of black masculinity. In the group with teenage mothers games, relaxation exercises, and the singing of songs were used to build rapport and group cohesion. Games were also used to facilitate discussion of sexuality, a topic that is typically regarded as taboo. One of the games that worked particularly well was the use of a sexual word game. Participants were asked to write all sexual words that they had heard others use on individual index cards. All cards were placed face down in the middle of the group. After the cards

were shuffled, each person had to pick a card and then read it out aloud. This produced much giggling, but it provided a perfect entrée for the theme sexual behaviour before pregnancy. Having an element of fun contributes towards making the experience both enjoyable and helpful.

Positive group experiences depend not only on the methods, but also upon appropriate material and logistical arrangements. Accessibility of the venue and the venue itself are important – comfort and privacy are just some of the factors to be considered. Facilitators and organizers usually arrange refreshments such as snacks, tea, coffee, and juice. Child care may have to be organised. The principle is that the conditions for both physical and psychological comfort must be optimal.

5.2.4 Co-facilitation

Having more than one facilitator is advisable. One of the key reasons concerns power dynamics within the group. Two facilitators sharing tasks helps ensure that a single person does not assume too much control and authority over others. Moreover, it is extremely difficult for a single facilitator to handle all the demands of group dynamics. Facilitating discussion is only one aspect of the task. It is important to observe group sessions to monitor participants' feelings, which are often expressed non-verbally. Depending on the theme or topic, sessions may become very intense and at these times it is useful to share the responsibility for what happens in the group. While respecting each other's work, it is also part of the process to have co-facilitators comment on each other, pointing out strengths and weaknesses. Because no two groups are alike, there are no fixed rules for facilitation, only guidelines. Furthermore, new exercises and methods are usually tried with each new group. Through mutual critique and observation, skills are developed.

Consciousness-raising groups attempt to embody collective power sharing and consensual decision making in the style and process of facilitation. Although the facilitators take on certain responsibilities, the idea is that everyone has an equal right to speak and be heard. Consensual decision making means that an issue is discussed until each participant is in agreement without duress (Home, 1991). Another aspect of power sharing is that deliberate efforts are made to minimize the 'expert' status of the facilitators. To this end facilitators often commit themselves to sharing personal information in the same way that participants do. Sharing of tasks through a system of rotation is yet another method that may be used to distribute power.

As work with a group progresses, participants may be encouraged to assume the role of co-facilitator with one of the trained or professional facilitators. This may be done after a few sessions during which participants would have had the opportunity to learn through observation such skills as listening without being judgmental, knowing when to ask questions, when to keep silent, and how to encourage equitable participation. Transference of skills is crucial to meet the objective of self-sustaining groups. De la Rey and Parekh (1996) reported that at the end of the weekly meetings of the group of teenage mothers, a one-day training workshop was arranged to impart skills that would enable the participants to act as co-facilitators for similar groups planned for a larger number of young mothers. The idea was that the initial group could, under the guidance of the programme co-ordinators, have a snowball effect so that several other groups would develop.

One of the obstacles that is especially relevant to women's groups is that most women's lives, especially in low-income communities, are heavily overburdened by the demands of both paid and unpaid labour. The processes involved in consciousness-raising groups is slow and when the focal issue is changing gender-related traditions and cultural practices, positive outcomes are not always easily measurable and visible. Very often gains are small but it is imperative that groups work within the limitations of their resources and skills. Many groups fall apart. But, as Home (1991) argues, it is better 'to succeed in a small project than to fail in a large one or to delay trying for fear of failure' (p. 168).

6 Group outcome, empowerment, and social change

The three levels of empowerment as explicated by Gutierrez and Ortega (1991) and presented earlier in this chapter may be used as a framework to assess the potential of consciousness-raising groups as an intervention strategy against gender oppression. It often happens that the outcome of group processes may be more apparent at one or two levels rather than at all three, but the interdependence of these levels must not be ignored.

While there is no formal, published evaluation study on the effectiveness of consciousness-raising groups in the South African context, Kravetz (1980) reviewed numerous United States' studies that sought to evaluate the outcome of consciousness-raising groups. In this review chapter, she cites several studies (e.g., Carden, 1974; Kirkpatrick, in Kravetz, 1980) that found that participation in such groups not only produced personal change but for some women also led to organized efforts to improve the position of women in the community. More recently, Home (1991) reviewed the outcomes of several different groups. Among the list of outcomes were a radio programme and a phone-in survey organized by an Australian 'women against rape' group, a women's art festival hosted by a Quebec group, and, again in Quebec, a group for single mothers in a low-income community who wrote a newsletter and a resource book.

Kravetz (1980) summarized the outcomes most frequently reported in the literature as follows:

- An improvement in self-esteem.
- Greater awareness of the effects of sexism.
- A greater sense of commonality with other women.
- More solidarity with other women.
- The development of a socio-political analysis of the nature of gender oppression.
- Change in interpersonal relationships and roles.
- Participation in work and/or community activities to improve the position of women.

Although more research is needed to examine the efficacy of consciousness-raising groups as a strategy to counter gender oppression, there is sufficient evidence in the literature to suggest that it can be usefully employed to critically examine gender roles and explore possible courses of change (Brannon, 1996).

7 Conclusion

Gender is a form of social inequality that impacts upon mental health and mental health service provision. This chapter has presented an argument for the use of consciousness-raising groups as an intervention strategy to overcome gender oppression. Feminist groupwork as explicated by Butler and Wintram (1991) is grounded in the conviction that collectivity among women is central to the struggle to end gender oppression. They show that in the context of a group, through sharing their individual experiences, women may break down the hegemony of individualism that constructs women's mental health problems simply as individual pathology without any linkages to structural and systemic oppression. By advancing the need for such groups to be community-based, and to be ultimately self-sustaining without any professional involvement, the potential relevance of this model to low- to middle-income countries like South Africa is elucidated. Not only do we need a model that challenges oppression and promotes social change, we also need a model that is feasible given the constraints on resources.

Although many benefits of groupwork have been highlighted, there are limitations.

Groupwork is slow; it requires careful planning, delicate negotiations, and consultation. While extolling the benefits of their approach, Butler and Wintram (1991) are careful to point out that it should not be seen as a 'panacea for all social ills; it can never be the sole answer to power imbalances and social injustice' (p. 27). The struggle to end gender oppression requires a multiplicity of strategies at both the individual and collective levels, in both civil society and in government across all sectors. Overall, research shows that consciousness-raising groups can lead to personal change, and for some participants, it also leads to organized efforts to improve the position of women in the community.

The potential contribution of consciousness-raising groups should be viewed in relation to other mechanisms and strategies in the broader struggle to end gender oppression. In South Africa, the potential contribution of such groups should be viewed in relation to the work of the Commission on Gender Equality, the coalition network to end violence against women, the alliances around reproductive rights, and the advocacy and lobbying initiatives of organizations and individual women and men in all sectors of society.

Ensure that the activities vary to promote interest and enjoyment. Some ideas for discussion are:

1.1 Examine the meanings associated with being a man or a woman;

1.2 Examine how these meanings enhance or restrict your behaviour;

1.3 Examine how being a man or woman affects your freedom;

1.4 Examine what connections there are between various structures and systems in society and gender.

2 Devise a list of some self-help groups in your community or region. Are any of these based on gender? If so, what is the main thrust? Does it challenge or maintain current gender relations?

3 Formulate a resource list of organizations that specifically deal with gender-related issues. Name the organization and list its contact details and main programmes. What role does consciousness raising play in their work?

Exercises

1 Form a consciousness-raising group with five to six of your friends/peers of the same gender as yourself. In the first session, devise a programme for the group.

References

AL-ISSA, I. (1980). *The psychopathology of women.* Englewood Cliffs, NJ: Prentice-Hall.

BRANNON, L. (1996). *Gender: Psychological perspectives.* Massachusetts: Allyn and Bacon.

BROWN, G. and HARRIS, T. (1978). *Social origins of depression: A study of psychiatric disorder in women.* London: Tavistock.

BROWNING, G. K. (1987). *Women and politics in the USSR: Consciousness raising and Soviet women's groups.* Sussex: Wheatsheaf Books.

BUDLENDER, D. (1995). *Health in our hands: Proceedings and policies of the Women's Health Conference.* Johannesburg: Women's Health

Project, Centre for Health Policy, University of the Witwatersrand.

BUTLER, S. and WINTRAM, C. (1991). *Feminist groupwork*. London: Sage.

CAVANAGH, K. and CREE, V. E. (Eds.). (1996). *Working with men: Feminism and social work*. London and New York: Routledge.

CONNELL, R. W. (1995). *Masculinities*. St Leonards, Australia: Allen & Unwin.

DE LA REY, C. and PAREKH, A. (1996). Community-based peer groups: An intervention programme for teenage mothers. *Journal of Community and Applied Social Psychology*, 6(5), 373-381.

DESJARLAIS, R., EISENBERG, L., GOOD, B., and KLEINMAN, A. (1995). *World mental health: Problems and priorities in low-income countries*. New York: Oxford University Press.

FRYE, M. (1992). Oppression. In M. L. Andersen and P. Hill Collins (Eds.), *Race, class and gender* (pp. 37-41). Belmont, CA: Wadsworth.

GOVE, W. R. (1972). The relationship between sex roles, marital status and mental illness. *Social Forces*, 51, 34-44.

GUTIERREZ, L. M. and ORTEGA, R. (1991). Developing methods to empower Latinos: The importance of groups. *Social Work with Groups*, 14(2), 23-43.

HOME, A. M. (1991). Mobilising women's strengths for social change: The group connection. In A. Vinik and M. Levin (Eds.), *Social action in group work* (pp. 153-173). New York: The Haworth Press.

KISEKKA, M. N. (1990). In E. D. Rothblum and E. Cole (Eds.), *Women's mental health in Africa* (pp. 1-13). London: Harrington Park Press.

KRAVETZ, D. (1980). Consciousness-raising and self-help. In A. M. Brodsky and R. T. Hare-Mustin (Eds.), *Women and psychotherapy: An assessment of research and practice (pp.267-283)*. New York: The Guilford Press.

LEE, C. C. (1994). *Mental health interventions for black adults: A consciousness raising group approach*. Keynote address at the Biennial Conference on Multicultural Counselling, 10-12 October 1994, Johannesburg.

LEWIS, E. (1991). Social change and citizen action:

A philosophical exploration for modern social group work. In A. Vinik and M. Levin (Eds.), *Social action in group work* (pp. 23-34). New York: The Haworth Press.

MAHARAJ, Z. (1994). Subversive intent: A social theory of gender. *Transformation*, 24, 40-54.

MAMA, A. (1995). *Beyond the masks: Race, gender and subjectivity*. London: Routledge.

MERCY, J. A., ROSENBERG, M. L., POWELL, K. E., BROOME, C. V., and ROPER, W. L. (1993a). Public health policy for preventing violence. *Health Affairs*, Spring, 7-29.

MERCY, J. A., ROSENBERG, M. L., POWELL, K. E., BROOME, C. V., and ROPER, W. L. (1993b). Public health policy for preventing violence. *Health Affairs*, 1, 112-131.

MILLER, J. and BELL, C. (1996). Mapping men's mental health. *Journal of Community and Applied Social Psychology*, 6(5), 317-327.

PARKER. W. M. (1988). *Consciousness-raising: A primer for multicultural counselling*. Springfield, IL: Charles C. Thomas.

SEGAL, L. (1990). *Slow motion: Changing masculinities, changing men*. London: Virago.

SHAPIRO, B. Z. (1991). Social action, the group and society. In A. Vinik and M. Levin (Eds.), *Social action in group work* (pp. 7-21). New York: The Haworth Press.

TAYLOR, E. D. (1991). The role of structure in effective agency advocacy. In A. Vinik and M. Levin (Eds.), *Social action in group work* (pp. 141-151). New York: The Haworth Press.

WALTERS, V. (1993). Stress, anxiety and depression: Women's accounts of their health problems. *Social Science and Medicine*, 36(4), 393-402.

WATSON, G., SCOTT, C., and RAGALSKY, S. (1996). Refusing to be marginalised: Groupwork in mental health services for women survivors of childhood sexual abuse. *Journal of Community and Applied Social Psychology*, 6(5), 341-354.

WILLIAMS, J. (1996). Social inequalities and mental health: Developing services and developing knowledge. *Journal of Community and Applied Social Psychology*, 6(5).

WILLIAMSON, G. (1997). *Notes: Recollections from a project*. Johannesburg: Centre for Peace Action.

16

Investing in the young for a better future: a programme of intervention

Norman Duncan
Ashley van Niekerk

Study objectives

This chapter will assist readers in a critical examination of:

- the development of a project that promotes the psychological development and well-being of pre-school children;
- the historical context and values within which this project evolved;
- its current status as a multi-levelled psycho-educational intervention; and
- an initial discussion of the shortcomings of this initiative.

1 Introduction

Children have historically constituted one of the most neglected and disadvantaged sectors of the South African population (Makan, 1996; National Institute for Economic Policy (NIEP), 1996). In this chapter we present an intervention programme that targets pre-school children as its primary beneficiaries. This programme has been hosted at the University of the Western Cape (UWC)[1] since 1990. The project, via a range of interlinking strategies, equips the caregivers of pre-school children with knowledge and skills to promote the psychological development of children. As an introduction to this programme, we consider, first, the importance of the current emphasis on pre-school children; and second, the conditions that constitute the context for the development of the majority of pre-school children in South Africa. An examination of these issues is crucial for understanding the need for and logic of the intervention programme proposed in this chapter.

2 Why the emphasis on pre-school children?

For a number of reasons, the pre-school years constitute one of the most important periods of psychological development. Firstly, this is a critical period for mental development and the acquisition of basic cognitive skills that are important in the development of the child both during this period, and later in life (Short, 1985). For example, various researchers (e.g., Hurlock, 1980; Thomas, 1987) argue that malnutrition during the pre-school years could seriously compromise cognitive development during this period, and during later periods of development. Indeed, according to Thomas (1987), the damage caused by malnutrition is in many cases irreversible, even when children are later provided with an adequate diet. It has also been reported that children who are not exposed to adequate stimulation in the form of structured pre-school education frequently experience difficulties at primary school (National Education Co-ordinating Committee (NECC), 1992; NIEP, 1996). Furthermore, it has been found that twice as many children who receive quality pre-school care, as opposed to those who do not, complete high school. Children who, for example, receive adequate pre-school care are also less likely to require special education[2] later in their scholastic careers. This is particularly true for children from low-income communities (Fair, 1996).

Secondly, various researchers and theorists also regard the pre-school years as a critical period for the emotional and social development of the individual. According to Fromm (in Ryckman, 1993), for example, it is during the pre-school years that the foundations for appropriate or inappropriate ways of adjusting to society are laid. Horney (1937) argues along similar lines that providing young children with a sense of security and safety during the early pre-school years is critical for positive emotional and social development later in life. A lack of a sense of security during early childhood, according to her, often lays the basis for emotional and social maladjustment both during childhood and later in life.

The importance of adequate pre-school care and nurturing for the social adjustment of the child is underlined by research findings cited by Fair (1996), which reveals that by the age of fifteen only 2 per cent of children who had received structured pre-school care and adequate nurturing had committed two or more criminal offences, as opposed to 15 per cent of children who did not receive such care.

In view of the above, Fair (1996) argues that the investment in the care of pre-school children benefits society in its entirety, for investing in the development of pre-school children contributes substantially to laying the foundations for the optimal development and well-being of future generations of adults. A healthier adult population, in turn, means better functioning communities less in need of costly psychological interventions (NIEP, 1996).

In view of the apparent benefits of investing in the psychological development of pre-school children, it is apposite at this point to explore the current position of pre-school children in South Africa.

3 The context of child development in South Africa

Despite the momentous political changes that South Africa has undergone in recent years (the most notable being the installation in 1994 of the country's first democratically elected government), the majority of South African children are still faced by enormous socio-economic problems, which could compromise their development (NIEP, 1996). These problems include poverty, homelessness, and exposure to violence.

An examination of the available indicators of young children's well-being, from the incidence of malnutrition, infant and child mortality rates, physical and sexual abuse, child labour, and missed education, all suggest that South Africa remains a particularly impoverished and hostile environment for most of its children (Lockhat and Van Niekerk, in press; NIEP, 1996). About 60 per cent of those in poor South African households, constituting just over half of the country, are children under the age of five (NIEP, 1996; South African Institute of Race Relations (SAIRR), 1996). Children living in these impoverished settings are significantly exposed to food shortages and consequently malnutrition. As reported in the Pillay and Lockhat chapter in this book, this situation has grave long-term implications for these children. They are regarded as being at considerable risk for impaired physical, mental, scholastic, and, in the longer term, occupational and social functioning (Lockhat and Van Niekerk, in press; NIEP, 1996; Pillay and Lockhat, see Chapter 6 in this volume).

The extent of this risk, as illustrated by recent reports on the rates of malnutrition, remain of concern. The Project for the Statistics on Living Standards and Development (PSLSD) (1994) has estimated that 16 per cent of African children under age five years are underweight, and between 20 per cent and 30 per cent are physically stunted (NIEP, 1996). The incidence of infant and child mortality are also still considerably higher than that of other countries with similar income levels (Duncan, 1997; NIEP, 1996; SAIRR, 1995). The consequences of this environment are mapped out in Pillay and Lockhat, particularly the disastrous impact on learning ability and school performance (Dawes and Donald, 1994; Lockhat and Van Niekerk, in press).

The above situation is most conspicuous in the poorer rural environments. In these areas, reports of child labour among especially African and 'coloured' children remain rife (SAIRR, 1995). Child abandonment and homeless children have also been reported with increasing frequency. It has been argued that these phenomena reflect the stressful and violent tensions associated with township life. The stresses on 'families have led to an increasing number of children joining "substitute families", such as criminal gangs, prostitute rings, and bands of street children' (NIEP, 1996, p. 18). Despite the decline of 'politically inspired' violence, criminal and domestic violence has continued to prevail in South African townships (Lockhat and Van Niekerk, in press). The levels of direct and indirect exposure to violence are reported to be high (Ensink et al., 1997). So too are the rates of sexualized violence, especially among girl children.

Children growing up under these or similar conditions are reported to exhibit a high prevalence of stress-related psychological symptoms, difficulties in cognitive development, lower levels of academic achievement, and higher rates of behavioural and antisocial disorders (Desjarlais, 1994). Pillay and Lockhat detail some of these consequences in Chapter 6 in this textbook.

Most researchers in the area of child development would argue that the above situation, if not addressed, would return to haunt South Africa in years to come (Dawes, 1994; Frankel, 1993; NIEP, 1996). Duncan and Rock (1994; 1997) assert that the situation facing young children could only be remedied by redressing the structural inequalities in our society, and by implementing legislation that offers greater protection to children. These measures for ensuring a more supportive context for child development will, however, not come into effect overnight, nor will they come into effect without strong advocacy from children's rights groups. In the meantime, the development of countless children will continue to be compromised.

The proposed intervention programme emanated out of the concerns about children's early development and well-being. The programme primarily deals with the training and empowerment of the care-givers of pre-school children, so that the former can (1) offer more effective support systems to children, and (2) have enough of an understanding of the principles of child development to vigorously advocate for the implementation of structural changes in our society, i.e. the structural changes that would bring about a decrease in the extant levels of child abuse and neglect. It is argued that this combination would ensure the optimal development of children. Furthermore, this intervention programme is structured to maximize the significant social support networks available to children.

4 Social support systems

Research conducted in South Africa during the early 1990s indicates that the deleterious impact of social stressors such as malnutrition and physical abuse can be significantly diminished if children have recourse to effective and stable support systems such as peer groups, the family, the community, religious institutions, and the school system (Letlaka-Rennert, 1990; Netshiombo, 1993; Simpson, 1993). While research shows that most of these support systems can mitigate the impact of environmental insults on the development of the child, we will only discuss the family and educational systems in this chapter. This choice is essentially based on the centrality of these systems to pre-school children (Papalia and Olds, 1989) and the intervention programme presented in this chapter.

4.1 The family

The family is often perceived as providing the ideal context within which child development can take place (Bonn, 1995; Poster, 1976). This perception basically derives from the belief that the family unit is pre-eminently suited to satisfy not only children's most basic physiological needs, but also their emotional, cognitive, and other higher order needs (Papalia and Olds, 1989).

Research on social support systems frequently also credits the family with the function of serving as one of the most effective buffers between children and social stressors. And indeed, to many children this social unit does provide significant support in situations that are essentially antagonistic to optimal development. For example, it has been found that children who can rely on a supportive family environment are less adversely affected by exposure to traumatic events than are other children (Netshiombo, 1993). This appears to be particularly true for pre-school children (Letlaka-Rennert, 1990).

However, in South Africa the legacy of apartheid and its attempts to destroy all viable black social structures have made it extremely difficult for the majority of families in this country to provide a supportive or protective context within which children's needs could be satisfactorily fulfilled. Through the decades, practices such as the migrant labour system, and legislation such as the Population Registration Act of 1950, the Group Areas Acts of 1950 and 1966, as well as a myriad of other calculated assaults directed against blacks by the apartheid system, effectively militated against countless families in providing the type of environment in which healthy children could be raised and that could offer support to children confronted by difficulties such as malnutrition, violence, and other forms of abuse (Robinson, 1994). As Cooper (1990) observes, apartheid 'steadily denuded [the black family] of its ability to provide a structured, nurturing ambience ... [for] the developing child' (p. 2).

Indeed, instead of offering children a supportive environment in which their needs can be adequately met and in which they can find nurturance, many families in this country, largely because of the legacy of apartheid, are frequently responsible for the further brutalization of children (Department of National Health and Population Development (DNHPD), 1993). As Dowdall (1990)

and the DNHPD (1993) observe, the location of the majority of families in severely overcrowded, underserviced, dreary, poverty-stricken, and crime-ridden townships are causing unbearable tensions in family life, often leading to intolerable levels of frustration and anger. This in turn frequently leads to the neglect and, at times, violent abuse of children within families (Angless and Shefer, 1997).

4.2 The educational system

According to the United Nations (1992) Convention of the Rights of the Child, adequate education should be considered the inalienable right of every child, because 'through education ... [children] gain knowledge and skills to survive, to learn and to contribute to the development of their communities' (UNICEF & NCRC, 1993, p. 53). Moreover, educational settings such as schools and pre-school centres can serve as important social support systems to children exposed to social traumata. Gibson (1989) argues that the school, by virtue of the calming influence of the everyday routine that it offers, can greatly enhance the resilience of children, thereby mitigating the impact of stressors to which children may be exposed. Obviously teachers are potentially also an invaluable source of support to children. Under the system of apartheid, however, South African children's education was severely compromised as a result of it being used primarily as a means to entrench gender, racial, and class inequalities rather than to ensure the optimal development of the child. In the process, the social support function of the educational system was also severely undermined. For a number of reasons, this remains one of the major shortcomings of the South African educational system – despite the fact that apartheid as formal state policy no longer exists.

Historically black schools to a large extent still represent the institutionalized neglect of children. As such, they are often incapable of offering children support when the latter are confronted with difficulties and trauma. Indeed, as illustrated in various reports published in recent years (e.g., NCRC, 1994; UNICEF and NCRC, 1993), these schools themselves are often the sites of child abuse.

As previously stated, it is largely in view of the inadequacies of the support systems available to children, particularly children from low-income black communities, as well as the myriad of problems frequently faced by the latter, that the following intervention programme was developed. Here it must perhaps be noted that this programme is still in the process of being developed and evaluated. Consequently, as the reader will in due course notice, it reflects several lacunae, some of which are discussed at the end of the chapter.

5 An intervention strategy: the early childhood development (ECD) programme

The early childhood development (ECD) programme was designed and piloted by the University of the Western Cape's Psychology Resource Centre (PRC) in 1990. The programme was initiated largely as a result of a spate of requests from pre-school educare workers from various working class communities in the Western Cape for the PRC to offer psychotherapeutic interventions to children in their care. According to these educare workers, a number of children at the pre-school centres where they worked presented with a range of what appeared to be psychological problems, which they felt ill-equipped to deal with. All these children were from extremely poor families and their parents could consequently not afford the services of professional psychologists; hence the request to the PRC, which works primarily in low-income communities and endeavours to offer mental health services free of charge.

After numerous meetings with the educare workers, as well as several assessments of all the children at the centres where they worked, it was established: (1) that there were indeed several children at these centres who showed signs of psychological and developmental difficulties, such as retarded language development, social adjustment problems, and various stress-related difficulties; and (2) that most of the difficulties experienced by the children appeared to be related to environmental factors, such as understimulation, poverty, and crime. Subsequently, it was decided that in view of the large numbers of children at these centres who appeared to present with problems, as well as the PRC's stated objective of spreading skills and expertise related to child psychology as widely as possible throughout the community, a community-based intervention programme would be the most appropriate way of addressing the educare workers' concerns regarding the children in their care. More specifically, it was decided to train pre-school educare workers in the basics of child psychology so that, where possible, they themselves could assist children in difficulty and then refer only their more serious cases to professional psychologists located in the PRC or elsewhere. Furthermore, it was decided that the training offered would first and foremost address preventive interventions, i.e. training that would enable care-givers to contribute to the optimal development of their charges so as to obviate the development of psychological problems among the latter. Ultimately, it was primarily on the basis of the above-mentioned decisions that the ECD programme was developed.

Here it should be noted that while the PRC's ECD programme aims at equipping child care-givers with the requisite skills and knowledge to assist in optimizing the development of children and to aid children in difficulty, it also endeavours to spread skills beyond those selected for inclusion in the programme. For this reason, it uses a 'multiplicator' model of training. Natural support resources and systems are a focus of the model. The programme aims to 'empower' care-givers to not only directly assist children, but to also impart the skills and knowledge they had acquired to other care-givers, thereby spreading the impact of the initial training.

The advantages of using the 'multiplicator' model of training

Training community-based child care-givers by means of the 'multiplicator' model of training has three important advantages:

1 This training model makes mental health care services directed at pre-school children more accessible to marginalized communities. Research undertaken by Simpson (1993), Peterson, Magwaza, and Pillay (in press), and Pillay, Magwaza, and Peterson(1992) reveals that there is currently an acute shortage of mental health care professionals to assist in dealing with the problems faced by South African children, particularly children in marginalized communities, such as black working-class communities. These researchers consequently argue that, rather than attempting to meet the needs of children on their own, professional mental health-care workers could put their skills to better use by training and supervising para-professional mental health care workers. This is in fact what the ECD programme attempts to do. Indeed, it endeavours to go beyond the strategy suggested by the above-mentioned researchers by training child care-givers to become trainers of other care-givers, thereby setting in motion a process whereby an ever-increasing number of care-givers within marginalized communities are equipped with a basic knowledge or skills in child psychology.

2 Unlike many professional health-care workers, the care-givers that will be trained by the PRC's multiplicator system will be familiar with the conditions within the communities targeted by the PRC. Research shows that children with difficulties are often best helped by those who understand and share their life experiences (Majodina, 1989; Orford, 1992; Rappaport, 1981; Serrano-Garcia, Lopez, and Rivera-Medina, 1987).

3 Various researchers suggest that involving members of marginalized communities, such as those targeted by the Psychology Resource Centre, in intervention programmes aimed at helping the children in their communities can enhance the entire community's sense of control over their lives (Dawes, 1992; Orford, 1992; Rappaport, 1981).

5.1 Theoretical framework

The ECD programme operates within the broad framework of community psychology. More specifically, it is centrally located within the framework of Rappaport's (1981) 'empowerment' model of community intervention. The primary principles of this approach can broadly be summarized as follows:

1 People's ability to provide their own solutions to their problems should be valued and utilized as the point of departure for community interventions (cf. Serrano-Garcia, Lopez, and Rivera-Medina, 1987).

2 The empowerment of people should be based on solutions using structures with which they are familiar and over which they can exert some control – structures such as the family, community, and pre-school centres.

5.2 The programme

Operating within the framework outlined above, and guided by the values discussed at the end of this section, the ECD programme consists of the following key components: (1) a basic course in child psychology; (2) an advanced course in child psychology; and (3) a parenting skills course. A description of these courses is presented below. However, here it must be noted that since the ECD programme is still in its pilot phase, these courses are still fairly fluid.

5.2.1 Basic course in child psychology

The primary objectives of the basic course in child psychology (BCCP) are to equip pre-school child care workers with the necessary skills to function at two levels: firstly, to assist in optimizing the development of children from marginalized communities; and secondly, to identify and assist children experiencing psychological and developmental problems. Assisting these children would include referring them to professional health care workers when necessary.

The course is primarily directed towards people who work with children in informal pre-school settings, as well as parents of pre-school children. The candidates normally selected for this course are pre-school care-givers who have had minimal opportunities to further their development via existing training programmes. The primary reason for this preference is linked to the PRC's goal of developing and spreading knowledge regarding child psychology and development beyond the (as yet relatively limited and privileged) group that normally has access to tertiary education and, therefore, to certain specialized information on child psychology and development.

In essence, the BCCP introduces care-givers to core concepts and skills aimed at facilitating an understanding of the psychological development of pre-school children. The topics dealt with include prenatal development, language development, emotional development, cognitive development, and social development during the pre-school years, concentrating on low-income communities in South Africa as the context for development. The course further provides a framework to understand, identify, and assist young children in difficulty. The course is essentially conducted by means of weekly two-hour workshops that take place over a full academic year, i.e. approximately thirty weeks. A tutor or facilitator accompanies the presenter of each session. The tutor, usually a postgraduate psychology student, provides both academic and personal support. The team of two or three tutors receives some initial training in adult education and groupwork. The tutors, along with the course participants, provide regular feedback to presenters and the PRC organizing team. The information shared in the workshops is integrated into a series of accessible booklets on child psychology, which are distributed among course participants for use in the course, as well as for later reference.

Currently, the ECD programme has facilities to present the BCCP course to three groups of thirty participants each.

5.2.2 Advanced course in child psychology

The advanced course in child psychology (ACCP) was developed as a follow-up to the BCCP. The course consists of approximately thirty workshops spread over one academic year and accommodates between thirty and fifty participants per year. The ACCP is primarily aimed at care-givers who had completed the BCCP. While the BCCP is essentially an introductory, general course on the basics of child psychology, the ACCP tends to concentrate on topics dealing with specific obstacles to optimal development faced by children in low-income communities. Ultimately, however, the topics dealt with are negotiated with pre-school care-givers participating in the ECD programme, and are primarily based on their interests and the needs of the children within their communities. Over the past few years, these have included topics such as: (1) the impact of malnutrition on development during the pre-school years; (2) racism and the pre-school child; (3) sexism and the pre-school child; (4) the effects of violence on the development of children in South Africa; (5) problems faced by differently-abled children in South Africa; (6) parentified children; and (7) the effects of single parenting on development of pre-school children. Thus, this programme is more concerned with the lived rather than theoretical problems experienced in targeted communities.

An important characteristic of the ACCP

is that it endeavours to examine the ways in which the communities in which the course participants are located are currently dealing with the obstacles to optimal development faced by their children. Successful community solutions to problems faced by children are integrated into subsequent ACCP courses.

Another important feature of the ACCP is that it attempts to provide participants with basic skills in training other adults in the basics of child psychology (i.e. the work dealt with in the BCCP). The ACCP, therefore, constitutes a crucial stage in the training of care-givers as potential trainers.

Training in the basics of adult education normally takes place as from the beginning of the second semester of the ACCP, by which stage course participants would have acquired an adequate repertoire of skills and knowledge in the basics of child psychology. As part of their practical training, participants in the ACCP are required to present, under the supervision of course tutors and other Psychology Resource Centre staff, at least one workshop dealing with one of the topics covered in the basic or advanced course in child psychology. Once it has been established that course participants have an adequate understanding of certain key issues pertaining to child psychology and child development in South Africa, and that they have the skills to share this knowledge with other adults, they are awarded a certificate. This certificate enables them to participate in the presentation of the next level of the programme.

5.2.3 Parenting skills course: training by the trainers

In terms of content, as well as structure, the parenting skills course is based on the basic course in child psychology. Furthermore, like the basic course in child psychology, the parenting skills course is also directed at parents and other care-givers of pre-school children. There are, however, two basic differences between these two courses, namely:

1 While the basic course in child psychology is presented by psychologists linked to the psychology resource centre, the parenting skills course is presented primarily by graduates of the advanced course in child psychology. Initially, they present the course under the supervision of tutors and psychologists attached to the Psychology Resource Centre.

2 The parenting skills course is presented within communities, rather than at the university-based Psychology Resource Centre.

Given the specific difficulties experienced by parents and other care-givers in the targeted communities, the parenting skills course also aims at enhancing course participants' skills in accessing community services and resources and in organizing parent support networks.

5.3 Values informing the ECD programme

All three components of the ECD programme are informed by the following values identified by Lazarus (1985) as the defining characteristics of community psychology:

1   *Commitment to marginalized communities:* In the above context, the term marginalized communities refers to: (1) black working-class communities and (2) children from these communities. The ECD programme is directed at communities historically marginalized from the mental health resources they require. The recipients of the programme are educare workers with the minimum of training in the area, and the ultimate beneficiaries of these programmes are children from impoverished communities in and around Cape Town.

2   *Ecological perspective:* Based on the objectives of community psychology and in keeping with its ideals of promoting optimal child development, the ECD programme attempts to intervene in the lives of the individuals targeted not merely at an individual/personal level, but also at a broader societal level. This does not mean that the ECD programme in any way wishes to de-emphasize the importance of the individual development of children and their care-givers. Rather, the programme stresses the inter-connectedness between children and their care-givers on the one hand, and the environment in which they are located on the other.

3   *Prevention:* As indicated earlier, the ECD programme endeavours to equip care-givers with the skills to optimize – and consequently obviate problems in – the development of children in marginalized communities. In this sense the programme is essentially preventive in nature, and by implication, therefore, future oriented. According to Lazarus

(1985), preventive programmes generally tend to be either person-centred or context-centred. The ECD programme can, however, be considered as both person-centred and context-centred. It is person-centred in the sense that it emphasizes the development of individual strengths and competencies (on the part of both children and their care-givers), and it is context-centred in that it endeavours to raise the awareness of course participants regarding the need to challenge the social conditions currently undermining the development of large numbers of children in our community.

4   *Empowerment:* As previously indicated, the ECD programme acknowledges and uses as its starting point the enhancement and promotion of existing human resources within communities. Indeed, the ECD programme departs from the premise that many of the skills that it seeks to develop are already present among course participants, albeit unacknowledged in many cases. The primary task of the programme therefore is to elicit and develop existing potential (cf. Rappaport, 1981; Seedat, Cloete, and Shochet, 1988), so as to enhance the capacity of communities to control their own lives.

5   *Social action:* Rappaport (1981) argues that many preventive programmes frequently do not change existing social problems. Indeed, to the extent that they often fail to challenge the root causes of these problems, they invariably add to the difficulties experienced by communities. It was with this in mind that the

ECD programme was designed to offer training to care-givers not only around optimizing children's development so as to prevent developmental problems, but also to empower course participants to challenge the conditions that give rise to the problems experienced by children from marginalized communities. In the final analysis, training child care-givers as activists for children's rights and social change is a key aspect of the ECD programme.

6 *Professional-client collaboration or citizen participation:* Rappaport (1981) argues that in order to be truly effective as activists for change, psychologists should play the role of collaborators working with, rather than for marginalized communities. This is an ideal that the ECD programme strongly identifies with, and adheres to in the training of child care-givers. Indeed, at the inception of the ECD programme, the PRC and its community-based partners agreed that full consultation (in terms of programme objectives and processes) on the part of all parties involved would be one of the non-negotiable principles of the programme.

7 *Self-reflection and critique:* Provision is made for all trainees and PRC staff participating in the ECD programme to regularly evaluate the content and development of the programme. The evaluation is facilitated by external agencies, who ensure that all feedback is minuted and made available to all stakeholders in the programme. This process is considered crucial to the development of the ECD programme.

6 An initial evaluation of the ECD programme

Given that it is still in its pilot phase, the ECD programme has until now been subjected to regular evaluations. These evaluations have primarily taken the form of focus group discussions and interviews with participants regarding programme objectives and processes, as well as a system of continuous evaluation of participants' understanding of, and their ability to apply, the various courses' content in their work settings. The focus group discussions and interviews took place at the end of each workshop and were facilitated by external evaluators. The evaluation of participants' understanding of the courses' content took the form of case studies and various other practical assignments introduced at regular intervals throughout the courses. The primary goal of the evaluations was to assess the quality so as to refine the three ECD courses.

Thus far, course participants' performance on continuous evaluation assignments have been remarkably good, with the annual pass rate for the various courses offered consistently exceeding 90 per cent. Furthermore, the feedback obtained from the focus group discussions and interviews has generally been fairly positive. For example, in the evaluations conducted thus far, participants have consistently commented that they had found the programme very valuable because it: 'allowed us to acquire valuable skills and information'; 'enhanced insight into childhood problems'; and 'allowed for personal growth' (PRC Annual Report, 1996/7). Based on comments such as these, as well as the high pass rates referred to above, it would appear as if the ECD programme has been reasonably successful in terms of one of its primary objectives, namely, to bring about the transfer of knowledge and skills to child care-givers working in the targeted communities.

In relation to its second objective, however, the ECD programme appears to have been less successful. Currently, there are few signs that the training offered to participants in the programme has led to significant social action on the part of the latter to bring about a change in the living conditions of children in the areas where they operate. Perhaps this is a result of a tendency detected among certain ECD trainees to view themselves as 'professional therapists-in-training', rather than as social activists. Tarail (in Orford, 1992: 221) comments on a similar trend, widely seen in the United States, where 'paraprofessionals [attempt to] out-professionalise the professionals,' to the point where they lose the 'natural helping skills' that had contributed most significantly to their effectiveness as paraprofessionals in the first place. On the other hand, the lack of social action to bring about significant changes in the lived reality of children from communities targeted by the ECD programme could be because there has not yet been sufficient time for the programme to have had the desired impact; or it might even be due to shortcomings in the training offered to participants. Nonetheless, this lack of visible social action is an issue that the PRC will have to address if the ECD programme is to have all the desired effects.

Other shortcomings identified by participants in the ECD programme include the following: Firstly, the programme is presented in English only, while the languages spoken in the areas targeted include Afrikaans and Xhosa. Secondly, the programme lacks a comprehensive monitoring system that can assess the real effects of the programme on the lives of the children in the care of the programme participants. Given the rationale for as well as the considerable resources invested in the ECD programme, this can be considered the most serious shortcoming of the programme.

At this stage, the only available measure of the impact of the programme on the lives of the targeted children is derived from reports obtained from the programme participants. According to the participants, the programme has had a very beneficial effect on their confidence and ability to deal with the developmental problems exhibited by their charges. This, according to them, has in turn had a positive impact on the functioning of the latter. *En passant*, various writers (see, for example, Chapter 3 in this volume) have observed that using paraprofessionals to deal with psychological problems frequently leads to 'role expansion' and 'job overload', in the sense that the latter now are called upon to deal with their primary jobs (for example, as pre-school educare workers) as well as serving as mental health workers. Surprisingly, none of the participant evaluations of the programme conducted thus far have indicated that the participants' training had augmented their work load. On the contrary. Most of the participants in the ECD programme have reported that having learnt something about child development has enabled them to deal more effectively with the problems experienced by the children in their care, thereby substantially reducing their work.

Another major shortcoming of the ECD programme relates to the issue of power. Despite the PRC's commitment to full and equal collaboration with its community partners in terms of developing and managing the ECD programme, very real power imbalances have developed between the ECD trainees and the PRC (see Seedat, Cloete, and Shochet, 1988; and Chapter 3 in this volume). At the moment, it is the PRC that largely determines the content of the programme and that manages trainee supervision and certification. There does not appear to be any sense of joint ownership on the part of the trainees involved in the programme. On the whole they see themselves as recipients of information and expertise rather than as co-formulators of the programme. If the PRC is to contribute to the empowerment rather than the disempowerment of communities, this issue will have to be addressed.

Despite these shortcomings, however, it has to be pointed out that the evaluations of the ECD programme conducted thus far have generally been positive. Regular evaluations have provided an initial format for feedback and input into the annual revision of course structures and material. The feedback from these evaluations, in conjunction with that from other formats (for example, conference and workshop presentations, and the writing up of this chapter), have assisted in the clarification of the ECD programme's theoretical framework, its objectives, and the programme structures. It is especially the writing up of the ECD programme that has not only allowed for a more explicit theoretical description of the programme, but also the identification of some of the inconsistencies and lacunae described above. Continuing feedback from programme participants and external observers ensure the dynamic and on-going development of the programme.

The last five years have witnessed a steadily increasing demand for the Psychology Resource Centre's ECD courses. Whether this is an indication of the need for courses such as these or whether it is merely a reflection of an increasing interest in child psychology remains to be examined.

7 Conclusion

Despite the advent of democracy, living conditions for the majority of South Africa's children remain bleak. The PRC has piloted a programme directed at promoting the psychological development of pre-school children from historically impoverished and oppressed communities. These children's development are reported to be particularly vulnerable to the poverty and violence that mark South African life. Seven million children are reported to belong to this category.

The PRC's ECD programme evolved in response to the threats facing these children. Formulated within the community psychology paradigm, the programme attempts to maximize the human and material resources available to the very young, so as to address the developmental problems frequently experienced by the latter. Care-givers working in and around Cape Town's poorer suburbs and townships are invited to participate in a two-year programme in children's psychological development. The training covers an array of issues pertaining to developmental processes and difficulties, and the skills needed to assist children. Participants in the programme provide similar though shorter inputs to parents and others in their neighbourhoods, thereby 'multiplying' the impact of the initial training offered via the ECD programme. The heightened awareness in communities of their children's physical, emotional, intellectual, and social needs is expected to contribute to safer communities and a living space more conducive to the optimal development of the very young.

Exercises

1 Develop an assessment/monitoring plan that can be used by the PRC to evaluate the efficacy of its ECD programme.
2 Discuss the advantages and pitfalls of using paraprofessionals in projects such as the ECD programme.
3 According to you, what are the ECD programme's major shortcomings? Devise appropriate strategies to deal with these shortcomings.

Notes

1 The University of the Western Cape is one of the three universities in the Western Cape region of South Africa. It is a historically black university.
2 Which is reported to be about four to five times as expensive as ordinary education (Fair, 1996).

References

ANGLESS, T. and SHEFER, T. (1997). Children living with violence in the family. In C. de la Rey, N. Duncan, T. Shefer, and A. Van Niekerk. (Eds.), *Contemporary issues in human development: A South African focus* (pp. 170-186). Durban: ITP.

BONN, M. (1995). Associations between peer relations in childhood and adversity. *Early Child Development and Care, 105,* 77-91.

COOPER, S. (1990). The violence of apartheid on the family. *PRC Bulletin,* 1(1), 2-3.

DAWES, A. (1992). *Children and political violence: Risk factors and management issues.* Proceedings of the Symposium on Child Mental Health: Present Status and Future Direction, Pietermaritzburg.

DAWES, A. (1994). The emotional impact of political violence. In A. Dawes and D. Donald (Eds.), *Children and adversity: Psychological perspectives from South African research* (pp. 177-195). Cape Town: David Philip.

DAWES, A. and DONALD, D. (Eds.). (1994). *Childhood and adversity: Psychological perspectives from South African research.* Cape Town: David Philip.

DEPARTMENT OF NATIONAL HEALTH AND POPULATION DEVELOPMENT (DNHPD). (1993). *Emosionele behoeftes van die slagoffers van geweld.* Unpublished report, Department of National Health and Population Development, Pretoria.

DESJARLAIS, R. (1994). *World mental health: Problems, priorities and responses in low income countries.* Draft paper, Harvard Medical School, Oxford.

DOWDALL, T. (1990). Working with children and their families in civil conflict situations. In Centre for Intergroup Studies, *The influence of violence on children.* Cape Town: Centre for Intergroup Studies.

DUNCAN, N. (1997). Malnutrition and childhood development. In C. de la Rey, N. Duncan, T. Shefer, and A. Van Niekerk (Eds.), *Contemporary issues in human development: A South African focus* (pp. 190-206). Durban: ITP.

DUNCAN, N. and ROCK, B. (1997). The impact of political violence on the lives of South African children. In C. de la Rey, N. Duncan, T. Shefer, and A. Van Niekerk (Eds.), *Contemporary issues in human development: A South African focus* (pp. 133-158). Durban: ITP.

DUNCAN, N. and ROCK, B. (1994). *Inquiry into the effects of public violence on children.* Preliminary report from the Commission of Inquiry regarding the prevention of public violence and intimidation.

ENSINK, K., ROBERTSON, B., ZISSIS, C., and LEGER, P. (1997). Post-traumatic stress disorder in children exposed to violence. *South African Medical Journal,* 87 (11), 1526-1529.

FAIR, J. (1996). *Corporate educare in South Africa.* Cape Town: Centre for Early Childhood Development.

FRANKEL, P. (1993). *Violence, traumatic stress and children: A short guide to therapeutic education.* Unpublished paper, University of the Witwatersrand, Johannesburg.

GIBSON, K. (1989). Children and political violence. *Social Science Medical Journal,* 28(7), 659-667.

HORNEY, K. (1937). *The neurotic personality of our time.* New York: Norton.

HURLOCK, E. B. (1980). *Developmental psychology: A life-span approach.* New York: McGraw-Hill.

LAZARUS, S. (1985). *The role and responsibility of the psychologist in the South African context: Survey of psychologists' opinions.* Unpublished paper presented at the Third National Congress of the Psychological Association of South Africa, Pretoria.

LETLAKA-RENNERT, K. (1990). Play therapy and family stability following detention. In Centre for Intergroup Studies, *The influence of violence on children.* Cape Town: Centre for Intergroup Studies

LOCKHAT, R. and VAN NIEKERK, A. (in press). South African children and mental health: A history of adversity, violence and trauma. *Social Science and Medicine.*

MAJODINA, Z. (1989). Exile as a chronic stressor. *International Journal of Mental Health,* 18(8), 87-94.

MAKAN, P. (1996). *The challenges of reconstructing early childhood development services from apartheid to democracy.* Cape Town: Centre for Early Childhood Development.

NATIONAL CHILDREN'S RIGHTS COMMITTEE. (1994). *Voiceless victims: The impact of political violence on women and children.* Braamfontein: National Children's Rights Committee.

NATIONAL EDUCATION CO-ORDINATING COMMITTEE. (1992). *Early childhood educare.* National Education Policy Investigation (NEPI). Cape Town: Oxford University Press.

NATIONAL INSTITUTE FOR ECONOMIC POLICY (1996*). Children, poverty and disparity reduction: Towards fulfilling the rights of South Africa's children.* A report commissioned by the Ministry in the Office of the President (Reconstruction and Development Programme).

NETSHIOMBO, K. F. (1993). *The psychological impact of political violence on South African black youths. Report 94/1.* Pretoria: Institute for Behavioural Sciences, University of South Africa.

ORFORD, J. (1992). *Community psychology: Theory and practice.* Chichester: Wiley and Sons.

PAPALIA, D. E. and OLDS, S. W. (1989). *Human development.* New York: McGraw-Hill.

PETERSEN, I., MAGWAZA, A.S., and PILLAY, Y. (in press). *The use of participatory research to facilitate a psychological rehabilitation programme for child survivors of violence in a South African community.*

PILLAY, A., MAGWAZA, A., and PETERSEN, I. (1992). Civil conflict in Mpumulanga: Some mental health sequelae in a sample of children and their primary care-givers. *South African Journal of Child and Adolescent Psychiatry,* 4(2), 42-46.

POSTER, M. (1976). *A critical theory of the family.* New York: Seabury Press.

PROJECT FOR STATISTICS ON LIVING STANDARDS AND DEVELOPMENT. (1994). *South Africans rich and poor: Baseline household statistics.*

PSYCHOLOGY RESOURCE CENTRE. (1996/7). *PRC annual report.* Unpublished report, University of the Western Cape, Bellville.

RAPPAPORT, J. (1981). In praise of paradox: A

social policy of empowerment. *American Journal of Community Psychology, 9*(1), 1-21.

ROBINSON, J. A. (1994). *An overview of the provisions of the South African Bill of Rights with specific reference to its impact on families affected by the policy of apartheid.* Unpublished paper, University of Potchefstroom, Potchefstroom.

RYCKMAN, R. M. (1993). *Theories of personality.* Pacific Grove: Brooks/Cole.

SOUTH AFRICAN INSTITUTE OF RACE RELATIONS. (1995). *Fast facts: State of the nation report.* Braamfontein: SAIRR.

SOUTH AFRICAN INSTITUTE OF RACE RELATIONS, (1996). *Fast facts: Household and child poverty.* Braamfontein: SAIRR.

SEEDAT, M., CLOETE, N., and SHOCHET, I. (1988). Community psychology: Panic or panacea? *Psychology in Society, 11,* 39-54.

SERRANO-GARCIA, I., LOPEZ, M., and RIVERA-MEDINA, E. (1987). Toward a social-community psychology. *Journal of Community Psychology, 15,* 431-445.

SHORT, A. (1985). *Seeking change: Early childhood education for the disadvantaged in South Africa.* Michigan: The High/Scope Press.

SIMPSON, M. A. (1993). Bitter waters: Effects on children of the stresses of unrest and oppression. In J. P. Wilson and B. Raphael (Eds.), *International handbook of traumatic stress syndromes.* New York: Plenum Press.

THOMAS, T. (1987). *Homelands psychosocial pathology: Impressions of a community doctor.* Paper presented at the Second National Conference of OASSSA, Mental Health in Transition, University of the Western Cape, Bellville.

UNICEF AND NATIONAL CHILDREN'S RIGHTS COMMITTEE. (1993). *Women and children in South Africa: A situation analysis.* Johannesburg: UNICEF and National Children's Rights Committee.

UNITED NATIONS. (1992). *Human rights in international law: Basic texts.* Geneva: Council of Europe Press.

17

Social policy and community psychology in South Africa

Sandy Lazarus

Study objectives

The key study objectives of this chapter are to assist the reader in understanding:

- the relevance of working at social policy level within the context of a community psychology perspective;
- one example of such an activity within the South African context (comprising a case study that will be used as a point of reference throughout the discussion;
- how the social policy process works, highlighting some of the key dynamics that need to be taken into account when working at this level;
- some key factors in the change process, to facilitate effective interventions at policy level;
- the roles and skills required of psychologists and others working in the social policy arena; and
- the training required to prepare psychologists and others to make a contribution at this level.

1 Introduction

1.1 The scope of community psychology

As outlined in other chapters in this book, community psychology reflects a paradigm shift that moves the focus from an individualistic towards a contextual analysis of problems and solutions. It also reflects a commitment to multi-level interventions aimed at addressing factors that impact on the mental health of all people. This includes a variety of strategies that relate to social change. With social change being a major focus within community psychology, interventions in the arena of social policy become important. The effect of social policies on the lives and therefore well-being of people has long been recognized (Rappaport, 1977) and, in South Africa, has become a living reality through, for example, the apartheid policy that has impacted so deeply on the lives of all citizens in this country.

1.2 Social policy

Jones (1991, p.505) defines public policy as a 'set of ideas and proposals for action culminating in a government decision'. These decisions are usually presented in the form of policy frameworks, which, in the South African government context, are usually referred to as 'white papers'. The legislative process is then usually pursued through the development of laws (acts) that both enable and inhibit particular developments within the country. Once the policy and legal framework are in place, specific regulations are usually developed. These are generally used as a basis for implementation, as they provide concrete guidelines for 'how things should be done', based on the policy framework. In this chapter, the term 'social policy' is used to include all these aspects.

Most of the literature on policy processes identify the following stages in policy development: initiation or agenda setting, formulation, implementation, and evaluation. The stage of formulation includes three important elements: a development of the philosophy or basic beliefs underpinning the policy, principles or broad guidelines emerging from this (specifics relating to the particular values underpinning the philosophical framework), and procedures or practical details outlining what the policy entails. The latter provides the practical guidelines used as a basis for implementation (Facherty, Howes, and Turner, 1992).

Within the context of these stages and phases of policy development, a number of factors play a role in the unfolding associated process. In reading general literature on the policy process, and when looking at issues highlighted within community psychology literature, three important dynamics are highlighted. The first relates to the complexity of the political process, and, in particular, the interests that the various stakeholders and contexts bring to the policy development process, and the need to understand the legislative process. The second relates to the way in which policy is developed, in particular, the challenges relating to facilitating citizen or community participation in the process. The third relates to the role of research in the policy process. These dynamics will be discussed in some detail below.

Although many psychologists in South Africa who struggled against apartheid were involved, albeit indirectly, in policy development processes, primarily through protesting against the apartheid laws, it is really only in the past few years that psychologists have, in a more organized way, become more directly linked to policy processes. In fact, many of the psychologists who were previously part of the struggle to dismantle apartheid are now involved in more formal policy formulation. This reflects a move from a 'protest' approach to social change to that of 'reconstruction and development'; or what could be seen as a move from a more 'conflictual' to a more 'consensual' approach. It also reflects a growing recognition in psychology in South Africa that psychology needs to relate more directly to social realities and problems and possibilities of the day. This shift has been influenced by a number of factors, one being the growing acceptance and development of a community approach to psychology in South Africa.

1.3 Scope and purpose

The purpose of this chapter is to look at social policy as a 'setting' for psychological practice – particularly within the South African context. The emphasis will be on a theoretical discussion of this particular strategy, locating it within the debates on policy development within and outside of community psychology circles so as to illuminate the processes and challenges involved.

In this chapter I provide a summary of a South African case study, which is used as a point of reference throughout the discussion (see Section 2). This case study outlines my own involvement in education policy development within South Africa, from 1991-1998. Although it serves as a personal reflection, it should be noted that many others were involved in the processes highlighted. It should also be remembered that reflecting on one particular case study in no way negates the many other initiatives that have emerged within South Africa. Although, at times, some of these initiatives may be referred to, I do not attempt to provide an overview of all relevant policy initiatives pursued by psychologists within South Africa.

In the chapter I also examine the relationship between social policy and community psychology. Some challenges relating to the policy process specifically, and social change more generally, are then identified and briefly discussed. An exploration of the possible roles that can be played by psychologists within the social policy arena is then pursued. The particular skills and knowledge required to do this, and the implications for the training of psychologists, are briefly out-

lined. In conclusion, I summarize the key points arising out of the above discussion.

2 A South African case study

In recent years, there have been various initiatives involving psychologists in public policy processes in an attempt to influence mental health policy development in South Africa. This has included the involvement of individual psychologists, groups of psychologists (see, for example, Foster, Freeman, and Pillay, 1997) as well as organized psychology (for example, the Psychological Society of South Africa). The case study, forming a focal point for the discussion in this chapter, is only one of these initiatives. It is offered as a focal point for reflection on a variety of issues pertaining to social policy development.

The case study includes (1) the National Education Policy Initiative (NEPI, 1993); (2) the development of position papers on education support services and lifeskills – referred to as a 'post-NEPI' project by some (De Jong et al., 1994; De Jong et al., 1995); (3) the National Commission on Special Needs in Education and Training (NCSNET); and (4) the National Committee for Education Support Services (NCESS) – a government commission set up by the Minister of Education to investigate issues relating to 'special needs and support' in education and training (Department of Education, 1997).

A South African case study

1 1991–92 NEPI experience

In anticipation of a change in government, the main public arm of the education struggle in South Africa – the National Education Coordinating Committee (NECC) – was instrumental in setting up a National Education Policy Investigation (NEPI), which involved approximately 160 academics, including a number of psychologists and other professionals who were asked to contribute to the development of policy options in one of the eleven focal areas of the investigation. My own involvement was in the Education Support Services Research Group, which examined the areas of school health, specialized education, and guidance and counselling. This work culminated in the NEPI Report on Support Services (1992).

A central aim of the NEPI initiative was to prepare for a 'new' South Africa, with the expectation that it would not be long before the apartheid government would be overturned and a new, probably African National Congress, government put in place. Within this context, the aim of the NEPI project was to: (1) identify existing conditions and needs in education; (2) explore comparative experiences in relevant areas; and (3) make proposals for the future in South Africa. These proposals were deliberately limited to identifying options rather than taking a particular position. It is

interesting to note that this was considered to be the particular role of policy research required at this point in the history of South African education policy development.

2 1992–1995: The Post-NEPI Project (Support Services and Lifeskills Education)

Members of the original Support Services Research Group, together with members of departments of educational psychology and specialized education of the three universities in the Western Cape province, and members from colleges and non-governmental organizations formed a local Western Cape Support Services Policy Research and Development Group. The group functioned to take the NEPI options further in the form of position papers. This team produced position papers in all areas relating to support services (De Jong et al., 1994). This included papers that discussed (1) a general vision, principles, and strategies for support services as a whole; (2) a strategic plan to achieve this vision; and (3) specific proposals regarding school health, social work, guidance and counselling, educational psychology, and specialized education.

Some of the above-mentioned team members were also commissioned by the national Centre for Education Policy Development (CEPD – the ANC's education policy unit located in Johannesburg) to develop proposals for lifeskills education in South Africa (De Jong et al., 1995).

The reports emerging from the above initiatives were widely circulated, and were used as one basis for the development of future policy and practice in education and training in South Africa. In addition, many of the authors participated in the development of general education policy through written submissions in response to draft policy documents, and through writing and sending articles to strategically placed people for consideration in the policy development process.

3 1996–1998: National Commission on Special Needs in Education and Training (NCSNET) and National Committee for Education Support Services (NCESS)

The developments outlined above culminated in the NCSNET/NCESS investigation, which was commissioned by the Minister of Education to investigate issues pertaining to 'special needs and support' in education and training in South Africa (Department of Education, 1997). The Report, which was handed to the Minister at the end of 1997, outlined a future vision, principles, and strategies required to build an integrated education system that is responsive to the diverse needs of the learner population, and is able to address barriers to learning and development. This included all aspects as well as all levels of education,

such as: early childhood, general and further education and training, higher education, and adult education. The emphasis was on identifying how all aspects of the curriculum and institutions could become more responsive to the full range of diverse needs of all learners, and the development of an integrated, community-based support system to assist in this process.

Although not couched in 'community psychology' terms, the content of the NCSNET/NCESS Report (Department of Education, 1997) reflects a clear move away from an individualistic, victim-blaming analysis, towards a systemic, developmental, preventive, and health-promotive approach to problems and solutions. The title of the report, 'Quality education for all: Overcoming barriers to learning and development', reflects this emphasis on understanding both problems and development challenges within 'context'.

Following from the work of the NCSNET/NCESS, the Department of Education has developed a policy paper to provide a national framework for education and training in South Africa (Department of Education, 1999).

3 Social policy and community psychology

Within the context of understanding problems and challenges 'in context', the need for work at multiple levels – including social

347

policy – to address these challenges is high-lighted within community psychology (Heller et al., 1984; Lazarus, 1988; Rappaport, 1977). Rappaport (1977) highlights the need for social interventions aimed at changing social systems such as education, mental health, the police, housing, the legal system, the economy, and labour. The purpose of such interventions is 'to facilitate rather than inhibit accomplishment of developmental tasks' (Rappaport, 1977, p.61). The assumption underlying these interventions is that there is a clear link between social factors and mental health. The goal of these interventions is to enhance the mental health or well-being of all citizens. Rappaport (1977) goes on to say that 'psychologists are urged to take responsibility for advocating public policy, even to the point of political debate and confrontation' (p.61).

Jason (1991) highlights the need for community psychologists to become more actively involved in projects that are designed to influence regulatory and legislative policies. He acknowledges the difficulties in working at this level, but emphasizes the need for community psychology to remain true and responsive to a more social action vision. He highlights some of the dilemmas of working at this level, as does the debate raised by Smail (1994) in the Journal of Community and Applied Social Psychology. This includes the question of whether or not psychologists should become involved in 'politics'- particularly when this involves a partisan approach; whether they in fact *do* have any power to influence things at that level; and whether and how to use research as a tool to influence social policies. Jason (1991) notes that community psychologists

have not been sufficiently involved at social policy level, despite the recognition by many in community psychology circles that there is a need to link research with public policy. He argues that 'this is perhaps the issue that most separates our rhetoric from our action, and it is a topic that needs more attention from our theorists and practitioners' (p.3). He argues for more emphasis on conducting social action research projects, ensuring that the outcomes enter the public policy arena where applicable.

A review of articles written, since 1990, in three internationally recognized journals on community psychology, namely, the *Journal of Community Psychology*, the *American Journal of Community Psychology*, and the *Journal of Community and Applied Social Psychology*, reveals that some of the research and action pursued within the context of a community psychology approach has either direct or indirect implications for public policy. However, there is very little debate about the role and activities of psychologists in terms of interventions at social policy level, either in terms of consensual strategies where researchers work with policy makers in the development process, or in terms of more conflictual approaches aimed at contesting policy through various community development and activist strategies.

The *Community Psychologist* (the official newsletter of the Society for Community Research and Action, American Psychological Association), has in recent years included a standing item for discussions on public policy. Articles in this journal have tended to highlight the different ways in which psychologists have engaged in social policy development. The role of community psychologists at this level has been reinforced, as one can see from Rickel's (1993) comment that:

> we community psychologists have much we can contribute to the formulation of public policy. My experience in Washington has taught me that we each have a responsibility to make our knowledge and expertise available to policymakers as often as possible. If they are ignorant of our areas of expertise, we have only ourselves to blame (p.13).

In addition to the importance of action at social policy level within community psychology itself, the general psychology profession has recognized the need to engage in policy-related activities beyond the discipline of community psychology. Solarz (1995) highlights a number of reasons why psychologists should become involved: (1) political decisions regarding funding on mental health affect the lives of psychologists whether they like it or not; (2) psychologists have 'substantive expertise' to contribute to the process and products of social policy; and (3) if psychologists do not address these pertinent issues, others, who are perhaps not as well equipped, will. The Psychologist's Guide to Advocacy (APA, undated), prepared by the American Psychological Association, also highlights the important tasks of psychologists in the social policy arena. These include:

- To strengthen psychology's role in the promotion of human welfare through the use of relevant psychological research and theory when public policy is formu-

lated to address public interest issues.
- To formulate and promote policies that address the needs of persons who are disadvantaged, who are subject to discrimination, or who have special needs related to developmental factors. These include women, children, youth, families, the aged, racial and ethnic minorities, people living in poverty, people with disabilities, and lesbians and gay men.
- To promote efforts to support the health of all people, especially those individuals with severe physical and mental disabilities, as well as other persons in need of health and mental health services.

The above discussion, which draws from general as well as community psychology sources, highlights the important role that psychologists can play within the social policy arena.

4 Challenges in social policy work

One of the points highlighted by those working within a community psychology approach is that it is important to understand the policy and social change process if one is to be effective. This section will highlight some of the key dynamics that need to be understood and engaged with at this level.

4.1 Research and social policy

Jason (1991), Solarz (1995) and the APA Guide to Advocacy for Psychologists (APA, undated) highlight the role of research or social science information in influencing social policy. Jason (1991) recognizes that there are many ways of influencing social policy, suggesting that the most subtle approach involves affecting regulations or policies that reflect the way laws are implemented. He argues that, to ensure that the best regulations are developed, studies should be undertaken. These studies 'can help shape regulations at the legislative level by providing decision makers timely and relevant data' (Jason, 1991, p.4). He highlights the strategy of documenting how non-legislative efforts are ineffective in correcting a social problem, thereby arguing for legislation to regulate the particular behaviour (for example, smoking). He then discusses the important role of evaluating legislation which he indicates is the most common activity of academics involved in social policy. While influencing and evaluating legislation, could be pursued as separate activities, Jason (1991) argues that a more comprehensive way of influencing social policy is to have an effect on the development of the legislation and subsequently be involved in the evaluation of the impact of the new legislation. This can be even more comprehensively developed to include involvement in influencing communities to abide by the new laws.

Jason (1991) raises a further important factor in social policy work: the need to respond to political issues in a timely fashion. He notes that data often needs to be collected and analysed quickly so that findings can be used when political decisions are being made. This requires one to be receptive to the often chaotic and unpredictable timetables of decision makers. The flexibility

required to meet these challenges highlights some important issues for researchers, particularly where time-consuming methodologies are required to ensure sufficient rigour and therefore accuracy in the research process.

Perkins (1995) highlights the importance of an 'empowerment research' approach within policy work where research is a collaborative process including researchers and the community and its citizens:

> Such a partnership among empowerment researchers, citizen/clients, and practitioners/administrators can improve the quality of the research, enhance its use, encourage greater public support for empowerment research, and ultimately improve empowerment applications in the community (p.784).

This refers to the action/community research approach, which constitutes a major intervention strategy within community psychology (Lazarus, 1988). Perkins (1995) highlights various advantages and disadvantages of such a research approach, but basically argues that it is an important strategy to pursue to ensure that the goals of empowerment are achieved.

Perkins (1995) notes that social researchers have always had difficulty applying their data to issues of public policy and communicating their data clearly and effectively to policy decision makers. He refers to Weis who identifies some of the difficulties. First, the logic and rationality of social scientists are not always compatible with how governments operate and with what politicians want to hear. Second, researchers often assume that they know best and that their views will be accepted, irrespective of the policy interests at stake. Third, research is used by policy makers in an expedient way, usually to support their political position. The point being made here is that policy making is not a rational process.

Caplan (cited in Perkins, 1995) identified five preconditions for social research being used by policy makers: (1) the policy maker must appreciate the scientific and other aspects of the policy issue; (2) the policy maker must value social direction and responsibility; (3) the policy issue must be well defined and require research knowledge to solve; (4) the research findings must be sound and have feasible implications; and (5) there need to be resources available to translate data into policy goals and objectives. Caplan makes the point that the two 'cultures' of researchers and policy makers need to be bridged if they are to work together. Scientific and political skills and interests need to be meshed, with scientists and politicians working together on both activities around a specific project (Perkins, 1995).

Perkins' (1995) recommendations to policy makers, programme planners, and 'empowerment' researchers are worthy of note. These include: (1) an emphasis on local grass-roots empowerment programmes; (2) an emphasis on both personal and collective strategies and multiple level interventions to foster empowerment; (3) becoming more familiar with the policy-making process, its complexity, and key players, and how to disseminate and directly apply their research – by working with executive, legislative, and judicial policy-making bodies and advocacy organizations at all levels; (4) planning effective policy research by identifying the relevant parties,

determining their interests, finding out what kinds of information are relevant to their interests, determining the best way to obtain this information, and determining how to report the research findings; (5) being proactive *throughout* the policy process (agenda formulation, policy adoption, policy implementation, and review); (6) playing the role of learner/collaborator; (7) learning how to disseminate more practical information; and (8) understanding the process of empowerment. Of course, a prerequisite for all of the above is an understanding and commitment to participatory democracy.

4.1.1 Research and social policy in South Africa

In the South African case study described in this chapter, research as a specific activity was pursued in both a proactive and reactive manner. It was proactive in that research was conducted in the early stages of 'agenda setting', before the formal policy processes had even begun. It aimed to influence the discourse as well as specific policy positions in the hope of these eventually becoming legislated. Some of the research conducted was reactive in that it was conducted in response to specific requests for input. The latter was particularly true for the NCSNET/NCESS, where research was commissioned around all relevant aspects of the policy. However, because much of this research had already been conducted within the proactive phase, it was able to be accessed and successfully used in the policy process itself.

Where research conducted before and during the NCSNET/NCESS was successfully used in the policy process, it related directly to particular policy *needs*. As mentioned above, some of these needs were correctly anticipated, while others were highlighted during the policy agenda setting and formulation phases. Those involved in the case study were able to identify and anticipate needs to the extent that they were aware of and sensitive to general political dynamics in the country, as well as developments within education itself. This seems to be a central requirement for psychologists or others who wish to make a contribution at social policy level.

4.2 The political arena

The above discussion on research and social policy highlights some of the dilemmas and challenges relating to bringing the 'scientific' and 'political' cultures together for the purposes of developing policy, and the need to acknowledge and work with the political interests within that context (Perkins,1995). The practical demands of such a context, particularly relating to tight time-frames and deadlines, was also highlighted (Jason, 1991).

Bowe and Ball (1992) provide a useful framework for understanding some of these dynamics, highlighting in particular the on-going conflict inherent in this process. They refer to different sources of influence on policy emergence. Specifically, they identify three contexts of policy process that must be taken into account when considering any attempts to influence or develop policy: (1) the context of influence; (2) the context of policy text production, and (3) the context of practice. The context of influence is the context within which public policy is normally initiated – including a variety of

political activities involving relevant stakeholders (for example, teacher protests and political party debates). The context of policy text production refers to the development of texts relating to the policy, including official legal texts, policy documents, commentaries by the media, or speeches by politicians or citizen groups. The context of practice refers to the interpretation of the policy texts and how this interpretation is translated into practice: the implementation of policy.

Bowe and Ball (1992) highlight the fact that all three of these contexts are characterized by some form of struggle. Each context is characterized by a 'push-and-pull' where different stakeholders attempt to achieve dominance and recognition. Interest groups struggle to influence the process, using various means at their disposal, for example, protests, submissions, personal interviews, and so on. The context of text production also reflects many tensions and struggles. The expression of policy in the form of policy documents lends itself to different interpretations and misunderstanding. The context of practice also lends itself to different interpretations and struggles. Implementers of policy interpret policies in the context of their own values and interest.

In the light of the above, the need for a comprehensive approach to policy development and implementation, which means a commitment to staying with the process from the beginning (initiation or agenda setting) to the end (evaluation of implementation) is important (Jason, 1991; Perkins, 1995). The above also highlights an important factor to be taken into account by psychologists who become involved at this level: public policy development is primarily a *political* process, and so when one chooses to work within a political setting, the dynamics and rules of the game must be understood and strategically worked with if successful influence is to be achieved.

In addition to understanding these informal dynamics, it is important that one understands how the legislative process works. It is interesting to note that the American Psychological Association's *Psychologist's guide to advocacy* (APA, undated) provides clear guidelines to help psychologists understand and therefore engage in the legislative process. This includes clarifying key terms within the legislative process, as well as identifying which committees, and key people, are involved in central issues relating to mental health and related issues. It also includes a description of the process by which legislators decide how to cast their votes, in order to sensitize psychologists to 'gaps' that should be taken to influence the policy. An overall outline of the legislative process – from beginning to end – is also provided. This 'short course in the legislative process' (p. 7) is followed by suggestions on how to provide effective communications for the purposes of affecting legislation. This includes (1) identifying and locating legislators; (2) understanding the role of congressional staff; (3) writing a constituent letter; (4) making a constituent telephone call; (5) meeting with your legislator; (6) and inviting your legislator to visit. This information is invaluable in assisting and equipping psychologists to become more involved, as citizens and as professionals, in the political and, in particular, legislative process. In addition to providing useful information in this regard, the APA also offers fellowships to psychologists wishing to specialize in the area of social policy work.

4.2.1 Engaging in the political arena in South Africa

The case study in this chapter reflects a potentially *comprehensive approach*, where I and others engaged in the process at the early stages of initiation and agenda setting, and pursued it through to policy formulation. The challenge now is to continue to engage with the implementation and evaluation phases. This point highlights the need for perseverance and long-term commitment to pursuing particular issues.

An interesting point to note is that much of the influence exerted by those involved in the case study was on the 'discourse' around the policy developments, and not only on the policy process itself. This is an important point for psychologists to note as they do have an important role in influencing the discourses around pertinent issues, whether or not they link directly with the policy process.

A factor that assisted in this case study was my and others' previous and continued involvement in the struggle and political development in the country. Such engagement resulted in an on-going awareness of political dynamics relating to the particular policy process being pursued. Engagement in the education context also proved to be a central factor that enabled the particular issues of 'special needs and support services' to be embedded in general education developments. Without sensitivity and knowledge of the specificities relating to this setting, this policy intervention would not have been possible.

The experience of the NCSNET/NCESS clearly highlighted the '*contexts of influence*' briefly discussed above. The different political and other interests of the many stakeholders influenced by this policy were very evident. First, within the Commission/Committee itself the members reflected the South African spectrum in a very representative way. Second, throughout the consultation process, different and often opposing positions became very clear.

Debate within the Commission/Committee and within various public forums highlighted the various political interests within the area of 'special needs and support services'. One of the key areas of contestation was around the retention or abolition of 'special schools' for learners with disabilities. Those schools that were particularly well resourced were particularly concerned about retaining these facilities, and revealed deep concerns that their resources would be diminishing in the face of extensive lack of resources among the historically disadvantaged, particularly black and rural communities, in South Africa. These and other tensions were resolved through compromises around opposing positions. These compromises arose out of political rather than educational interests.

The people involved in the initiatives in this case study were not informed about legislative procedures. Initially, this was not considered to be appropriate given the illegitimacy of the pre-1994 government. Thereafter, the legislative processes were being reconstructed within a democratic framework. I and others involved had to learn about these procedures as we progressed in the process, drawing from our own and others' 'on-the-ground' experiences. Now that parliamentary and legislative processes are more settled, it would be beneficial to develop simple manuals that could help psychologists and others to engage in the different aspects of the social policy process.

4.3 Facilitating citizen participation

Perkins (1995) and Heller et al. (1984) emphasize the need for psychologists to be involved in 'bottom-up' processes such as facilitating citizen participation in public policy decision-making processes. They identify the need for ordinary citizens to receive training and facilitation so that policy formulation and debate reflect the needs of the people.

A recent article in one of the international journals of community psychology provides an interesting case study of the involvement of service providers in the development of policy (Kingfisher, 1998). Kingfisher highlights the central role that service providers such as social workers can play as co-producers of relevant and workable social policy. He shows how they can potentially play an important role in mediating policy development both upwards and downwards. That is, they can assist in developing policy that meets the real needs of the community concerned, and they can play a central role in the implementation of this policy. The study highlights that this will only occur if the important role of service providers is properly recognized and optimally utilized by policy formulators.

Facilitation of citizen participation in policy processes is an important aspect within the context of South Africa, where a concerted effort is being made in most ministries and government departments to pursue the development of policy in a democratic way. Social policy development usually occurs within the context of commissions, government committees, or task teams, and can include limited or extensive consultation of some or all relevant stakeholders – those people who have a 'stake' in the outcome of the policy. Various government departments in South Africa have developed consultative structures and forums for the purpose of including all relevant stakeholders in policy development and other relevant business of the departments concerned. Most of these bodies – for example, the National Education and Training Council – provided for in the National Education Policy Act, 1996 have a central role in advising ministers on key policy and practice matters. This is an expression of the commitment to democracy enshrined in the new Constitution of South Africa.

The way in which policy is developed has a major impact on the successful implementation of the policy. There seems to be some evidence that where people feel some sense of ownership of the product they are more likely to put it into practice. This suggests that, in addition to the promotion of democratic practices in social life, citizen participation in policy processes should be fostered wherever possible. It should be noted, however, that there are clearly times when conflictual rather than consensual tactics should be pursued. Where citizens' interests are diametrically opposed, consen-

sual strategies pursued through stakeholder forums are less likely to succeed.

The empowerment agenda of a participatory approach to policy formulation has been highlighted within community psychology literature (Heller et al., 1984; Perkins, 1995). The goal of facilitating maximum participation is therefore not only to ensure that the policy is implemented successfully, but also to foster the empowerment of citizens: to provide them with real opportunities to take control of their own lives. While this should be a general goal within a democratic society and within the values and aims of a community psychology approach, it is not without its tensions.

4.3.1 Facilitating citizen participation in South Africa

The NCSNET/NCESS reflected a serious attempt to foster citizen participation within the policy process. Various strategies were pursued to enable citizens, particularly the key stakeholders, to express their views and engage in debates. These included requests for written submissions, public hearings (where verbal submissions were made), workshops (particularly around the vision and principles acting as a basis for the policy), stakeholder meetings (set up by stakeholders themselves), site visits, as well as informal communication. The composition of the NCSNET/NCESS team was also, in itself, an attempt to include the voices of key stakeholders. In this regard the team reflected a fair representation of South Africa's demography, particularly in terms of geographical area, race, gender, and key stakeholders. The composition of the Reference Group, which supported the process throughout, was also fairly representative of the various stakeholders.

However, all of the above did not result in full participation within the country. In particular, teachers and parents of learners who did not consider 'special needs and support' to be of concern to them did not participate well in the process, despite various attempts to involve them. The lack of an adequate media campaign during this policy process was one negative factor impacting on this. From comments received, it seems that a further factor that impeded a fuller citizen participation in this particular policy process was the 'future shock' experienced by so many South Africans during this transition period. All government departments have been in the process of developing policy for the 'new' South Africa, and most of them have attempted to involve citizens – particularly through requests for submissions on draft policy papers. In recent years, therefore, people have been inundated with such requests, making it practically impossible to comment in any meaningful way on all policy developments concerned.

The evaluation of the NCSNET/NCESS (Department of Education, 1998) highlighted the important role of conflict management, and, in particular, the extent to which conflict should be resolved through compromise, *or* retained for the purposes of furthering more radical positions. This evaluation revealed that, despite problems experienced, the gains of working within a democratic framework outweighed the losses. These gains related to a 'better product' as well as a process of stakeholder ownership that will hopefully assist in the implementation process.

5 Understanding the change process

One major aspect of understanding and working within the social policy arena is understanding the process of change and, in particular, how this impacts on the policy process.

5.1 Approaches to change

One needs to be aware of the different approaches to change and how these serve the particular interests or goals one is trying to pursue. One useful way of categorizing different approaches is a model suggested by Burrell and Morgan (in Hewton, 1982, p.9), which is based on two major dimensions that help us to determine a particular approach to change: the subjective-objective dimension, which either emphasizes or de-emphasizes peoples' perceptions, views, and wishes in the process, and the regulation-radical dimension, which favours either a consensual or conflictual approach to change. An intersection of these two dimensions produces a matrix that results in four typical paradigms of change: radical humanist, radical structuralist, interpretive, and functionalist approaches (see Hewton, 1982 for details of this framework).

In understanding social policy processes, Hewton's (1982) framework provides a useful point from which to understand the particular approaches to change that could be pursued. For example, within the context of the subjective-objective dimension, approaches to social policy that examine the subjective element would emphasize the importance of citizen participation in the process. The radical humanist approach, which reflects an empowerment principle favoured by many in community psychology, would include various bottom-up approaches. Such bottom-up approaches aim to empower people to participate in and strongly influence the development of policy within the context of a critical understanding of the policy process and content. The interpretive approach would also aim at fostering participation, but would accept the contributions without critical examination of these within the context of power relations in society. Approaches, such as radical structuralist and functionalist approaches, that are more concerned with *objective* factors, would be less concerned with people's perceptions and views, reflecting a more top-down approach to policy development.

The *radical-regulation* dimension refers to the extent to which the policy process and product work within existing frameworks, and emphasise cohesion and consensus. This relates to an important issue within community psychology itself: the extent to which, and when and how one pursues either consensual or conflictual strategies to achieve particular social ends.

5.1.1 Approaches to change in the case study

The case study reflects both a bottom-up and top-down approach to social policy development, with a major emphasis being on the facilitation of citizen participation in the process.

The particular approach to the inclusion of citizens' views in the NCSNET/NCESS

process seems to have been located primarily within the critical radical humanist approach. That is, while the public's views *were* taken seriously in formulating the proposed policy (NCSNET/NCESS, Department of Education, 1997), these views were not uncritically accepted. They were tested against the framework of principles, which reflected a clear commitment to a human rights approach, and, in particular, redress and equity. These principles, emerging directly from the new Constitution of South Africa, acted as an objective, top-down framework for the NCSNET/NCESS policy process.

5.2 Factors that influence the change process

Within the context of understanding and working within a particular approach to social change, the factors that affect the change process should also be understood for the purposes of strategic planning and action within the public policy arena (Lazarus, 1997). The following eighteen factors are worthy of note in this regard.

1 *Planning:* Although change is a fundamentally unpredictable process, intentional forward planning certainly aids in the possibility of reaching goals set.
2 *A clear vision, principles, and procedures:* It is important to have a clear target towards which implementation strives. Policies should include a philosophy, principles, and guidelines, as well as some clear procedures that need to be followed.
3 *Managing the complex and dynamic nature of change:* While planning for

change can and should occur, the unpredictable and complex nature of the process should not be underestimated. The dynamic nature of change implies a need to adopt a comprehensive or multiple-level approach, where various aspects of the system are targeted for transformation. In order to manage the complexity of the process, planned change should incorporate step-by-step goals, strategies, and tasks that facilitate some sense of control and direction.

4 *Successful experiences:* Small-but-successful approaches to change are important. This is one reason why many policy innovations include pilot programmes in the initial phases of implementation. Openness to change is reinforced by observed success in related initiatives. It is also important to understand the history of previous experiences of change. If people have experienced negative effects of previous efforts to change a particular aspect of society, or are 'burnt-out' as a result of 'change-overload' (future shock), this acts as a barrier to their openness to change.

5 *Readiness to change:* The main impetus for change usually comes from peoples' dissatisfaction with the existing order. It is important, therefore, to develop readiness or a 'ripe environment' for change by, for example, highlighting contradictions or points of conflict and developing these into clearly identified needs and priorities for action. Changes being suggested must link to real needs and interests in some way.

6 One aspect of change that relates to the concept of readiness is the idea that we move through cycles of being in a 'frozen', to an 'unfrozen', to a newly 'frozen' state. It is in the 'unfrozen' states that we are most susceptible and able to make major changes in our lives. We become 'unfrozen' through personal crises and major changes, and also through social processes, such as a the transition being experienced in South Africa at present.

7 *Balancing safety with challenge:* While conflict and being in an 'unfrozen state' is conducive to change, too much of this can be overpowering and counterproductive. It is important, therefore, to provide or support a sufficient sense of safety and security, from which people can move into new spaces.

8 *The mind and the body:* Changing people's minds (for example, through education strategies) is an acceptable part of any change strategy, but this should not exclude the 'feeling' level of people. If people's basic needs and interests are not in some way involved in the change process, there is likely to be extreme resistance and possible sabotage.

9 *Reflective practice:* Critical social theories emphasize the importance of reflection, for the purposes of achieving insight, in the process of development or change. The principle here is that if we provide people and institutions with opportunities to reflect on their practices, they can, if provided with appropriate guidance and stimulus, learn from their practices and make new choices for the future. This involves building a culture of change. In the process of policy development, this aspect is most pertinent in the

phases of monitoring and evaluation.

10 *Involving strategic people:* It is important to involve strategic people in the process: leaders, competent enthusiasts, and those who will be centrally involved in implementation. Engaging leadership in this process is important given the critical role played by key stakeholders and leaders in facilitating the adoption, implementation, management, and maintenance of innovations (Fullan, 1992). Engaging key representatives of those most affected by the change is just as important. Without their support and ownership of the process, change is likely to be resented, and possibly sabotaged.

11 *Control and ownership:* We need to acknowledge the need of people to have a sense of control. This could be through participation in the decision making and therefore the ownership of, and commitment to, the policy process and outcome. This participation could be facilitated in various ways. In policy development processes, this could entail extensive consultation with key stake-holders. There is a need for both a 'top-down' and 'bottom-up' approach to change, and therefore policy develop-ment. This means that there needs to be authoritative actions at the top of the system to facilitate and ensure implementation, while at the same time, development of ownership of the initiative 'on the ground'.

12 *Addressing resistance to change:* It is important to understand and work with the dynamics of resistance in order to facilitate change. This could involve fanning the resistance, for the purposes

of achieving a particular outcome, or attempting to lower the resistance towards acceptance of a change process and outcome. Much resistance is generated from the fear of loss, for example, loss of security, loss of identity, loss of autonomy, loss of role certainty, loss of job and income, loss of resources, or even loss of life. These fears need to be recognized and addressed.

13 *Resource distribution:* The recycling of resources highlighted in ecological theories (Heller et al., 1984) may be helpful in promoting the adaptation that is necessary in any change process. This could mean, for example, using existing personnel in new ways, or using existing structures in new ways. This requires a major focus on the reorientation of people to facilitate the development of new roles, skills, and forms of practice. Most policy development recognizes this aspect in their emphasis on training and retraining of personnel who are affected by the policy.

14 *Re-education:* Related to the above, a major concern in the change process should be the re-education of people. Educational programmes and media campaigns are important strategies in this regard.

15 *Legislative pressure:* Unless some changes are enacted constitutionally and through committed policy initiatives, the lives of those affected are unlikely to change in real terms. Legislation needs to provide both the pressure and the support for changes being pursued.

16 *Political factors:* As discussed in some detail in the previous section, one needs

to understand factors in the political arena that both enhance and obstruct the policy development process. The struggle around policy development needs to be recognized. The inevitability of compromise that arises out of the clash of different spheres of influence needs to be accepted if disappointment is to be avoided.

17 *Finances and sustainability:* A central aspect relating to political factors is that of financial resources. Policy formulation, implementation, and evaluation can be blocked or enhanced by the lack or availability of sufficient financial resources. Linked to this is the issue of sustainability. For continuity to occur, structures and processes should be set in place to ensure the on-going life of the innovation. This means that the changes need to be institutionalized. This is important to note when considering donor funding in the initial stages of implementing policy.

18 *Time-factors:* Sufficient time needs to be allocated to policy-development processes. Given that time is money, this can be a problematic factor in ensuring adequate engagement with any or all of the stages of policy development.

5.2.1 Working with the change process in South Africa

The case study as a whole reflects an intuitive rather than formally planned process, where I and others involved hoped to influence policy and strived to do this with an intuitive sense of the strategies to pursue.

The NCSNET/NCESS process was formally planned, but it was only approximately halfway through the process that the actual dynamics relating to policy development and the social change process were formally reflected upon by the entire Commission/Committee (Lazarus, 1997). Had this been done earlier, the process could have been improved.

The development of the NCSNET/NCESS policy included the articulation of a vision, principles, and procedures. The philosophy, however, was contentious and required circular strategies to facilitate the paradigm shift required by all concerned. This impacted on the 'neat' unfolding of the process.

The policy proposals emerging from the NCSNET/NCESS reflect clear strategies aimed at both structural and people change. The strategies reflect a comprehensive or multiple-level approach that targets all aspects and levels of the education system.

One clear problem relating to this policy is its *comprehensive* nature, in that it poses challenges to all aspects and levels of education, and another problem is the *timing* of its promulgation – at a time when the country, and the education system in particular, is reeling from 'change-overload'. The current conditions therefore seriously challenge the immediate practicability of the policy guidelines. Unless this is adequately taken into account in the implementation plan, it could result in serious implementation failure.

The implementation plan of the NCSNET/NCESS reflects a phasing-in, developmental process which, in the initial stages, relies on pilot programmes and projects, and draws from best practices that already reflect the principles of the new policies. This may assist in addressing the feelings of being overwhelmed by so many challenges relating to the transformation process.

During the NEPI and post-NEPI processes, some consultation was pursued but this was limited in scope. The involvement of strategic people in this process related mainly to service providers (Kingfisher, 1998). The NCSNET/NCESS process formally attempted to include all major stakeholders in the process. However, perhaps the most important stakeholders – teachers and parents who historically have not considered special needs and support to be their business – were minimally involved, despite the involvement of teacher unions and departments in the process. The consultation processes and wide distribution of documents resulting from all the activities in this case study assisted in enabling all relevant stakeholders to feel part of and own the outcomes of the process. One of the ways in which this ownership has revealed itself is the way in which local initiatives have gone ahead with policy implementation even in the absence of the official policy. For example, many district support centres have been developing their competencies to work in new ways since the days of NEPI. The policy is only confirming what they have been part of developing. Furthermore, many provinces have already begun to implement policy guidelines as a result of the NCSNET/NCESS. This has caused some problems from a national perspective, however, as the NCSNET/NCESS report is *not* policy.

Some attempt was made to address resistance to change within the NCSNET/NCESS, primarily through citizen participation, negotiation, and compromise, and through showing people how they can transform their roles in a positive way. Where there was resistance to the basic principles, such as redress and equity, attempts were made to indicate the moral obligation relating to pursuing these principles, but where resistance continued in the face of this, this was not resolved.

The NCSNET/NCESS emphasizes the optimal use of existing resources and the need to find creative and constructive new roles for personnel and even institutions (for example, specialized schools). Training of personnel to support the restructuring of roles is also emphasized. The need for public communication campaigns also highlights a recognition of the need to re-educate the public as a whole.

The NCSNET/NCESS implementation plan reflects a commitment to on-going monitoring and evaluation for the purposes of informing future policy and practice. The NCSNET/NCESS itself attempted to include a reflective aspect to its work, with evaluations of the process occurring within the investigation period, and then a final evaluation at the end (Department of Education, 1998).

Those involved in the initiatives outlined in this case study had to become and remain aware of broader political dynamics and developments within education throughout the process. Learning how to 'play the political game' was also necessary. The interests of the different stakeholders were clear, particularly during the public consultation process pursued within the NCSNET/NCESS. These interests were not always obvious, however. They required analysis within the context of understanding broader political and social dynamics. While most people involved in the NCSNET/NCESS process were able to make such an analysis, there was a tendency at times to discount any opposing view as unacceptable political interests and ignore it. A critical approach to this hidden text of policy development is important but can become counterproductive if not worked with strategically.

Lack of sufficient funds to engage in policy research and consultation processes was clearly felt during the NEPI and post-NEPI process. This lack seriously impeded the extent of the projects, and meant that there was a heavy reliance on the goodwill of some academics and service providers to engage in such work. This raises a question about how practically possible it is for citizens to engage more formally in the policy process. Lack of funds during the NCSNET/NCESS process also created barriers to that process. This included limited citizen participation, particularly relating to those who have been historically disadvantaged and have minimal financial means to travel to meetings/hearings, or make submissions. The budget did not allow for a more realistic time-frame for the investigation, nor did it allow for adequate research to be conducted. Concerns have been raised as to whether the Ministry of Education will commit sufficient resources to facilitate implementation of the policy paper emerging from the NCSNET/NCESS process. This concern arises out of real fiscal constraints and budget cuts being experienced in South Africa at present – usually at the expense of social services of one sort or another.

A consistent complaint within the NCSNET/NCESS (Department of Education, 1998) related to the extremely limited time-frame of the investigation. The Commission/Committee eventually agreed to abide by the time-frame in the light of the need of the country for clear policy guidelines relating to special needs and support services in education and training. The product was, however, compromised through this decision. As highlighted in previous discussion in this chapter, this is a compromise that often has to be made when working within the demands and pressures of political life.

It is interesting to note that many of the factors in the social change process were, wittingly or unwittingly, taken into account in both the *processes* that were pursued, and in the *content* of the actual publications emerging from the processes identified in the case study (for example, Department of Education, 1997). Many weaknesses relating to these factors have also been highlighted. The evaluation of the NCSNET/NCESS (Department of Education, 1998) was an important process in assisting the government and members of the Commission/Committee to address these factors more adequately in the future.

6 Roles and activities of psychologists working in a policy context

While traditional psychological issues are obvious points of focus for policy work, all aspects of social life constitute a potential focus. This means that while most psychologists involved in this work may concentrate on issues relating *directly* to mental health, particularly in the areas of health and welfare, other areas of public life also need to be monitored and pursued. These include areas such as housing, sport and recreation, safety and security, education, as well as those identified by Rappaport (1977) earlier in this chapter.

The earlier discussion on the relationship between community psychology and social policy highlighted a number of activities that could be pursued within the context of social policy. These included: (1) policy analysis; (2) evaluation of policy outcomes/implementation; (3) diffusion of information and innovations; (4) conducting research to impact directly on policy; and (5) facilitating citizen participation in the policy process.

Within the context of initiatives undertaken by the American Psychological Association (APA, undated; Solarz,1995), and an anonymous handout presented at a workshop on policy at a conference of the Society for Community Research and Action (Anonymous, 1996), a number of roles and activities that are relevant to social policy work are identified:

- Identifying policies that can be informed by psychology.
- Educating politicians on the value of input from psychology.
- Communicating effectively with politicians.
- Translating research information so that it is relevant to the policy concerned.
- Understanding the legislative process, identifying when you can have most influence in this process, and following the course of legislation.
- Identifying key legislators and political representatives, and developing on-

going relationships with them.
- Mounting grass-roots campaigns.
- Working with professional organizations and coalitions.

A few of these roles are highlighted in some detail in the box below.

One of the ways for psychologists to make direct connection with policy processes is through the existing policy units currently located in South Africa. This includes the Education Policy Units located in Johannesburg, Durban, and Cape Town, as well as the Centre for Health Policy, and Centre for Social Policy in Johannesburg. Another way is to become active in the Psychological Society of South Africa (PsySSA), the professional association of psychologists in this country, which is attempting to make more direct connections with relevant policy processes when and where appropriate.

Psychologists' roles within policy context

1 *Policy analysis:* A psychologist can influence policy through monitoring the development of policy by analysing policy texts, submitting responses following such analyses, attending public hearings, and observing policy in practice.

2 *Policy formulation:* One direct way of being involved in the policy formulation process would be as a member of a commission, committee, or department that is responsible for the formulation of policy . This would entail a comprehensive range of activities.

3 *Monitoring and evaluation of policy implementation and new initiatives:* One key role for a psychologist would be to monitor and evaluate the way in which policy is being implemented. This could include evaluating pilot projects, which are often used as a form of 'kick-starting' various policies, as well as conducting periodic evaluations of espoused policies.

4 *Conducting research:* A major role for psychologists in policy processes is to conduct studies that inform the content and process of the social policy concerned. This includes conducting research and building theories that influence relevant discourses. The traditional and innovative research knowledge and skills developed by psychologists can play an invaluable role in the policy process.

5 *Facilitating community participation:* The primary role of the psychologist here would be to work with others, within the context of organized groupings, to influence the policy context. This may be for the purposes of exerting pressure around a particular issue, or it may be a particular effort to facilitate citizen involvement and participation in policy development processes generally, for the purposes of general empowerment.

6 *Advocacy:* Advocacy around issues pertinent to various social policies is a well-recognized role for psychologists working within a community perspective. This could be done through individual activities (such as speaking at forums or writing letters to the newspaper), or within the context of organized groupings (for example, working with a group against abuse of women).

7 *Lobbying:* Direct lobbying of policy makers and others in strategic positions is a major business in the United States of America, constituting full-time jobs for thousands of people, including psychologists. This activity entails keeping key policy makers and politicians informed of the issues being lobbied for, and trying to persuade them of a particular position.

While an individual psychologist may choose to be involved in only one or two of the above-mentioned activities, it is important to note the point made by Jason (1991) and Perkins (1995) that a comprehensive strategy that involves involvement in *all* phases of policy development and implementation is the most effective strategy to ensure that one's goals are pursued. The case study outlined in this chapter reflects such a comprehensive approach, albeit still incomplete.

7 Training for policy work

Much of the traditional knowledge-base and skills of psychology are relevant to social policy work. This includes research skills as well as skills in conflict management, facilitation, and general interpersonal skills. It also includes all psycho-social theories that assist in understanding the relevant issues relating to the social policy concerned, and which point to ways of intervening for the purposes of promoting the well-being of all citizens.

Moving into the political arena does, however, demand more than what traditional psychology training programmes prepare one for. Community psychology programmes could, however, provide opportunities to engage with theoretical frameworks that assist in understanding and working within political settings (for example, frameworks to assist in 'systems-thinking' and critical approaches to psychology).

Although it is necessary to learn new skills and insights in order to work effectively within the social policy arena, the process and the abilities to respond in appropriate ways should not be mystified. Besides the fact that many of the skills required can be generalized from the core skills of all psychologists, many of the skills needed to work at this level are and have been learnt through experience on the ground. In South Africa, for example, the struggle against apartheid over the past few decades has prepared many, including psychologists, to engage in political processes. Training in social policy interventions should therefore draw upon existing competencies, and assist in drawing out the ways in which these competencies can be generalized to include work in political settings.

Training in community psychology can play a major role in preparing one to participate in public policy processes. Learning how to conduct action research, which includes a wide range of research and other skills, is one major area of knowledge and skills that can prepare one for this work. Other courses that could be offered within

pre-service or continuing education programmes include (1) theories and practice regarding policy development; (2) information about the legislative process in South Africa, such as names of committees and people relating to specific issues; (3) community development and empowerment relating to facilitating citizen participation in policy development; and (4) research for social policy.

8 Conclusion

In this chapter I have argued the relevance of working at social policy level within the context of a community psychology perspective. Within this context I have highlighted specific factors and dynamics that need to be taken into account when working at the level of social change, with a particular emphasis on social policy processes. Possible roles and activities of psychologists working at this level were then briefly outlined, with a brief discussion on the implications for the training of psychologists. A thread running through all of the above is a particular case study of my involvement in policy development within education from 1991-1998. This was used as a basis for reflecting on the theoretical issues raised in the discussion.

I hope that this chapter has highlighted the importance of social policy interventions within a community psychology approach in South Africa. Psychologists need to recognize their potential power *and* their humble place in influencing social policies. We need to work closely with politicians, and also with other relevant disciplines, professions, and community sectors to ensure a holistic and comprehensive approach to social policy development. It is important, however, that, in our attempt to contribute to the reconstruction and development of South Africa, we do not lose the critical edge that has been sharpened by the struggle against apartheid and for democracy in South Africa. A critical stance should be brought to bear on the policy development processes at all stages. This is a major challenge facing those of us who are engaged in this area of work.

It is also important that policy work does not become a panacea for community work. While good participatory policy development should involve extensive grassroots work, it is easy to become distanced from the day-to-day realities of ordinary citizens as one engages in the often idealistic nature of public policy work.

Within the context of South Africa at present, our immediate challenge is to help develop new policies that improve the quality of life of all citizens, maximizing individual potential and collective well-being. In the medium and long term, the challenge is to monitor policy developments to ensure that they continue to strive towards the principles enshrined in the country's Constitution; to participate in pilot programmes for the purposes of feeding practical learnings into the development of further policy; to conduct solid research work to keep the issues and debates alive and linked to social policy; and to be involved in community work to ensure that the needs of people are always kept at the forefront of the development of social policy, and therefore, social life in South Africa.

Exercises

1 What skills do you need to equip yourself to engage in social policy processes? How can you gain these skills?

2 Identify the skills and insights or theoretical understandings that you *already* have that could be generalized into the social policy setting.

3 What existing bodies of knowledge in psychology do you think can equip you to engage at this level? What other bodies of knowledge, at present ouside psychology, could help you to develop a deeper understanding of the process?

4 Draw up a programme outline for the training of psychologists for policy work, indicating the courses that should be included in such a programme.

5 Identify specific activities that you could engage in to influence social policy.

6 Identify what you consider to be priorities for social policy interventions in South Africa at present.

7 Identify specific activities that could be pursued to foster citizen participation in policy processes.

8 Draw up a simple manual explaining to your colleagues how to engage in the different aspects of the social policy process in South Africa at local, provincial, and national levels. (The APA manual, undated, could assist you in this exercise.

References

AMERICAN PSYCHOLOGICAL ASSOCIATION (APA). (undated). *Psychology in the public interest: A psychologist's guide to advocacy.* Washington: APA Public Policy Office.

ANONYMOUS. (1996). *Becoming an advocate: Legislative strategies for community psychologists.* Handout presented at workshop on public policy at the fifth biennial conference of the Society of Community Research and Action, Chicago.

BOWE, R., BALL, S. J., and GOLD, A. (1992). *Reforming education and changing schools.* London: Routledge & Kegan Paul.

DE JONG, T., GANIE, L., LAZARUS, S., NAIDOO, T., NAUDE, L., and PRINSLOO, E. (1994). *Education support services in South Africa: Policy proposals.* Cape Town: Education Policy Unit, University of the Western Cape.

DE JONG, T., GANIE, L., LAZARUS, S., and PRINSLOO, E. (1995). Proposed general guidelines for a lifeskills curriculum framework. In A. Gordon (Ed.), *Curriculum framework for the general phase of education.* Gauteng: Centre for Education Policy Development.

DEPARTMENT OF EDUCATION. (1997*). Quality education for all: Overcoming barriers to learning and development.* Report of the NCSNET/NCESS. Pretoria: Author.

DEPARTMENT OF EDUCATION. (1998). *Evaluation of the NCSNET/NCESS process.* Pretoria.

DEPARTMENT OF EDUCATION. (1999). *Consultative paper: Special education.* Pretoria.

FACHERTY, A., HOWES, J., and TURNER, C. (1992). What you need is a policy ...! *Educational Psychology in Practice,* 7(4), 237-238.

FOSTER, D., FREEMAN, M., and PILLAY, Y. (Eds.). (1997). *Mental health policy issues for South Africa.* Cape Town: MASA Multimedia.

FULLAN, M. G. (1992). *Successful school improvement: The implementation perspective and beyond.* Buckingham: Open University Press.

HELLER, K., PRICE, R. H., REINHARZ, S., RIGER, S., WANDERSMAN, A., and D'AUNNO, T. A. (1984). *Psychology and community change: Challenges of the future.* Humewood: Dorsey Press.

HEWTON, E. (1982). *Rethinking educational change:* *A case for diplomacy.* England: Society for Research into Higher Education.

JASON, L. A. (1991). Participating in social change: A fundamental value for our discipline. *American Journal of Community Psychology,* 19(1), 1-16.

JONES, B.(1991). *Politics UK.* Hartfordshire: Philip Allan.

KINGFISHER, C. P. (1998). How providers make policy: An analysis of everyday conversation in a welfare office. *Journal of Community and Applied Social Psychology,* 8, 119-136.

LAZARUS, S. (1988). *The role of the psychologist in South African society: In search of an appropriate community psychology.* Unpublished Ph.D. dissertation, University of Cape Town.

LAZARUS, S. (1997). *Discussion paper on the implementation process.* Paper presented to Task Group 6 (Implementation Plan) of the NCSNET/NCESS. Pretoria: Department of Education.

LAZARUS, S. and SEEDAT, M. (1996). *Community psychology in South Africa.* Paper presented at fifth biennial conference of the Society for Community Research and Action, Chicago.

NATIONAL EDUCATION POLICY INITIATIVE (NEPI). (1992). *Support Services.* Report of the NEPI Research Group on Support Services. Cape Town: Oxford.

NATIONAL EDUCATION POLICY INITIATIVE (NEPI). (1993). *Framework Report.* Cape Town: Oxford.

PERKINS, D. D. (1995). Speaking truth to power: Empowerment ideology as social intervention and policy. *American Journal of Community Psychology,* 23(5),765-794.

RAPPAPORT, J. (1977). *Community psychology: Values, research, and action.* USA: Holt, Rinehart & Winston.

RICKEL, A. (1993). Congressional fellowship: Psychology's chance to influence health policy. *The Community Psychologist,* 26(3),13.

SMAIL, D. (1994). Community psychology and politics. *Journal of Community and Applied Social Psychology,* 4, 3-10.

SSLARZ, A. L. (1995). *Psychologists and public policy: What are we to do?* Paper presented at the XXVth Interamerican Congress of Psychology, Puerto Rico.

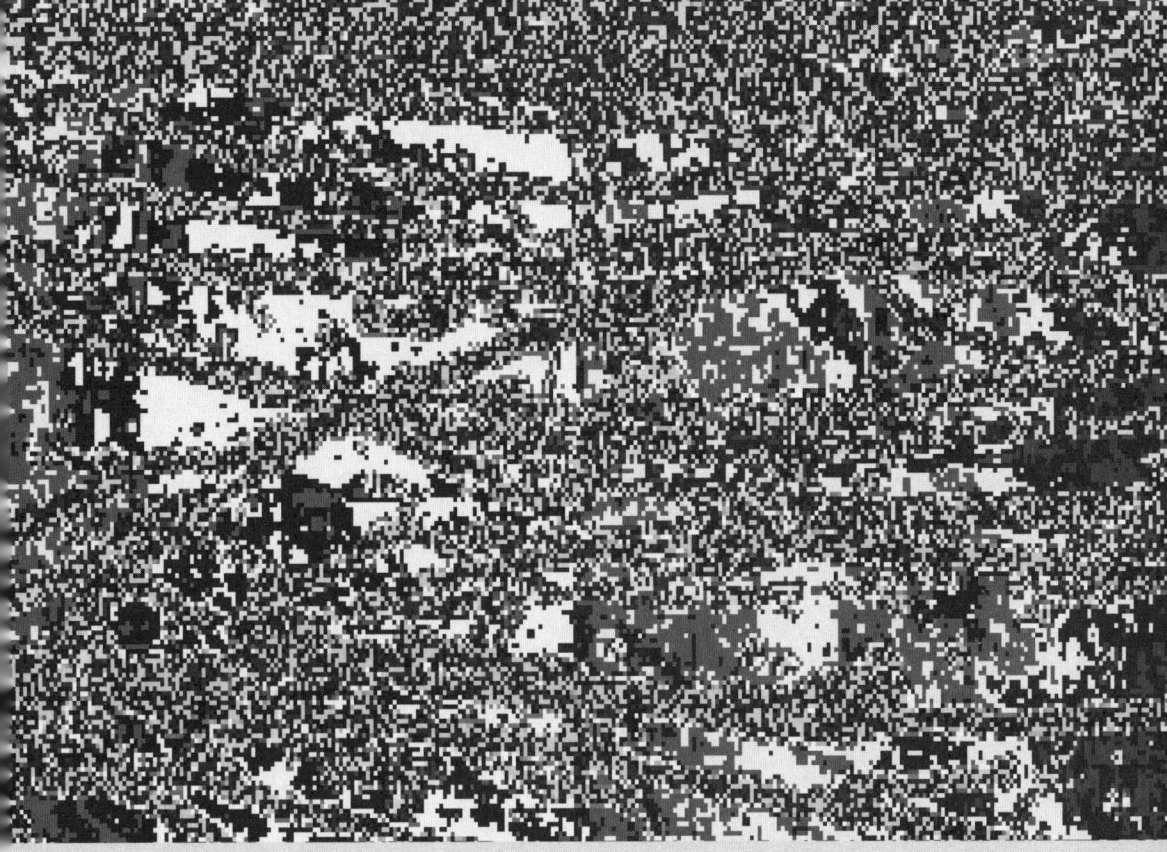

SECTION IV

Perspectives
from elsewhere

18

Community-based community psychology: perspectives from Australia

Brian John Bishop
Christopher Conrad Sonn
Adrian Thomas Fisher
Neil Murray Drew

Study objectives

At the conclusion of this chapter you should be able to:

- describe the history and development of community psychology in Australasia;
- the key principles of community psychology in Australia, particularly Western Australia; and
- understand how community psychology theory and practice can be integrated.

1 Introduction

Community psychology has had a presence in Australasia for two decades. While its educational directions emerged from North America, it has developed a regional distinctiveness. The discipline's development has not been consistent; rather it has lurched from pillar to post. It is only in the past few years that it has started to develop a consistent profile, with a local text book and the development of professional bodies such as the Australian Psychological Society (APS).

The local distinctiveness of community psychology reflects the social and political structures that have underpinned the nature, types, and locations of psychological services. The movement in Australia towards community-based health and mental health services from the 1970s provided a strong foundation of practice based on, and philosophical alignment to, community psychology principles. Much of this had a strong emphasis on the community development, psycho-educational, and community management initiatives and interventions.

There are regional differences in the practice of community psychology in Australia. Community psychology started in Queensland with the arrival of two Americans. They developed a community psychology programme in the 1970s, but it was discontinued (Gardner and Veno, 1979). Community

371

psychology next emerged in Victoria. The Board of Community Psychologists, a professional specialization board within the Australian Psychological Society, was based there, and many informal educational activities developed around it. A strong group was active in Western Australia for many years and was influenced by the community mental health orientation of the late Robyn Winkler at the University of Western Australia. Later, however, Curtin University and more recently Edith Cowan University (ECU)

have become increasingly influential in the field of community psychology. Members in areas of Queensland are now also beginning to reclaim some of the ground that was lost in earlier years.

There are now four graduate programmes in Australia and New Zealand. The earlier programmes at the University of Queensland and at Curtin are no longer running. The current educational opportunities are shown in Table 1.

Table 1 Community psychology programmes in Australia, 1998

UNIVERSITY	STARTED	REQUIREMENTS	DEGREE	EMPHASIS
University of Waikato	1982	Undergraduate degree in psychology	Postgraduate diploma (years 4 to 6), research masters, and Ph.D.	Indigenous issues, social change, and evaluation
Curtin University of Technology	1986	Postgraduate diploma or honours	Masters and Ph.D. by research	Social change, community development, and rural issues
Edith Cowan University	1990	Postgraduate diploma or honours	M.Psych. (year 5 & 6), research masters, and Ph.D.	Community, environmental participatory research, and cultural issues
Victoria University of Technology	1993	Postgraduate diploma or honours	M. Psych. (years 5 & 6), research masters, and Ph.D.	Action research, evaluation, policy and social issues
University of Southern Queensland	1994	Postgraduate diploma or honours	M. Psych. (years 5 & 6), research masters, and Ph.D.	Clinical and community

2 Approaches to community psychology and conceptual principles

The initial intellectual thrust came from North America. Both New Zealand and Australian community psychology theory was based on ecological principles, ecological fit, prevention and, later on, empowerment (Bishop and D'Rozario, 1990; Thomas and Robertson, 1992). While acknowledging the intellectual debt to the United States of America, local historical developments have meant that the current theory and practice are distinctive.

Whereas community psychology in North America developed from clinical psychology, in Australia its origins are broader based. Although influenced by clinical psychology (Curry and Farhall, 1995), community psychology has been shaped by a variety of disciplines within psychology. The range of disciplinary backgrounds of those who came to see themselves as community psychologists were broad. They came from clinical psychology (Curry and Farhall, 1995; Pretty, Andrews, and Collett, 1994), cross-cultural and indigenous psychology (Hamerton et al., 1995; Sonn and Fisher, 1996), from gender equity (Robertson, 1996), and applied social and environmental psychology backgrounds (O'Connor, Pooley, and Cohen, 1997; Syme and Bishop, 1993). The disparate backgrounds of these individuals provided for the integration of differing world views and values that in turn energized the development of new perspectives. These new perspectives are reflected in the following theoretical issues and two associated examples.

2.1 Ecological focus and levels of analysis

The ecological focus has been a central feature of community psychology. For example, Reiff (1968) used six levels of analysis to include individual, family, group, organization, community, and society, while Bronfenbrenner (1977) described four ecological systems to embrace the micro-, meso-, exo-, and macrosystems. These conceptual tools have been used to develop the ecological framework within community psychology at large. We would argue that these tools have come to be seen as more than analytical devices, just as it has been argued that research and statistical methods have moved from being used to purely answer questions to being used as metaphors to frame questions (Girgerenzer, 1988; McCall, 1977). The divisions between systems or levels have become conceptual boundaries where none exist. In the Australian conceptualization of society, individuals exist at all levels and the levels exist in humans. That is, people constitute social systems and social systems are people. Social structures, history, politics, and culture are carried and transmitted from person to person. The structure exists because of the common world views that are so powerful that we do not recognize the extent to which we are prisoners of this socially constructed reality (Sarason, 1984).

A similar argument can be made about Dokecki's (1992) ecological model of research practice. He argues that psychology needs to put more emphasis on research at the qualitative macro-level as depicted in Table 2.

373

Table 2 Dokecki's (1992) methodological framework

LEVEL/ TYPE OF ENQUIRY	MICRO	MACRO
Qualitative/personal	Interpretive studies	World-view studies
Quantitative/ impersonal	Experimental and functional studies	System analytic studies

However, it can be argued that this perpetuates the concept of dichotomies that do not exist. It is argued that the model provides the community with a metaphor that is easily understood. In reality, research needs to address all aspects simultaneously as people operate in all phases. They behave in ways that can be assessed quantitatively and qualitatively and that has meaning at both the micro- and macro-level, and all points in between. This is consistent with Wicker's (1989) notion of substantive theorizing, which encourages in-depth exploration of issues in context.

The implication is that there is an emphasis on process as well as outcome. The de-emphasis on outcomes is a consequence of taking a holistic approach. Attempting to work with people at all levels simultaneously and in an integrated fashion means that it is very difficult, or impossible, to get a grasp on the whole picture. Moreover, the picture changes with time and the particular perspective it is viewed from. Emphasizing a process perspective acknowledges the apparent complexity of social phenomena or processes, and forces us to adopt a tolerance of ambiguity and uncertainty. Accepting that we must work with ambiguity and uncertainty teaches us that

we need to behave much more humbly than positivistic psychology encourages. We do not have better answers than others, but have another perspective of a particular social situation. In attempting to bring about change, recognition of the uncertainty and ambiguity inherent in communities forces us to recognize the political nature of change. The 'objective and dispassionate' role of the professional, 'the polisher of mirrors', is necessarily forgone and we have to join the hurley-burley of social life (Gergen, 1988). 'Scientific purity' is necessarily compromised by the political and social context of community decision making. This is not a weakening of the position of psychological research. Rather what is possibly lost in methodological rigour is gained in ecological validity and relevance. Rigour is compromised, but must be countered by increased effort. As the research process is weakened, the conclusions must be strengthened by observations from a variety of perspectives (Drew and Bishop, 1997; Newbrough, 1995).

2.2 Roles and rhetoric

Throgmorton (1991) extended such argument to the role of the professional who needs to be aware of the rhetoric of those involved in decision making. He argues that the rhetoric of the politicians, the professionals, and the community are different enough for considerable misunderstanding to occur. To be effective in working with decision makers, we need to appreciate their rhetoric and to understand the context in which they work. (See Lazarus's Chapter 17, in this volume.) Throgmorton advocates a role for professionals to work at the place where the roles and rhetoric of the politicians, the community, and the professionals intersect, and to be translators and mediators (see Case study 1).

The process of working at the interface of politicians, the community, and the professionals requires that change is viewed in the longer term and that the ethics and values of the researcher must be frequently questioned. In this role, there is an acknowledgement of the agendas of other parties and acknowledgement of one's own agendas. For example, public consultation in decision making is currently in vogue and has offered community psychologists the opportunity for consultancies (see Case study 2). The motivation of the decision makers in allowing the community some input may well be considerably different from that of encouraging platonic democracy. Similarly, the motivation of the community psychologists may well be about giving the community voice and creating the expectation that the community should be consulted more frequently, whereas the psychologists' rhetoric may be more about making better decisions and easing the process of change.

While the motivations of the parties may be quite different, and while the com-munity psychologists may not approve of the motives of the decision makers, this is the political reality. The decision makers want change for their own reasons and the community psychologists want change for other reasons. We have found it pragmatic to attempt to bring about change by working with decision makers. By implementing their agendas we can also use the opportunity to realize ours. By learning their rhetoric and jargon we can also expose them to ours and slowly attempt to change their frames of reference. (See Lazarus's Chapter 17, in this volume.)

2.3   Knowledge and theorizing

A final issue has been the emphasis put on integrating practice with theory. It has been recognized that objective knowledge is only one component of knowledge (John, 1994; Schön, 1984). Professional knowledge, knowledge that arises from reflecting on professional practice and action research, is seen as a neglected area within much of positivistic psychology. The reflective-generative approach of Dokecki (1992, 1996), or the iterative-generative approach, representing a fusion of professional and objective knowledge, is common. This approach involves valuing local knowledge and building understanding of local contexts and competencies through a process of reflecting on observation and action. This is reflected in the emphasis on narratives as a means of communicating aspects of knowledge that cannot be articulated or are difficult to articulate in terms of objective knowledge. While not endorsing all that postmodernists have written, a social-constructionist position on knowledge has been valuable in conceptualizing community psychology theory in Australia (Gergen, 1988). Similarly, Polkinghorne's (1983) concept of 'assertoric knowledge', and recognition of the relativity of knowledge have also served to inform the idea of integrating practice and theory.

3 Case studies

The following two case studies are included as illustrative examples of the theoretical and applied developments within community psychology in Australia.

3.1 Case study 1 – involvement of communities in research agendas

Substantive theorizing involves grounding the research in a local community context (Wicker, 1989). However, it is possible to go further and involve local communities in setting the research agenda. The following example was part of a larger research project based in rural Western Australia and involving five local government districts. The issues to be researched were negotiated with these communities.

The first aspect of the research was to 'scope' issues: to identify what the communities thought were the major issues confronting them. This was done by identifying the key people in the community. These people were interviewed. The major issue facing the five communities was the sustainability of their communities. This issue was not restricted to these communities, but

rural Australia is facing major problems of survival (Lawrence, 1995). There has been a steady withdrawal of services, such as banking, education, and health.

A major local concern was health services. Four of the shires were serviced by a local hospital. There had been attempts to downgrade the hospital. The communities were very concerned that their hospital was under threat of further downgrading or even closure. The community asked the research team to look at the health issues.

The investigation of the health issues involved a range of activities in collaboration with the communities and the health department. For example, the research team collaborated with the health department to conduct a needs assessment for the region. As there was considerable mistrust between the communities and the health department, a community-based research committee was established to monitor the needs assessment.

The needs assessment survey was very good and the results were not threatening to the health department. It was decided to run a workshop to discuss the outcome of the survey. The health department suggested that two days would be required to provide the appropriate epidemiological information and the needs assessment results. The research team had been asked to facilitate the workshop as they had the trust of the communities. After initially planning fourteen hours of lectures to inform the community, the health department settled for ninety minutes, allowing the community more opportunity to express their concerns. It was obvious that the health department officials were apprehensive about being confronted by hostile members of the communities.

The workshop was well patronized, with over 100 community members attending, as well as state and federal health departments' senior officials. While the health department officials were initially defensive and the communities aggressive, after a period of time the real issues emerged and were discussed. What was clear was that the health department's mistrust of the communities caused a situation where they felt embattled and expected the community would want more than it was possible to provide. By the end of the workshop they appreciated that the community was realistic about the limited funding that was available and simply wanted some input into the broader policy issues. What the research team became aware of was that the community and the health department's world views were different. The health department saw a need for a broader concept of health, including prevention and community health delivery. In the interest of prevention other services would have to be restricted. On the other hand, in the minds of the communities, health was closely associated with the hospital and the local doctor. Thus much of the conflict arose from the parties talking at cross purposes.

This example shows that the role of community psychologists can be one of mediating between the rhetoric of the community and the health department (Throgmorton, 1991). It also shows that working with decision makers can be emancipating for both the community and the professionals. Professionals frequently express considerable surprise in the levels of knowledge of the community, the value of negotiating with the community, and the ease with which they can maintain their professional power if they are prepared to work with the community openly and fairly (Johnson, 1992).

3.2 Case study 2 – community involvement in developing waste minimization programmes

In 1995 the Community Environmental Research Team (CERT) at Edith Cowan University, in Perth, were invited to contribute to the development of a waste minimization and recycling policy for the City of Wanneroo in Perth. Wanneroo is one of the largest and fastest growing local authorities in Western Australia (WA). The committee charged with authorizing the development of the policy had stipulated that there should be public involvement in policy development. From its inception, CERT had been involved in community programmes and intervention in local issues and problems (Wicker and Sommer, 1993). The project illustrates many of the principles discussed earlier in the chapter. This brief review will examine those elements of our approach that were found to be particularly useful.

3.2.1 The context

In many Western democratic countries there has been a marked loss of trust and confidence in politicians, politics, and public officials, which was evident in Case study 1. Laird (1989) called this the 'decline of deference', a decline in the community's willingness to defer important decisions to public officials. This has been linked to a loss of support for the system of government. The evidence indicates that there has been a marked shift towards demands for more participatory democratic processes. There is evidence that in Australia there has been just such a decline of deference (Drew and Bishop, 1997).

Community involvement programmes have the opportunity to re-invest trust in governmental agencies, as community involvement promotes procedural fairness, if done well. Potential benefits include community empowerment and the development of a collaborative relationship between governmental agencies and the community (with lessened conflict).

A risky methodology was proposed. This included an openness to the community; importance of beginning from the ground up; trusting the process; and iterative-generative practice in which the researcher is enriched and informed by the process of being in the community. A substantive approach was also adopted in all its ramifications, and we have attempted to go further by elaborating aspects of the macroclimate, such as the decline of deference.

The proposed strategy consisted of three stages, including the initial scoping exercise to explore ways in which the community wanted to be involved (Drew, O'Connor, and Pooley, 1996). In the first stage the issue of public involvement in the City of Wanneroo was scoped and the community profiled. The scoping exercise identified over three hundred potential stakeholder groups in the community. Information was obtained in a number of ways, including an archival search of local community newspapers and community documents, and a media release

soliciting participation. Stakeholder groups were contacted, asked to complete a brief survey, and invited to participate in a semi-structured interview. A telephone survey of a random sample of 200 residents was also included in this phase. Based on the information provided by the key stakeholders and community members, a detailed involvement strategy was proposed. We were particularly pleased that decision makers provided funding for this stage as this is often not the case. Communities are typically offered a range of involvement strategies selected by the project team.

In stage two, a series of focus groups was used to examine a range of waste minimization and recycling options. The results were summarized and returned to participants for comment as part of the reflective process. A final report including a range of options for the development of the strategy was forwarded to the city officials, who engaged a consultant to conduct a cost benefit analysis of the various alternatives. A discussion paper was distributed to all residents as an insert in the local community newspaper. The discussion paper detailed the community input and the consultants' report on the feasibility of options for waste management and recycling. The final element of stage two was a large-scale community survey and a series of qualitative interviews to explore community preferences and priorities.

Based on the results, a draft policy was drawn up for public review, thus constituting stage three of this project. Overall, the process was designed to be open, transparent, iterative, reflective, procedurally fair, and empowering. This project is another example where community psychologists find themselves at the interface between decision makers and the community (Throgmorton, 1991). Although the initial time line was six months for the entire project, it took a little over eighteen months; the project team worked hard to persuade the decision makers that speed was a false economy. To rediscover trust and confidence takes time. (Also see Lazarus's Chapter 17, in this volume.)

4 Conclusion

In this chapter the history, development, and conceptual underpinnings of community psychology in Australia have been briefly described. While the intellectual heritage can be traced to North America, socio-historical, cultural, and political imperatives have led to a community psychology with a distinctly regional flavour. This is not surprising, in that generally, as seen in the case studies, community psychologists have immersed themselves in the context. They have indeed become active participants in the construction of their social world (Gergen, 1988). This requires a genuine willingness to relinquish power and control in the interests of establishing a meaningful dialogue with a broad range of interpretive communities (Throgmorton, 1991).

The theoretical and conceptual bases are derived from an ecological framework that acknowledges the embeddedness of people in social structures, history, politics, and culture. In common with counterparts in North America there is a general rejection of the positivist worldview and call for the integration of quantitative and qualitative approaches in research and practice. In particular, there is an emphasis on process as well as outcomes. Another important feature of community psychology has been the recognition that community psychologists find themselves working with different groups. Where these groups intersect, there is potential for communication problems, which are exacerbated by the different rhetoric used by each group. It was suggested that the community psychologist then becomes an active translator and mediator.

The shift in emphasis from outcomes to process has heightened the need for tolerance of uncertainty and ambiguity. There are elements of 'suck it and see' in research and practice, where the community psychologist often enters the field without any pre-conceptualizations. The questions and answers emerge as the process unfolds. The temptation to reassert authority and ownership over the process is often strong, and requires confidence in and adherence to the principles of ecological focus, world-view analysis, and empowerment, as described earlier.

The growth and development of community psychology in Australia have waxed and waned over the years. The process has nevertheless yielded a relatively robust, if diverse, identity, and the field continues to expand its horizons. Those in the field are bound by shared beliefs about the process of community research and action. Iterative-generative practice has enriched not only the communities in which we work but also the development of the field. Most community psychologists operating within the iterative-generative framework also find the process liberating. By divesting themselves of the dominant positivistic discourse of psychology, community psychologists can more easily be involved in a transformative process (Prilleltensky and Nelson, 1997; Sampson, 1983), rather than being dispassionate reporters of social change.

Exercises

1 Carefully review Case study 1 and then answer the questions that follow:

1.1 A number of assertions have been made about the motivations and actions of government agencies and officials, yet this is largely speculative. How can these assertions be validated?

1.2 What is the ethical stance of helping a community get its housing needs met, when there are many other communities requiring housing? Were the actions of the research team and the community tantamount to queue jumping, thus disadvantaging some other community?

2 After carefully reviewing Case study 2, consider the following questions:

2.1 Is working with a shire council on middle-class environmental concerns appropriate for community psychologists, when there are more pressing issues, such as oppression, that need to be dealt with?

2.2 Discuss the risks for community psychologists working at the interface between communities and decision makers.

3 Part of the continued oppression of Aboriginal people comes from mining companies' need to access land for exploration and exploitation. Community psychologists have been involved in conducting social impact assessments, in which the impact of major developments on local people is assessed. Part of this process involves 'scoping and profiling' (Taylor, Bryan, and Goodrich, 1990) (see Case study 2). While these techniques can be somewhat complicated, the following exercise is intended to help you understand the potential benefits of careful scoping and profiling.

Imagine yourself as a consultant to the Community Environmental Research Team (CERT), studying the impact of the mining giant Global Uranium's proposed development of a uranium mine in the north-west of Australia. There are three affected communities that may have to be relocated. The company is also promising possible employment for Aboriginal people. In groups or individually:

3.1 Identify the issues that may be of concern to the communities.

3.2 Generate a list of sources of information about the communities, such as community newspapers, local histories, and census data. Also identify who may be influential people and institutions.

3.3 Having generated a list of local factors, evaluate the qualitative costs and benefits of the proposed development.

References

BISHOP, B. J. and D'ROZARIO, P. N. (1990). The contextual effects on the development of community psychology in Australia. *The Community Psychologist*, 24(1), 15-17.

BRONFENBRENNER, U. (1977). Toward an experimental ecology of human development. *American Psychologist*, 32, 513-531.

CURRY, L. and FARHALL, J. (1995). The shift from psychiatric nurse to manager: The design, implementation and evaluation of an action learning program. *Therapeutic Communities – International Journal for Therapeutic and Supportive Organisations*, 16(4), 215-228.

DOKECKI, P. R. (1992). On knowing the community of caring persons: A methodological basis for the reflective generative practice of community psychology. *Journal of Community Psychology*, 20, 26-35.

DOKECKI, P. R. (1996). *The tragi-comic professional: Basic considerations for ethical reflective-generative practice*. Pittsburgh, PA: Duquesne University Press.

DREW, N. M. and BISHOP, B. J. (1997). *Methodology in applied social and community psychology*. ReCAP Research and Technical Report, 97/1. Perth, Australia: Curtin University of Technology, School of Psychology.

DREW, N. M., O'CONNOR, M., and POOLEY, J. A. (1996). *Public involvement in waste minimisation and recycling in the City of Wanneroo*. Local Government Report. City of Wanneroo, Australia.

GARDNER, J. M. and VENO, A. (1979). An inter-disciplinary, multilevel, university-based training program in community psychology. *American Journal of Community Psychology*, 7, 605-620.

GERGEN, K. J. (1988). *Towards a postmodern psychology*. Paper presented at the 23rd International Congress of Psychology, Sydney.

GIRGERENZER, G. (1988). *From tools to theories: The art of theory construction in cognitive psychology*. Paper presented at the 23rd International Congress of Psychology, Sydney.

HAMERTON, H., NIKORA, L. W., ROBERTSON, N., and THOMAS, D. (1995). Community psychology in Aotearoa/New Zealand. *The Community Psychologist*, 28(3), 21-23.

JOHN, I. D. (1994). Constructing knowledge of psychological knowledge: Towards an epistemology for psychological practice. *Australian Psychologist*, 29, 158-163.

JOHNSON, P. T. (1992). *How I learned to harness public controversy to make better decisions*. Paper presented at the Annual Conference of the International Association of Public Participation Practitioners, Portland, Oregon.

LAIRD, F. (1989). The decline of deference: The political context of risk communication. *Risk Analysis*, 9, 543-550.

LAWRENCE, G. A. (1995). *Future for rural Australia: From agricultural production to community sustainability*. Rockhampton, Australia: Central Queensland University Press.

MCCALL, R. B. (1977). Challenges to a science of developmental psychology. *Child Development*, 48, 333-344.

NEWBROUGH, J. R. (1995). Toward community: A third position. *American Journal of Community Psychology*, 23, 9-38.

O'CONNOR, M., POOLEY, J. A., and COHEN, L. (1997). *Service system innovation with Western Australian communities*. A paper presented at the 6th Biennial Conference on Community Research and Action, Columbia, SC.

POLKINGHORNE, D. (1983). *Methodology for the human sciences: Systems of inquiry*. Albany: State University of New York Press.

PRETTY, G. M., ANDREWS, L., and COLLETT, C. (1994). Exploring adolescents' sense of community and its relationship to loneliness. *Journal of Community Psychology*, 22, 346-358.

PRILLELTENSKY, I. and NELSON, G. (1997). Community psychology: Reclaiming social justice. In D. Fox and I. Prilleltensky, *Critical psychology: An introduction* (pp. 166-184). London: Sage.

REIFF, R. (1968). Social intervention and the problem of psychological analysis. *American Psychologist*, 23, 524-531.

ROBERTSON, N. (1996). Reforming institutional responses to violence against women: A comprehensive community intervention project. In D. Thomas and A Veno (Eds.), *Community psychology and social change: Australian and New Zealand perspectives* (pp. 81-104). Palmerston North, New Zealand: Dunmore.

SAMPSON, E. (1983). *Justice and the critique of pure psychology*. New York: Plenum Press.

SARASON, S. B. (1984). If it can be studied or developed, should it be. *American Psychologist*, 39, 477-485.

SCHÖN, D. (1984). *The reflective practitioner: How professionals think in action*. New York: Basic Books.

SONN, C. C. and FISHER, A. T. (1996). Psychological sense of community in a politically structured group. *Journal of Community Psychology*, 24, 417-430.

SYME, G. J. and BISHOP, B. J. (1993). Public psychology: Planning a role for psychology. *Australian Psychologist*, 28, 45-51.

TAYLOR, C., BRYAN, C., and GOODRICH, C. (1990). *Social assessment: Theory, process and techniques*. Canterbury: Centre for Resource Management.

THOMAS, D.R. and ROBERTSON, N. (1992). A conceptual framework for the analysis of social policies. In D. R. Thomas and A. Veno (Eds.), *Psychology and social change: Australian and New Zealand perspectives* (pp. 37-54). Palmerston North, New Zealand: Dunmore.

THOMAS, D. and VENO, A. (Eds.). (1992/1996). *Community psychology and social change: Australian and New Zealand perspectives*. Palmerston North, New Zealand: Dunmore.

THROGMORTON, J. (1991). The rhetorics of policy analysis. *Policy Sciences*, 24, 153-179.

WICKER, A. (1989). Substantive theorising. *American Journal of Community Psychology*, 17, 531-547.

WICKER, A. W. and SOMMER, R. (1993). The resident researcher: An alternative career model centred on community. *American Journal of Community Psychology*, 21, 469-482.

19

Community mental health in the USA: challenges to urban community mental health centres[1]

Elizabeth Sparks

Study objectives

The main objective of the chapter is to acquaint you with the current challenges facing community mental health centres (CMHCS) in the United States of America. After reading and studying this chapter you will:

- have an understanding of the development of the CMHC movement in the United States;
- be able to identify three major challenges facing CMHCS in urban, low-income communities in the United States;
- have a basic understanding of the socio-political forces surrounding urban CMHCS; and
- be able to use the experiences of urban CMHCS in the United States to consider ways in which community mental health in other cultural contexts can avoid becoming marginalized.

1 Introduction

The community mental health movement in the United States has had a difficult history. It began in the early 1900s when reformers struggled to establish humane practices in the treatment of the mentally ill (Sarason and Sarason, 1993). Early reformers believed that psychiatric care for the poor could best be provided in institutions that removed the mentally ill from society. By the 1950s, however, it became clear that these institutions were not effective (Levy, 1969). They were costly, demonstrated poor treatment outcomes, and reflected the discriminatory practices against people of colour[2] that were, and often still are, prevalent in the United States (Prudhomme and Musto, 1973; Wilson and Lantz, 1957). Community mental health was seen as a remedy to the problems in the existing mental health system. The movement gained momentum during the civil rights era in the 1960s, and in 1963 the United States Congress passed legislation establishing the community mental health centres (CMHCS). These centres were located in low-income and rural communities with the goal of improving mental health care for the poor (Bentley, 1994; Ray and Finley, 1994). Their primary goal was to provide comprehensive mental health services to all, regardless of age, psychiatric diagnosis, ethnicity, or socio-economic status.

In this chapter, I discuss three current challenges to urban CMHCS in the United States. The first challenge is the need for these centres to maintain fiscal stability during this period of shrinking government resources and changes in the way mental health services are being funded. I review thirty years of federal legislation on CMHCS, and discuss the impact of these policy changes on the centres' current fiscal difficulties.

The second challenge facing urban CMHCS is the need to provide care to an ever-growing number of seriously ill and uninsured clients. The de-institutionalization of the chronically mentally ill, which began in the 1970s, and the social problems they encounter living in unsupervised, often dangerous community situations have contributed to this problem.

The third challenge is one that is being experienced throughout the entire health care system in the United States, the introduction of managed care. Managed care is a term that has many different meanings. However, it is generally defined as the action of any entity that pays for health care services, public or private, to contain costs while maintaining an established standard of care (Minkoff, 1994). Using the state of Massachusetts as an exemplar, I discuss problems that can result when managed care is implemented in a community mental health system.

I conclude the chapter by identifying ways in which the experiences of urban CMHCS in the United States can be instructive to practitioners in other cultural and political contexts to help them prevent the type of marginalization that occurred in the United States as they develop community mental health systems in their countries.

2 Mental health funding for the poor

The United States has a comprehensive health care system that includes different types of health care providers and delivery systems. One way of categorizing this system is by dividing it into the 'private' and 'public' sectors. The term 'private sector' refers to those services that are paid for either by the individual or through private medical insurance. Services for clients in the private sector tend to be readily available, and represent what is considered to be the most efficient and state-of-the-art medical care available in the United States. The term 'public sector' refers to services that are paid for by one of the two government insurance programmes for those who are elderly, or low-income and/or indigent (Medicaid for the poor/indigent; Medicare for the elderly). Services in the public sector are often provided by the same practitioners and health care facilities that service private sector clients; however, many public sector clients are also serviced by community health care facilities. Within the public sector, CMHCS are an essential component for service delivery, and a majority of their clientele are Medicaid recipients.

2.1 The Medicaid programme

The Medicaid programme was established in 1965 as a federal programme to provide health insurance for persons living at or below poverty level. In order to receive Medicaid assistance, recipients must meet eligibility requirements based on income and undergo re-assessment at regular intervals to determine continuity of coverage in the programme. Contrary to common perception, Medicaid is not a broad entitlement programme that assures access to health care for all poor persons (Dutton, 1981). Eligibility regulations are complex and can vary across the fifty-two American states. For example, most state regulations support Medicaid eligibility for all families who receive public assistance and whose incomes place them below poverty level. However, in certain states, once a family's income rises above this level, but below a certain ceiling, Medicaid coverage is provided only for children under six years of age. And, in some states a family loses its Medicaid coverage entirely when it has annual earnings of $10 000, day-care benefits of $2 528, and food stamp benefits with a cash value of $2 208 (US House of Representatives, 1994).

In 1975 approximately 63 per cent of the United States population with incomes below poverty level were eligible for Medicaid. This number dropped to 50 per cent by 1981 due to changes in eligibility requirements, which left approximately 12,5 million poor

people, including 5 million poor children, with no health care insurance coverage (Center for the Future of Children, 1992; Dutton, 1981). By 1994, the number of persons receiving Medicaid in the general population was down to 40 per cent (Douglas and Torres, 1994).

2.2 The increasing problem of the uninsured

Most individuals who are ineligible for Medicaid remain uninsured (Council on Ethical and Judicial Affairs, 1994). In addition, the ranks of the uninsured have been steadily growing as large numbers of employed persons are unable to either afford health insurance or to obtain it because of pre-existing medical conditions, a situation that leads to denial of coverage by many insurers. Between 1988 and 1991, the number of persons without health insurance rose from 13,4 per cent to 14,1 per cent. This represents approximately 2.8 million people in the United States (Coughlin, Ku, and Holahan, 1994). By 1991, this figure rose to 16,1 per cent. Most uninsured individuals are young adult ethnic minorities (black and/or Hispanic) living in families where no one is employed (US Department of Health and Human Services, 1991). As is the case in other low-income contexts around the world, a person who is without insurance coverage is expected to pay for health care services. Most of the uninsured in the United States cannot afford the cost of routine medical services, and tend to use hospital emergency rooms for critical care.

Thus, funding for medical and psychiatric care for the poor in the United States is provided by Medicaid for those who meet eligibility requirements. For those who do not, or who are unable to obtain private health insurance coverage, medical costs must be personally financed or covered by free care resources that are made available to hospitals and clinics through government funding. In recent years, the growing number of uninsured people requesting services has outstripped available free care resources, making it increasingly difficult for cmhcs and other community-based centres to respond to the need.

3 The socio-political context surrounding urban community mental health care centres

There have been significant differences in the rates of serious illness, both physical and mental, and mortality between European Americans and ethnic minorities in the United States for most of its history (Otten et al., 1990). When community health centres were originally developed, it was expected that they would improve services to such an extent that the existing differentials in health care status between the affluent and the poor, and between European Americans and ethnic minorities would be reduced or eliminated. Unfortunately, the cmhcs have been unable to live up to their early promise, and these differentials have continued. The development of community mental health in the United States has taken place within a socio-political context that is characterized by institutional racism and inequities in the

distribution of resources to the poor. Most ethnic minority groups in the United States experience some degree of oppression and discrimination. However, the discrimination towards African Americans has been particularly virulent since they were first brought to the United States as slaves during the 1700s. In the mental health system, African Americans and other ethnic minorities have historically received inadequate diagnostic and treatment services. While gross abuses of the human and civil rights of ethnic minorities have mostly disappeared due to changes in federal and state laws, racism and discrimination remain beneath the surface and continue to have an effect on the physical and mental health of the ethnic-minority poor in the United States (Campinha-Bacote, 1991; Hutchinson, 1992; Jenkins-Hall and Sacco, 1991; Jones and Corchin, 1982; Wade, 1993).

3.1 The impact of race on health status

Currently, statistics indicate that the overall health status of African Americans and other ethnic minorities has continued to decline, relative to European Americans, despite general improvements in health care standards and practices (Dutton, 1981; Mullings, 1989; Payne and Ugarte, 1989; Starr, 1986). African Americans have been found to have a shorter life expectancy than European Americans (69,6 years compared with 75,2 years, respectively). There are also striking gaps between African Americans and European Americans with regards to infant death rate and mortality due to heart disease, cardiovascular disease, and cancer

(Mullings, 1989; Rice and Winn, 1990; Sullivan, 1989). Ethnic minorities also suffer from higher rates of debilitating and chronic diseases and have been found to have less protection against infectious diseases, a situation that is seen most clearly in the racial differences in the epidemiology of the acquired immune deficiency syndrome (Hutchinson, 1992).

Differences between ethnic groups have also been noted in mental health. Prior to the 1960s, the psychological functioning of African Americans received considerable negative attention in the research literature (e.g., Moynihan, 1965). The personality characteristics of African Americans were perceived as deficient, and little effort was made to identify strengths and resilience (Billingsley, 1968; Hill, 1972). Most theories of counselling have been based on the experiences of European American, middle-class clients and therapists, which has led to the development of a mental health system that uses a restrictive, Eurocentric, and ethnocentric orientation (Carter, 1991; Jones and Korchin, 1982; Ridley, 1984; Sue and Sue, 1990). Many believe that this has contributed to the underutilisation of mental health services by ethnic minorities (Campinha-Bacote, 1991; Sue, 1977; Sue and Zane, 1987).

There also appears to be racial bias in psychiatric assessment and diagnosis (Mukherjee et al., 1983; Wade, 1993). Research has suggested that African Americans are rated as more psychologically impaired by European American therapists. They are also more likely to be labeled as having a chronic syndrome, rather than an acute episode, when diagnosed with psychotic or affective disorders (Jenkins-Hall and Sacco, 1991; Jones and Korchin, 1982; Sata, 1990). The 1980s explosion of social ills, including family disintegration, drug abuse, and increased urban violence, produced a dramatic increase in demand for free and reduced-cost mental health services in low-income communities.

3.2 The face of poverty

Of the 33,6 million individuals living in poverty during 1990, approximately 11 per cent were European American, 32 per cent were African American, and 28 per cent were Hispanic; the remaining 29 per cent were from other ethnic groups (United States Bureau of Census, 1992). The United States Department of Health and Human Services has concluded that both African American and Hispanic female heads of households are more than twice as likely as their European American counterparts to have incomes below poverty level, with more than one-half of the former living below poverty level (United States Department of Health and Human Services, 1990). These families live with various stresses associated with poverty, and as a result have a disproportionate number of both physical and mental health concerns. Unfortunately, they are also disproportionately represented in the 15 per cent of the United States population who do not have access to adequate health care (us Bureau of Census, 1991).

4 Current challenges to community mental health

For over thirty years, cmhcs have struggled to provide services to the poor and the chronically mentally ill from a marginalized position within the larger health care delivery system, largely as a result of limited economic resources. CMHCs located in urban communities, which primarily service ethnic-minority populations, have had to face not only problems with funding, but also institutionalized racism, inequities in the distribution of resources within the health care system, and disproportionately higher numbers of individuals with serious physical and mental health concerns.

In recent years, this task has become increasingly difficult and urban CMHCs are currently facing three major challenges: (1) the need to secure adequate funding in order to maintain their fiscal viability; (2) providing co-ordinated and effective services for a growing number of uninsured individuals; and (3) responding to the national trend in the United States towards the increasing management of health care services.

4.1   Securing adequate funding

Beginning with the Kennedy administration, the federal government assumed leadership for a number of public sector social and health care initiatives, including the establishment of CMHCs in low-income and rural communities. Federal legislation provided funding for the building and implementation of over 2 000 CMHCs across the country, and allowed for four and a half years of federal funding for initial staffing purposes. There was a clear federal expectation that CMHCs would develop alternate sources of funding and become self-sufficient at the end of this initial start-up period. It was also expected that these centres

would be mainstreamed with other health care services, thereby integrating the public and private sector health care systems.

The CMHCs have been plagued with funding difficulties ever since their inception. The expectation that they would become self-supporting within five years was never fully realized, and most, if not all, continued to rely heavily on federal funding. Over the ensuing twenty years, the United States Congress fluctuated in its funding commitment to the CMHCs. In 1976, the original legislation was amended to expand the core of services that CMHCs were able to provide. However, they were not allowed to receive Medicaid reimbursements for providing services to recipients, which was a significant source of lost revenue for the urban CMHCs. By 1981, the U.S. Congress passed legislation that effectively ended large-scale federal support for comprehensive, community-based mental services. However, in the late 1980s, this position shifted once again when legislation was passed that encouraged community care through the expansion of the allowable uses of federal funds in community programmes. This change in the federal mandate was the result of the de-institutionalization movement that was occurring in the United States at that time.

De-institutionalization of the mentally ill began in the late 1970s when thousands of clients who had been hospitalized for years within large public institutions were discharged to community residences and programmes. There was the belief that de-institutionalization would be beneficial to the mentally ill because it would: (1) improve staff-patient ratios; (2) eliminate inappropriate hospital admissions; (3) transfer services to local communities; and (4) facilitate the development of alternatives to institutionalization (James, 1987).

The State Mental Health Planning Act of 1986 (P.L. 99-660) and amendments to Medicare and Medicaid made these two critical programmes more accessible to community-based providers. This Act restored federal leadership in the co-ordination of community-based services to the seriously mentally ill, and enabled CMHCs to obtain Medicaid reimbursements for services to this population.

The Omnibus Budget Reconciliation Act of 1990 (P.L. 101-508) further established federal leadership by mandating that government funding be used primarily for out-patient, community-based services to individuals with serious mental illnesses (Bentley, 1994). This legislation expanded residential support, day support, therapeutic consultation, and case management for the seriously, chronically mentally ill. By the 1990s, most of the federal funding to CMHCs was targeted to services for the chronically mentally ill. This subgroup, however, represented only 1 per cent of the total mentally ill population. The federal funding priority on services for the chronically mentally ill brought about a complex fiscal situation for urban CMHCs. At the time of writing this chapter, they were being forced to seek alternative sources of funding in order to provide services to the non-chronic and uninsured populations in their communities. Most centres have turned to grant funding for this revenue.

Generally, grants are solicited from private foundations and state and federal en-

tities. At times, securing such funding can be difficult, especially when there is a theoretical and ideological 'mismatch' between funders and the CMHCs. This can happen when there are differences in the conceptualization of the problem. For example, one urban CMHC located in a neighbourhood where the rate of violence was quite high had long recognized the need to provide a programme for children living in a low-income housing development. When the request for proposals (RFP) was issued by the federal government for programmes that would 'gang proof' young children, the staff decided to respond. The RFP outlined the government's conceptualization of the problem; however, the CMHC staff had a somewhat different perspective. The government cited research suggesting that gang activity could be prevented in young children by strengthening their decision-making skills and by providing structured, alternative activities. The CMHC staff viewed the problem from a more ecological perspective, and although they agreed with the need to boost children's internal resources, they also recognized the importance of poverty and environmental conditions as contributing factors to youth involvement in gangs. The programme designed by the CMHC was not only aimed at the children, but also included training workshops for parents and job placement assistance to increase their feelings of control over the environment. This approach highlighted the important role played by parents in deterring gang involvement in their children, and targeted significant programme resources to enhance their skills.

Even when grant funding is successfully acquired, there are often restrictions on this funding that can present additional problems. Most grant funding is short-term (one to three years in duration), making it difficult for programmes to have sufficient time to impact complex, multifaceted problems. Also, the total amount of funding and limits on the types of activities that are reimbursable can sometimes restrict the scope of the programmes to such an extent that their effectiveness in ameliorating the targeted problem is questionable. Thus, the federal focus on services for the chronically mentally ill has resulted in a problematic situation for CMHCS. It has forced them to secure alternative funding in order to provide programmes for their non-chronic and uninsured clientele, a task that can sometimes be difficult to accomplish.

4.2 Providing comprehensive and culturally sensitive mental health care

In addition to complexities surrounding funding, urban CMHCS must also contend with providing services to clients who have multiple problems and are more difficult to maintain in the community. During the 1970s and early 1980s, the prototypical CMHC client was an adult of forty years and older, with a major mental illness, who had spent a considerable amount of time in a public institution. He or she had entered the community out-patient mental health system during the period of de-institutionalization, and was maintained relatively successfully in a staffed residential living situation, which was typically a half-way house or group home. Today, this prototypical client has changed. He or she is younger than twenty

years old and becomes mentally ill under a public health care system that provides for only short-term, acute hospital care. The available out-patient treatment has often been uncoordinated and the client has difficulty remaining stable in the community (Pepper, 1987). Many of these young clients exhibit a range of social disabilities that often accompany severe psychiatric disorders, and have been exposed to drug and alcohol use. This has resulted in a dramatic increase in the number of dual-diagnosis (substance abuse and a major mental disorder) patients seeking treatment. Regrettably, public policy and practice in the last decade have not contributed to enhancing the interconnections between substance abuse treatment services and mental health (Pepper, 1987). Family networks for these patients are often overwhelmed, and the community-based systems of care responsible for providing services continue to be underfunded. A brief case vignette presented in the box below helps to illustrate some of the challenges CMHCS face in attempting to provide comprehensive services to this population of young, dual-diagnosis patients.

The case of Sam illustrates the complexities involved in providing comprehensive, community-based mental health care for dual-diagnosis patients. The CMHCS are attempting to meet the needs of these clients, but their funding difficulties, coupled with the complex nature of these clients' service needs, make this an extremely challenging situation.

The case of Sam

Sam is a thirty-year-old African American man who has a twelve-year history of hospitalizations and residential placements. He suffered his first psychotic break when he was a freshman in college at age eighteen, and has been diagnosed with schizophrenia. Sam's first hospitalization was in a small, private general hospital, where he remained for approximately five days. He was transferred to a private psychiatric hospital when he became uncooperative with treatment and refused medication. Sam's course of treatment in the psychiatric hospital was difficult, and it was necessary to obtain an involuntary commitment in order to administer medication. He was subsequently transferred to a public institution, where he remained for another month. Sam's condition eventually stabilized and he was discharged. He was referred for services to his local CMHC and, as a priority-status client, he was placed at the top of the waiting list for assignment to a case manager.

Sam did receive a case manager within a month after discharge. However, it soon became clear that he was unable to continue living at home with his mother. He began using drugs, primarily marijuana and cocaine, and his behaviour was too difficult for his mother to manage. He was arrested by the police at one point, which led to his re-admission to the hospital. There was a waiting list for the residential facility in his home

community, and his case manager was unable to locate a suitable alternative living arrangement. Sam was discharged from the hospital, after being once again stabilized on medication, to his mother's home to await placement in the residential facility. The cycle continued for the next six months while Sam awaited placement; he would stay home for a few weeks; use drugs; become unmanageable at home; wander the streets and get arrested. His mother and other extended family members attempted to monitor his behaviour; however, this became increasingly difficult. Sam often became angry with their efforts to control him and he would 'act out' by using drugs. This led to this repetitive cycle of hospitalizations.

4.3 Responding to public sector managed care

The third challenge facing community mental health is recent and its full impact on service delivery has yet to be realized. This challenge is the implementation of public sector managed care. All managed care plans involve some form of administrative review to measure the amount and appropriateness of health services used by plan members, and a case management procedure to co-ordinate and assure continuity of care. Currently, approximately two-thirds of all individuals with private health insurance are enrolled in managed care plans (Minkoff, 1994).

391

Proposals are also being considered by the United States Congress that would, if enacted, require many millions of individuals, currently covered by Medicare and Medicaid, to join managed health care plans (Minkoff, 1994). Massachusetts is one state that has already entered into such an arrangement for its Medicaid programme.

The trend towards more intensive management of health care services by the insurance industry began in the 1980s as a response to rising health care costs. In 1965, health expenditures in the United States were $39 billion, representing only 6 per cent of the gross national product (GNP). In 1981, this figure rose slightly to 9,8 per cent. By 1991, however, a total of $738 billion was spent on health care, nearly 14 per cent of the GNP (Council on Ethical and Judicial Affairs, 1994). This increase represented both federal government and corporate expenditures. The Federal government's expenditures for health care grew by 20 per cent from 1987 to 1989, faster than social security increases (12,4 per cent), military spending (5,7 per cent), and interest on the national debt (17,8 per cent) (Freudenheim, 1988). In the corporate world, 34 per cent of pre-tax expenses was spent on employee health benefits in 1984, and by 1988, this figure rose to 52,6 per cent (Broskowski, 1991; Califano, 1986).

In general, managed care plans are thought to contain costs through arrangements by which health providers agree to provide a full range of health care services to a set population of patients for a pre-paid sum of money. The provider is responsible for managing the care of these patients, and risks losing money if total expenses exceed the predetermined amount of funds. Under

Managed care plans in the United States

There are primarily two types of managed care plans currently in use within the United States health care system. One type is characterized by health maintenance organizations (HMOs). HMOs are health plans that contract with medical groups to provide a full range of health services for their enrollees for a fixed pre-paid, per-member fee. The second type of plan is called preferred provider organizations (PPOs). These are health plans that encourage savings by establishing a network of preferred providers – health professionals who agree to provide medical services to plan members for discounted rates. Plan members may go 'out of network' to seek medical services from non-affiliated providers; however, they must pay a larger out-of-pocket cost for this option.

the traditional fee-for-service system, only the insurer bore the risk of losing money if costs were excessive. With managed care, this risk is shared by the providers and the insurance companies. These plans are also structured so that both share profits if health care costs are contained. Managed care supporters argue that these plans provide higher quality care, promote preventive medicine, and meticulously monitor quality. Opponents characterize them as bureaucratic systems that diminish choice for all and force health care providers to place saving money before saving lives. The reality of managed care probably lies some-where in between these two positions. Yet, both advocates and opponents agree that managed care has re-shaped the private and public health care delivery systems in the United States.

To gain a better sense of the ways in which managed care has impacted on com-munity mental health, I will outline what has occurred in the urban CMHCs in Boston, Massachusetts since the introduction of pub-lic sector managed care in 1992. The state of Massachusetts entered into a contract with a private managed care company, Massa-chusetts Health Management Association (MHMA), to co-ordinate and manage its Medicaid programme. Facilities providing services to Medicaid recipients were required to have contracts with MHMA that specified the services that would be provided and their reimbursement rate. In order to monitor services, MHMA mandated the length of treatment an individual client could receive, and determined which medical procedures, medications, and mental health services would be reimbursable.

Initially, the CMHCs and Medicaid recip-ients experienced little change in the health care delivery system. Clients were allowed to select providers from a list that included most of the hospitals, private out-patient clinics and CMHCs in the state, and many were able to remain with the facilities that had previously provided their care. Although there was competition between facilities for new clients, the CMHCs were able to negoti-ate reasonable contracts with MHMA and most weathered the initial implementation phase of managed care fairly well. However, some CMHCs did lose a substantial portion

of their funding, and at least one centre in the Boston area closed its doors.

The contract with MHMA ended in 1996, and it was awarded to another managed care company, known as the Partnership. Although it is too early to determine the impact that this transition will have on service delivery, it appears that the Partner-ship plans to conduct a more tightly-con-trolled system. Like all managed care com-panies, the Partnership supports brief treat-ment models; however, it has introduced very strict controls, including the require-ment of an administrative review after the second session with a client. There is also an expectation that clients will receive an array of services, with less reliance on individual psychotherapy and more on day treatment programmes, therapeutic housing, and com-munity supports. These services are typical-ly not provided by CMHCs.

One of the most significant aspects of managed care that urban CMHCs will have to face in the future is capitation. Capitation is the process by which treatment facilities are paid a fixed amount of money on a monthly basis to provide full medical and mental health care to individuals. At the present time, it is unclear whether contracts between the Partnership and CMHCs will take into account the severity of illness among the clientele serviced by a particular facility. For example, Centre A and Centre B may each have a contract with the Partnership where they will be paid $500 per individual per year to provide mental health services for that individual. If both facilities provide care for 1 000 patients, this would mean that the managed care contract would pay a total of $500 000 to each centre for all of the mental health needs for every person serviced during that year. But, if Centre A is a CMHC whose patient population is 70 per cent chronically mentally ill, while Centre B has only 30 per cent of its clientele in this category, the expense-per-individual could vary significantly between the two sites. Centre B may save money during the year, since many of its clients may not exhaust the $500 capitated amount. Centre A, however, is likely to lose money because the level of care needed by its large number of chronically ill patients would more than likely exceed the capitated amount.

A seemingly obvious solution to this situation would be to develop managed care contracts that provide sufficient funding to cover the average cost of care to the clientele serviced by a facility. The difficulty, however, is that competition exists between facilities and each must attempt to provide effective care at the lowest cost. If Centre C indicates to the managed care company that it can provide the same level of care as Centre A for $20 000 less, it is likely to win the contract and Centre A will no longer be a reimbursable site for Medicaid recipients. Thus, CMHCs and other community-based mental health facilities must stay competitive by keeping the cost of their service delivery within a certain range. For urban CMHCs this task can become quite complicated because they often treat clients who have multiple problems and who are seriously ill by the time they seek services. This can make the provision of adequate care costly, forcing these facilities to come up with creative ways to contain costs in order to remain competitive in the health care marketplace.

Another area of concern in public sector managed care is the role that culture will play in the determination of capitation contracts. The urban CMHCs strive to be culturally sensitive in their approach to treatment. However, this sensitivity may necessitate the use of treatment models that are not consistent with brief psychotherapy approaches. For example, the establishment of trust within a therapeutic relationship may take longer with some ethnic-minority clients due to feelings of mistrust and suspicion of institutional systems. Similarly, clients who are recent immigrants may require longer term assistance because of complications resulting from war-related traumas, refugee flight experiences, and re-settlement in the United States. Such experiences have an impact on psychological functioning and must be addressed if clients are to be effectively treated. The extent to which cultural issues and the specific needs of ethnic-minority individuals will be reflected in managed care contracts is unclear at the present time. Hopefully, managed care companies like the Partnership will be sensitive to these issues and will establish capitated rates and administrative procedures that are responsive to the needs of diverse populations.

The final impact of public sector managed care deals with the moral and ethical values inherent in the provision of health care for the poor and chronically mentally ill. Most individuals in the United States believe that health care is a 'right' of every citizen and that the government should provide adequate care for those who are poor and uninsured (Council on Ethical and Judicial Affairs, 1994). Yet, there is less agreement on who deserves to receive this care, and how the government should pay for it. The American democratic system tends to support a decision-making process that protects and promotes the rights of the majority, which can be detrimental to ethnic-minority groups and lead to marginalization. For example, the state of California recently passed legislation by popular vote that made illegal immigrants ineligible to receive public services, including financial assistance, free education, and public-funded medical care. In this instance, the democratic process was used to promote the values and rights of the majority at the expense of a disenfranchised minority group. What occurred in California should make us wary of fully embracing a managed care system that may undermine whatever gains have been made in the provision of community mental health services to the ethnic-minority poor. Care must be taken to insure that benefits for the poor and seriously ill will not be eroded over time, and that all individuals will continue to have access to an adequate level of health care regardless of their ability to pay.

Guaranteeing such a public sector mental health system may be difficult. The United States has long had an ambivalent relationship with its ethnic-minority poor and chronically mentally ill citizens. As recently as 1992, research indicated that the most insoluble problem facing public health systems was the difficulties individuals have in accessing health care when providers refuse to treat those who are not covered by Medicaid (Center for the Future of Children, 1992). Many health care facilities have policies and practices that pay little attention to issues of access, resulting in barriers

to care for many ethnic-minority and poor individuals. Also, providers may have negative attitudes towards groups of patients defined by race or ethnicity, or economic status that interfere with their ability to provide effective services. These non-financial, institutional barriers to care must be addressed by managed care companies if there is to be equity between the private and public health care systems.

Urban CMHCs are currently facing a number of serious challenges that will affect their ability to provide comprehensive, culturally-sensitive, and effective services to the ethnic-minority poor and seriously mentally ill in the future (Baler, 1994; Broskowski and Eaddy, 1994; James, 1987). If they are to remain effective providers in a mental health system characterized by managed care, they must find creative ways to keep their costs competitive while also providing the services needed. Some of the urban CMHCs and other community-based centres are attempting to address this challenge through developing effective time-limited treatment approaches. Others are also considering the possibility of mergers, or partnerships, as a means of maximizing resources and co-ordinating services.

5 Lessons that can be learned

The current challenges impacting urban CMHCs in the United States can be instructive for mental health workers in other cultural and political contexts who are developing community-based services for the poor. The experiences of these centres are particularly relevant to South Africa because both countries share a history of racism and discrimination against people of colour.

Each country is also currently facing the challenge of establishing equity in health care services for the poor. The CMHCS in the United States were based on a mental health model of community psychology, and their focus has been on prevention and intervention with the sorts of mental health problems that affect large numbers of community residents. Although the environment was taken into account in the conceptualization of mental health problems, urban CMHCS have tended to allocate most, if not all, of their resources to services for the individual and his or her family. In thinking about the model of community psychology that should be used to develop a community mental health system, the experiences of the CMHCS in the United States suggest that it is necessary to expand beyond a mental health model (see also Chapters 2, 5, and 6 in this volume for a more complete discussion of these models). It will be important to allocate a substantial portion of the system's resources to interventions that change not only the psychological state of individuals, but also the environmental conditions that affect their lives, such as housing, employment, and transportation. In this way, the system will incorporate the mental health model with the ecological and social action perspectives.

A second lesson that can be drawn from the experiences of CMHCS in the United States is related to the complexities surrounding funding. The sources of funding for CMHCS have historically been conditional and restrictive. It will be important

for community mental health systems in other cultural contexts to have multiple and varied sources of funding. In this way, centres will be able to maintain a measure of flexibility in the direction and intent of their services. Efforts should also be made to secure funding that allows for a range of prevention, intervention, and social action programmes so that mental health services for the poor will not become individually focused and marginalized as they did in the United States.

6 Conclusion

Urban CMHCS in the United States are currently facing three major challenges: (1) maintaining adequate funding to meet the mental health needs of community residents; (2) providing comprehensive and culturally-sensitive care for a growing number of seriously ill and uninsured clients; and (3) responding to the national trend towards public sector managed care. This latter challenge is the most significant, and has forced urban CMHCS to re-examine their service delivery systems.

The experiences of urban CMHCS in the United States can be instructive to those in other cultural contexts who are developing community mental health systems. In the United States, the mental health model of community psychology was used almost exclusively, resulting in a system characterized by individualized treatment approaches. It is important to think critically about the model of community psychology that will be used to frame the community mental health system, and to consider using a more ecological perspective. This will enable the community centres to address the environmental and structural factors that negatively impact the lives of clients. It is also important for such a system to have diverse sources of funding that can support comprehensive efforts in prevention, intervention, and social activism. It is hoped that community mental health systems in other cultural contexts can avoid the marginalization of services for the poor that was experienced in the United States.

the mental health workers and determine whether they are facing similar problems in their programmes. If they are, discuss what is being done to address them. If they are not, determine what may be helping the centres avoid these problems.

Exercises

1 Using the community mental health system in the United States as an example, discuss the possible pros and cons of developing a mental health system in low-income situations that primarily relies on government funding.

2 In South Africa and the United States, there are a large number of individuals without health insurance or the financial resources necessary to pay for health care services. Review the section in the chapter pertaining to the problem of the uninsured in the United States. Discuss whether the situation is similar in your context, and if so, think about ways that the community health system might respond to this challenge.

3 The chapter highlights three current challenges facing urban CMHCs in the United States. Conduct a site visit to a community mental health centre (or its equivalent) in your area. Talk with

Notes

1 I would like to thank Drs Herbert Joseph, Jr. and Janet Anderson for sharing their experiences as directors of urban, community-based mental health facilities. They are successfully steering their centres through public sector managed care in Massachusetts, and their thoughts and insightful observations were instrumental in helping to make sense of the current and future challenges to CMHCs in the United States.

2 Throughout this chapter, the terms 'people of colour' and 'ethnic-minorities' are used interchangeably. In the United States, both terms refer to individuals who are of other-than-European descent and who represent a numerical minority in the population. The most recent census (1996 data) reports that whites (European Americans) constitute 75 percent of the United States population; 11 percent are black; 10 percent are Hispanic; and 4 percent are 'other', which includes American Indian and Asian/Pacific Islanders.

References

BALER, S. G. (1994). Community mental health in the year 2001: Is there a place for CMHCs? *Administration and Policy in Mental Health,* 21(4), 325-333.

BENTLEY, K. J. (1994). Supports for community-based mental health care: An optimistic review of federal legislation. *Health and Social Work,* 19(4), 288-294.

BILLINGSLEY, A. (1968). *Black families in America.* Englewood Cliffs, NJ: Prentice-Hall.

BROSKOWSKI, A. (1991). Current mental health care environments: Why managed care is necessary. *Professional Psychology: Research and Practice,* 22(1), 6-14.

BROSKOWSKI, A. and EADDY, M. (1994). Community mental health centers in a managed care environment. *Administration and Policy in Mental Health,* 21(4), 335-352.

CACI (1991). *The sourcebook of zip code demographics.* Washington, DC: US Department of Public Health.

CALIFANO, J. A., JR. (1986*). America's health care revolution: Who lives? Who dies? Who pays?* New York: Random House.

CAMPINHA-BACOTE, J. (1991). Community mental health services for the underserved: A culturally specific model. *Archives of Psychiatric Nursing,* 5(4), 229-235.

CARTER, R. T. (1991). Cultural values: A review of empirical research and implications for counselling. *Journal of Counselling and Development,* 70, 164-173.

CENTER FOR THE FUTURE OF CHILDREN. (1992*). The future of children: U.S. health care for children.* Los Altos, CA: The Packard Foundation.

COUGHLIN, T. A., KU, L., and HOLAHAN, J. (1994). *Medicaid since 1980: Costs, coverage and shifting alliance between the federal government and the states.* Washington, DC: The Urban Institute Press.

COUNCIL ON ETHICAL AND JUDICIAL AFFAIRS. (1994). Ethical issues in health care system reform. *Journal of the American Medical Association,* 272(13), 1056-1062.

DOUGLAS, R. L. and TORRES, R. E. (1994). Evaluation of a managed care programme for the non-Medicaid urban poor. *Journal of Health Care for the Poor and Underserved,* 5(2), 83-98.

DUTTON, D. (1981). Children's health care: The myth of equal access. In U.S. Department of Health and Human Services (Ed.), *Better health for our children* (pp. 357-441). Washington, DC: Public Health Service.

FREUDENHEIM, M. (1988, November). US health care spending continues sharp rise. *New York Times,* p. A1.

HILL, R. B. (1972). *The strengths of black families.* New York: Emerson Hall.

HUTCHINSON, J. (1992). AIDS and racism in America. *Journal of the National Medical Association,* 84(2), 119-124.

JAMES, J. F. (1987). Does the community mental health movement have the momentum needed to survive? *American Journal of Orthopsychiatry,* 57(3), 447-451.

JENKINS-HALL, K. and SACCO, W. P. (1991). Effect of client race and depression on evaluations by white therapists. *Journal of Social and Clinical psychology,* 10, 322-333.

JONES, E. E. and KORCHIN, S. J. (1982). *Minority mental health.* New York: Praeger.

LEVY, L. (1969). Financing, organisation and control: The problem of implementing comprehensive community mental health services. *American Journal of Public Health,* 59, 40-47.

MINKOFF, K. (1994). Community mental health in the nineties: Public sector managed care. *Community Mental Health Journal,* 30(4), 317-321.

MOYNIHAN, D. P. (1965). *The Negro family: The case for national action.* Washington, DC: Government Printing Office.

MUKHERJEE, S., SHUKLA, S., WOODLE, J., ROSEN, A.M., and OLARTE, S. (1983). Misdiagnosis of schizophrenia in bipolar patients: A multiethnic comparison. *American Journal of Psychiatry,* 140, 1571-1574.

MULLINGS, L. (1989). Inequality and African-American health status: Policies and prospects. In W. V. Horme (Ed.), *Race: Twentieth century dilemmas – twenty-first century prognoses* (pp. 155-182). Madison, WI: University of Wisconsin Institute on Race and Ethnicity.

OTTEN, M. W., TEUTSCH, S. M., WILLIAMSON, D. F., and MARKS, J. (1990). The effect of known risk factors on the excess mortality of black adults in the United States. *Journal of the American Medical Association,* 263, 845-850.

PAYNE, K. W. and UGARTE, C. A. (1989). The office of minority health resource center: Impacting on health related disparities among minority populations. *Health Education*, 20, 6-8.

PEPPER, B. (1987). A public policy for the long-term mentally ill: A positive alternative to reinstitutionalisation. *American Journal of Orthopsychiatry*, 57(3), 452-457.

PRUDHOMME, C. and MUSTO, D. F. (1973). Historical perspective on mental health and racism in the United States. In B. M. Willie (Ed.), *Racism and mental health* (pp. 45-63). Pittsburgh, PA: University of Pittsburgh Press.

RAY, C. G. and FINLEY, J. K. (1994). Did CMHCS fail or succeed? Analysis of the expectations and outcomes of the community mental health movement. *Administration and Policy in Mental Health*, 21(4), 283-293.

RICE, M. F. and WINN, M. (1990). Black health care in America: A political perspective. *Journal of the National Medical Association*, 82, 429-437.

RIDLEY, C. R. (1984). Clinical treatment of the nondisclosing black client. *American Psychologist*, 39, 1234-1244.

SARASON, I. G. and SARASON, B. R. (1993). *Abnormal psychology: The problem of maladaptive behavior*. Englewood Cliffs, NJ: Prentice Hall.

SATA, L. (1990). *Working with persons from Asian backgrounds*. New York: Hahnemann University.

STARR, P. (1986). Health care for the poor: The past twenty years. In D. Weinberg (Ed.), *Fighting poverty: What works and what doesn't* (pp.107-132). Cambridge, MA: Harvard University Press.

SUE, D. (1977). Community mental health services to minority groups. *American Psychologist*, 32(8), 616-624.

SUE, D. W. and SUE, D. (1990). *Counselling the culturally different*. New York: John Wiley and Sons.

SUE, S. and ZANE, N. (1987). The role of culture and cultural techniques in psychotherapy: A critique and reformulation. *American Psychologist*, 42, 37-45.

SULLIVAN, L. W. (1989). Shattuck lecture: The health care priorities of the Bush administration. *New England Journal of Medicine*, 321, 125-128.

US BUREAU OF CENSUS (1991). *Current population reports: Poverty in the United States – 1991*. Washington, DC: Government Press.

US BUREAU OF CENSUS (1992). *Statistical abstracts of the United States: 1992*. Washington, DC: Government Press.

US DEPARTMENT OF HEALTH AND HUMAN SERVICES (1990). *Health status of minorities and low income groups*. Washington, DC: Public Health Services.

US DEPARTMENT OF HEALTH AND HUMAN SERVICES (1991). *Health status of the disadvantaged*. Washington, DC: Public Health Services.

US HOUSE OF REPRESENTATIVES (1994). *Commission on ways and means: Green Book*. Washington, DC: US Government Press.

WADE, J. C. (1993). Institutional racism: An analysis of the mental health system. *American Journal of Orthopsychiatry*, 63(4), 536-544.

WILSON, D. and LANTZ, E. (1957). The effect of cultural change in the Negro race in Virginia as indicated by a study of state hospital admissions. *American Journal of Psychiatry*, 14, 25-34.

glossary

Advocacy

To speak up; to plead the case of oneself and/or others; to champion a cause. Also refers to speaking and acting on behalf of people whose rights may be in jeopardy.

Alienation

From a Marxist perspective it refers to the mechanism whereby capitalists expropriate the surplus value of workers' labour, and the condition of having one's creative work treated as a commodity.

Alternative psychology

For the purposes of this book alternative is used synonymously with 'critical' and 'relevant' to refer to those perspectives that are critical of the positivist approaches in psychology and attempt to present social contextual understandings of psychology.

Analytic epidemiology

Studies causal and protective factors to explain why health-related outcomes occur and whether interventions work.

Assertoric knowledge

Neither universal nor objective, it is perspectival and offered to the community of interest as a contribution to the public discourse or debate. Its value is in the contribution it makes to the debate about issues of concern, not the extent to which it is irrefutable.

Bracketing

A mental exercise in which the researcher identifies and then sets aside taken-for-granted assumptions in a social context.

Capitalism

A form of economic organisation, prevalent especially in the West since the industrial revolution, in which some own the means of production while others have to sell their labour.

Civil society

This notion is drawn from the work of the Italian Marxist, Gramsci. He broadened the Marxist ideas of class struggle to include a public space outside of the state where there is a struggle to assert ideological dominance.

Communicative action

Dialogue can take place if there is no domination by one participant or perspective, and all have equal opportunity to express themselves.

Conscientization

The process whereby an individual or group develops a critical understanding of their situation, what constructs it, and what the root cause of problems is.

Consciousness-raising

The process that leads women and men to see the connections between individual experiences, gender, societal structures, and social processes so that there is an understanding of how the personal is political.

Descriptive epidemiology

Describes the occurrence of disease and other health-related characteristics in human populations in terms of person (the who: age, sex, social class), place (the where: geographic location), and time (the when: season, day of week, time of day, day of month).

Dialogue

The exchange of views and reciprocal interaction between the researcher and the community.

Distanciation

Improving one's understanding of a situation by standing outside it and viewing it from a distance.

Diversity

Diversity can be in terms of gender, sexuality, ethnicity, religion, and physical and mental condition.

Dual-diagnosis clients

These are individuals who meet DSM-IV criteria for both a major mental illness diagnosis, usually schizophrenia or some

other psychotic disorder, and a substance-related disorder.

Empowerment

Reflects the idea that people and communities can actively manage or control their own lives. Implicit in this belief is the recognition that many social arrangements and institutions are inherently disempowering.

Epidemiology

Applied research that studies the distribution and determinants of health-related conditions and events in populations, and applies this information to the control of health problems.

Epistemology

A branch of philosophy concerned with how we know what we know and the justifications made for knowledge claims.

Experimental evaluation

A study in which the experimenter has some control of the conditions in which the study takes place and some aspects of the independent variables being studied, including assignment of study participants.

External validity

An evaluation design is externally valid if it is effective in a specific experimental instance.

False consciousness

According to the Marxist perspective this refers to the incorrect ideas people have about their relations to other people, particularly a failure to see this as a relationship of economic exploitation.

Formative evaluation

Focuses on ensuring that a programme is carefully planned and designed, and that the objectives and implementation phases are carefully defined.

Gender

The characteristics and practices that are regarded by society to be appropriate to women and men; also refers to the socially constructed meanings of femininity and masculinity.

Gender oppression

The power relationship between women and men as groups, which manifests in structured inequality of access to material and social resources so that men have privileged access over women.

Human agency

At the broadest level it refers to the fact that humans create and are able to change social reality. This view challenges the idea that humans are passive and is related to the concept of collective agency, which refers to the ability of a class of people to decide on a course of action and to carry it out.

Human subjectivity

This refers to an understanding of how humans interpret and construct their own reality. It suggests that there is an interaction between ideological and political structures and the lived experiences of humans.

Idealism

Treating everything as if it were words or ideas.

Ideology

A system of ideas or norms that direct social or political action. The Marxist usage of this term is more specific in that it refers to those processes that distort reality by disguising class conflict and inequality. Thus ideology operates as false consciousness.

Impact evaluation

Evaluating the net effects. Impact may refer to programme effects for the larger community and is in this sense wider than outcome evaluation.

Incidence

Incident cases are the number of new cases reported during a specified period in a defined population, such as the number of head injuries among males living in Johannesburg during 1997.

Internal validity

An evaluation design is internally valid if it is effective in a specific experimental instance. Internal validity shows that the intended programme outcomes are a result of the programme and not of influences outside of the programme.

Interpellation

The process through which ideologies 'call out' or 'hail' individuals to occupy certain social positions.

Interpretative communities

These are the different groups in society, each with a different set of rules and conventions that govern the way they communicate within the group. When the rules and conventions differ between groups there is the potential for poor communication, or what researchers call abnormal discourse.

Interpretative evaluation

Refers to an evaluation approach that does not judge the nature of what is evaluated as good or bad, valuable or unworthy, but recognizes that these judgements are entirely relative to the people making the judgements, coming from their own viewpoints and contexts.

Local knowledge

The collection of ideas and assumptions that are used by a community to guide, control, and explain actions within a specific setting.

Marxism

There is a large body of literature drawing on the work of Karl Marx, variants of which are referred to as neo-Marxism. It is a critique of capitalism, suggests a method for the analysis of society (historical-materialism), and argues for a new social order that is not exploitative and oppressive.

Means of production

The property, machines, and money needed to produce goods, typically owned by capitalists.

Model

This refers to a representation of reality, or a framework for understanding and conducting research and interventions.

Morbidity

Refers to non-fatal instances of a disease.

Mortality

Refers to fatal cases of a disease. Mortality data (fatalities) often do not fully reflect the extent of a particular problem, as many serious social problems, such as injuries due to violence, occur widely but are mostly non-fatal.

Needs assessment

An analysis of a situation in which one determines what the problems and needs are in a community and how problems are linked together.

Ontology

A branch of philosophy concerned with existence and the nature of things that exist.

Outcome evaluation

A study of whether or not a programme produced the intended effects.

Paradigm

A set of principles and beliefs either implicit or explicit that provides a framework for understanding social reality. It often refers to assumptions about knowledge, human nature, and science.

Participation

The capacity for influencing the decision-making process or the involvement of community members in the research process.

Participatory evaluation

Refers to the inclusion of some or all parties to an evaluation, as opposed to having an external, 'objective' expert doing the major part of the research.

Participatory research (PR)

Involves a dialogical relationship between researcher and community, in which the community's needs and problems form the reference point to which the entire research process is accountable.

People-centred development

An approach where development is seen as a process whereby members of a society increase their personal and institutional capacities to mobilise and manage resources, which leads to participation in the intervention and implementation processes.

Philosophy

The rational investigation of questions about the existence of knowledge and ethics.

Positivistic evaluation

A positivistic perspective assumes that the subject matter is independent of the observer-researcher as a true factual world 'out there'. The evaluator therefore strives to capture this truth objectively without bias or contamination and does this by remaining separate and uninvolved.

Post-modernism

It is both a philosophy and a theory of society and focuses on the interpretation of text and discourse. It emphasizes the local and specific context of knowledge.

Praxis

The circular relationship between understanding and practice; a form of social intervention that is at one and the same time an idea and an action.

Prevalence

Prevalent cases are all cases of a particular disease or phenomenon and therefore include existing and new cases, but exclude people that have died or recovered. For instance, prevalent cases of brain injury include everyone injured in a particular year, plus all who had sustained brain injury prior to that time and had not yet died.

Problematizing

The process of beginning to see that one's understanding of a situation is limited, and that this in turn is limiting effective action, thereby creating the opportunity for alternative ways of understanding and action.

Process evaluation

A study of what goes on while a programme is in progress. It usually incorporates a process of programme monitoring to establish whether the intervention is being implemented as planned, and so can serve as an early warning system.

Progressive

Sometimes used as a synonym for Marxist. In South Africa commonly used to distinguish liberals from socialists or Marxists. Also used interchangeably with critical.

Proletariat

Those who do not own the means of production; the working class.

Quasi-experimental evaluation

In a quasi-experimental evaluation the treatment and comparison groups are selected non-randomly, but some controls are introduced to minimise threats to validity.

Reflective-generative or practice

A process of theory and practice development in which theory informs practice and practice informs theory. It is a reflective process in which both conceptual and experiential knowledge are advanced.

Reflexivity

The way in which understanding and theories have an efct on the conditions they are trying to describe.

Social movements

Refers to groupings outside the formal parliamentary structures that arise in response to social issues. They operate in the space outside of political parties and serve as a mechanism for highlighting a range of social concerns.

Surplus value

Only part of the wealth produced by a worker is needed to provide in his/her needs and keep him/her happy. The rest is surplus value and is expropriated by the capitalist.

Summative evaluation

This form of evaluation has a retrospective focus, and involves an attempt to establish the outcomes, effects, or impact of the programme by observation or measurement.

Systematic evaluation

Systematic approaches to evaluation conceptualize social programmes as entities reflecting a number of different stages or phases in planning and implementation.

Thematic universe

The ideas, values, hopes, and concepts by which people live.

Totalitarian state

A state that allows very little freedom, seeking to control all aspects of behaviour. Most so-called Marxist states were of this sort.

Trauma counselling

Refers to interventions in which traumatic events are re-experienced and worked through.

recommended readings

APPIGNANESI, R. (1994). *Marx for beginners.* Cambridge: Icon Books.

BERGLUND, A. I. (1976). *Zulu thought patterns and symbolism.* Cape Town: David Philip.

BIN-SALLIK, M. (1991). *Aboriginal tertiary education in Australia* (2nd ed.) Underdale, South Australia: Aboriginal Studies Key Centre, University of South Australia.

BISHOP, B. J. and D'ROZARIO, P. N. (1990). The contextual effects on the development of community psychology in Australia. *The Community Psychologist,* **24**(1), 15–17.

BRONFENBRENNER, U. (1977). Toward an experimental ecology of human development. *American Psychologist,* **32**, 513–531.

BULHAN, H. A. (1985). *Frantz Fanon and the psychology of oppression.* New York: Plenum Press.

BUTCHART, A. and SEEDAT, M. (1990). Images of community and implications for South African psychology. *Social Science and Medicine,* **31**, 1093–1102.

CURRY, L. and FARHALL, J. (1995). The shift from psychiatric nurse to manager: The design, implementation and evaluation of an action learning program. Therapeutic communities. *International Journal for Therapeutic and Supportive Organisations,* **16**(4), 215–228.

DAWES, A. R. L. (1986). The notion of relevant psychology with particular reference to Africanist pragmatic initiatives. *Psychology in Society,* **5**, 28–48.

DIXON, J. (1995). Community stories and indicators for evaluating community development. *Community Development Journal,* **30**(4), 327–336.

DOKECKI, P. R. (1992). On knowing the community of caring persons: A methodological basis for the reflective-generative practice of community psychology. *Journal of Community Psychology,* **20**, 26–35.

DOKECKI, P. R. (1996). *The tragi-comic professional: Basic considerations for ethical reflective-generative practice.* Pittsburgh, PA: Duquesne University Press.

DONALD, D. R. and HLONGWANE, M. M. (1989). Issues in the integration of traditional African healing and Western counseling in school psychological practice: Three case studies. *School Psychology International,* **10**, 243–249.

DREW, N. M. and BISHOP, B. J. (1997). *Methodology in applied social and community psychology.* ReCAP Research and Technical Report, Curtin University, 97/1.

DREW, N. M., O'CONNOR, M., and POOLEY, J. A. (1996). *Public involvement in waste minimisation and recycling in the City of Wanneroo.* Perth: School of Psychology, Edith Cowan University.

DUFFY, K. G. and WONG, F. Y. (1996). *Community psychology.* Boston: Allyn and Bacon.

EDWARDS, D. J. A. (1991). Duquesne phenomeno-
logical research method as a special class of case
study research method. In Van Vuuren, R.,
Dialogue beyond polemics. Pretoria: HSRC.

ELDEN, M. and LEVIN, M. (1991). Cogenerative
learning: Bring participation into action research.
In W. Foote Whyte (Ed.), *Participatory Action
Research*. London: Sage.

FANON, F. (1967). *The wretched of the earth*.
Ringwood, Australia: Penguin.

FERREIRA, M., MOUTON, J., PUTH, G., SHURINK,
E., and SHURINK, W. (1988). *Introduction to qualitative research methods*. Pretoria: HSRC.

FISHER, E. P., OWEN, R. R., and CUFFEL, B. J.
(1996). Substance abuse, community service use,
and symptom severity of urban and rural residents
with schizophrenia. *Psychiatric Services*, **47**(9),
980–984.

FREIRE, P. (1972). *Pedagogy of the oppressed*.
Ringwood, Australia: Penguin.

GARBARINO, J. (1992). *Children and families in the
social environment* (2nd ed.). New York: Aldine de
Gruyter.

GARDNER, J. M., and VENO, A. (1979). An interdisciplinary, multilevel, university-based training
program in community psychology. *American
Journal of Community Psychology*, **7**, 605–620.

GILLILAND, B. E. and JAMES, R. K. (1997). *Crisis
intervention strategies*. Pacific Grove, CA:
Brooks/Cole.

GOOSEN, M. and KLUGMAN, B. (Eds.). (1996). *The
South African women's health book: The women's
health project*. Cape Town: Oxford University Press.

GUMEDE, M. V. (1990). *Traditional healers: A medical
doctor's perspective*. Cape Town: Skotaville.

HAMERTON, H., NIKORA, L. W., ROBERTSON, N.,
and THOMAS, D. (1995). Community psychology
in Aotearoa/New Zealand. *The Community
Psychologist*, **28**(3), 21–23.

HENGGELER, S. W., and SANTOS, A. B. (Eds.).
(1997). *Innovative approaches for difficult-to-treat
populations*. Washington, DC: American
Psychiatric Press.

HOLDSTOCK, T. (1979). Indigenous healing in South
Africa: A neglected potential. *South African
Journal of Psychology*, **9**, 118–124.

HUMPHREYS, K. and RAPPAPORT, J. (1993). From
the community mental health movement to the
war on drugs: A study in the definition of social

problems. *American Psychologist*, **48**, 892–901.

IVEY, A. E., IVEY, M. B., and SIMEK-MORGAN, L.
(1997). *Counseling and psychotherapy: A multicultural perspective*. Boston: Allyn and Bacon.

JAGGER, A. M. and ROTHENBERG, P. S. (1995).
*Feminist frameworks: Alternative accounts of the
relations between women and men* (3d ed.). New
York: McGraw-Hill.

JOHN, I. D. (1994). Constructing knowledge of psychological knowledge: Towards an epistemology
for psychological practice. *Australian Psychologist*,
29, 158–163.

KAMENKA, E. (Ed.). (1987). *The portable Karl Marx*.
London: Penguin.

KITSHOFF, M. (1996). *Kaleidoscope of African independent churches*. Lewiston: Edwin Mellen.

LAIRD, F. (1989). The decline of deference: The
political context of risk communication. *Risk
Analysis*, **9**, 543–550.

LAWRENCE, G. A. (1995). *Future for rural Australia:
From agricultural production to community sustain-
ability*. Rockhampton, Qld.: Central Queensland
University Press.

LAZARUS, A. (Ed.). (1996). *Controversies in managed
mental health care*. Washington, DC: American
Psychiatric Press.

LEVINE, M. and PERKINS, D. V. (1997). *Principles of
community psychology: Perspectives and applications*
(2nd ed.). New York: Oxford University Press.

LEWIS, J. A. and LEWIS, M. D. (1989). *Community
counseling*. Pacific Grove, CA: Brooks/Cole.

LINNEY, J. A. (1990). Community psychology into
the 1990's: Capitalizing opportunity and promoting
innovation. *American Journal of Community
Psychology*, **18**, 1–19.

MANN, P. A. (1978). *Community psychology: Concepts
and applications*. New York: The Free Press.

MCCALL, R. B. (1977). Challenges to a science of
developmental psychology. *Child Development*,
48, 333–344.

MCFARLAND, B. H., BIGELOW, D. A., and SMITH,
J. M. (1997). Community mental health program
efficiency. *Administration and Policy in Mental
Health*, **24**(6), 459–474.

MEYERS, L. J. (1993). *Understanding on Afrocentric
world view: Introduction to an optimal psychology*.
Dubuque: Kendal/Hunt.

NATIONAL INSTITUTE OF MENTAL HEALTH.
(1987). *Toward a model plan for comprehensive,*

community-based mental health. Rockville, MD: US Public Health Service, Alcohol, Drug Abuse, and Mental Health Administration.

NEWBROUGH, J. R. (1992). Community psychology in the postmodern world. *Journal of Community Psychology*, **20**, 10–25.

NEWBROUGH, J. R. (1995). Toward community: A third position. *American Journal of Community Psychology*, **23**, 9–38.

NEWMAN, W. L. (1997). *Social research methods: Qualitative and quantitative approaches.* Massachusetts: Allyn and Bacon.

NIXON, C. T. and NORTHRUP, D. A.(Eds.). (1997). *Evaluating mental health services: How do programs for children 'work' in the real world?* Children's mental health services, Vol. 3. Thousand Oaks, CA: Sage.

O'DONELL, L., COHEN, S. and HAUSMAN, A. (1996). The evaluation of community-based violence programmes. In M. Terre Blanche, A. Butchart, and M. Seedat, *New perspectives in community psychology.* Pretoria: UNISA.

OGBU, J. U. (1992). Cultural mode, identity, and literacy. In J. W. Stigler, R. A. Shweder, and G. Herdt (Eds.), *Cultural psychology: Comparative essays on human development* (pp. 520–541). New York: Cambridge University Press.

OOSTHUIZEN, G. C., EDWARDS, S. D., WESSELS, W. H., and HEXAM, I. (1989). *Afro-Christian religion and healing in southern Africa.* Lewiston: Edwain Mellen.

ORFORD, J. (1992). *Community psychology: Theory and practice.* Chichester: Wiley and Sons.

POLKINGHORNE, D. (1983). *Methodology for the human sciences: Systems of inquiry.* Albany: State University of New York Press.

PRETTY, G. M., ANDREWES, L., and COLLETT, C. (1994). Exploring adolescents' sense of community and its relationship to loneliness. *Journal of Community Psychology*, **22**, 346–358.

PRILLELTENSKY, I. and GONICK, L. (1996). Polities change, oppression remains: On the psychology and politics of oppression. *Political Psychology*, **17**, 127–148.

PRILLELTENSKY, I. and NELSON, G. (1997). Community psychology: Reclaiming social justice. In D. Fox and I. Prilleltensky, *Critical psychology: An introduction* (pp. 166–184). London: Sage.

RAPPAPORT, J. (1987). Terms of empowerment/ exemplars of prevention: Toward a theory of community psychology. *American Journal of Community Psychology*, **15**, 121–144.

RAPPAPORT, J. (1994). Empowerment as a guide to doing research: Diversity as a positive value. In E. J. Trickett, R. J. Watts, and D. Birman (Eds.), *Human diversity: Perspectives on people in context* (pp. 359–382). San Francisco: Jossey-Bass.

REIFF, R. (1968). Social intervention and the problem of psychological analysis. *American Psychologist*, **23**, 524–531.

ROBERTSON, N. (1996). Reforming institutional responses to violence against women: A comprehensive community intervention project. In D. Thomas and A Veno (Eds.), *Community psychology and social change: Australian and New Zealand perspectives* (pp. 81–104). Palmerston North, New Zealand: Dunmore.

SAMPSON, E. (1983). *Justice and the critique of pure psychology.* New York: Plenum Press.

SARASON, S. B. (1974). *The psychological sense of community: Prospects for a community psychology.* San Francisco: Jossey-Bass.

SARASON, S. B. (1981). *Psychology misdirected.* New York: Free Press.

SARASON, S. B. (1984). If it can be studied or developed, should it be? *American Psychologist*, **39**, 477–485.

SCHNETLER, J., STOKER, D J., DIXON, B. J., HERBST, D., and GELDENHUYS, E. (1989). *Survey methods and practice.* Pretoria: HSRC.

SCHÖN, D. (1984). *The reflective practitioner: How professionals think in action.* New York: Basic Books.

SERRANO-GARCIA, I., LOPEZ, M., and RIVERA-MEDINA, E. (1987). Toward a social-community psychology. *Journal of Community Psychology*, **15**, 431–445.

SEVE, L. (1978). *Man in Marxist theory.* Sussex: Harvester Press.

SHERMAN, H. J. (1995). *Reinventing Marxism.* Baltimore: Johns Hopkins University Press.

SOLOMON, J., ZIMBERG, S., and SHOLLAR, E. (Eds.). (1993). *Dual diagnosis: Evaluation, treatment, training and program development.* New York: Plenum Press.

SONN, C. C., BISHOP, B. J., and HUMPHRIES, R. (1997). *Dealing with dominant cultural paradigms: Indigenous students in mainstream higher education.*

Perth: Curtin Indigenous Research Centre.

SONN, C. C. and FISHER, A. T. (1996). Psychological sense of community in a politically structured group. *Journal of Community Psychology*, **24**, 417–430.

SPRADLEY, J. P. and MCCURDY, D. W. (1972). *The cultural experience: Ethnography in complex society.* Chicago: Science Research Associates.

SUSSKIND, E. C. and KLEIN, D. C. (1985). *Community research methods, paradigms and applications.* New York: Praeger.

SYME, G. J. and BISHOP, B. J. (1993). Public psychology: Planning a role for psychology. *Australian Psychologist*, **28**, 45–51.

TAYLOR, C., BRYAN, C., and GOODRICH, C. (1990). *Social assessment: Theory, process and techniques.* Canterbury: Centre for Resource Management.

TELESFORD, M. C. (1996). Implementing community mental health programs: Lessons learned from the mental health initiative for urban children. In C. A. Heflinger and C. T. Nixon (Eds.), *Families and the mental health system for children and adolescents: Policy, services, and research.* Children's mental health services, Vol. 2 (pp. 63–74). Thousand Oaks, CA: Sage.

TERRE BLANCHE, M. and SESELI, L. (1996). Tracking programme efficacy: The development of an outcome assessment model. In M. Terre Blanche, A. Butchart, and M. Seedat, *New perspectives in community psychology.* Pretoria: UNISA.

THOMAS, D. and VENO, A. (Eds.). (1992/1996). *Community psychology and social change: Australian and New Zealand Perspectives.* Palmerston North, New Zealand: Dunmore.

THOMAS, D. R. and ROBERTSON, N. (1992). A conceptual framework for the analysis of social policies. In D. R. Thomas and A. Veno (Eds.), *Psychology and social change: Australian and New Zealand perspectives.* (pp. 37–54). Palmerston North, New Zealand: Dunmore.

THROGMORTON, J. (1991). The rhetorics of policy analysis. *Policy Sciences*, **24**, 153–179.

TOLAN, P., KEYS, S. C., CHERTOK, F., and JASON, L. (1990). *Researching community psychology.* Washington, DC: American Psychological Association.

WALLEN, J. (1992). Providing culturally appropriate mental health services for minorities. *The Journal of Mental Health Administration*, **19**(3), 288–295.

WEHRLY, B. (1995). *Pathways to multicultural counseling competence: A developmental journey.* Pacific Grove, CA: Brooks/Cole.

WEISSBERG, R. P., GULLOTTA, T. P., HAMPTON, R. L., RYAN, B. A., and ADAMS, G. R. (Eds.). (1997). *Establishing preventive services.* Thousand Oaks, CA: Sage.

WICKER, A. (1989). Substantive theorising. *American Journal of Community Psychology*, **17**, 531–547.

WICKER, A. W., and SOMMER, R. (1993). The resident researcher: An alternative career model centred on community. *American Journal of Community Psychology*, **21**, 469–482.

ZINN, M. B., HONDAGNEU-SOTELO, P., and MESSNER, M. A. (1997). *Through the prism of difference: Readings on sex and gender.* Boston: Allyn and Bacon.

index